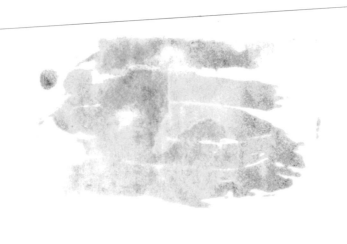

Upper Gastrointestinal Surgery

Other titles in the series:

Emergency Surgery and Critical Care
Simon Paterson-Brown

Hepatobiliary and Pancreatic Surgery
O. James Garden

Colorectal Surgery
Robin K. S. Phillips

Breast and Endocrine Surgery
John R. Farndon

Vascular and Endovascular Surgery
Jonathan D. Beard and Peter A. Gaines

Transplantation Surgery
John L. R. Forsythe

A COMPANION TO SPECIALIST SURGICAL PRACTICE

Series editors

Sir David C. Carter
O. James Garden
Simon Paterson-Brown

Upper Gastrointestinal Surgery

Edited by

S. Michael Griffin

Consultant Surgeon
Oesophago-Gastric Cancer Unit
Newcastle General Hospital
Newcastle Upon Tyne

Simon A. Raimes

Consultant Surgical Gastroenterologist
Department of General Surgery
Cumberland Infirmary
Carlisle

W B Saunders Company Limited
London · Philadelphia · Toronto · Sydney · Tokyo

W. B. Saunders Company Ltd 24–28 Oval Road
London NW1 7DX

The Curtis Center
Independence Square West
Philadelphia, PA 19106-3399, USA

Harcourt Brace & Company
55 Horner Avenue
Toronto, Ontario M8Z 4X6, Canada

Harcourt Brace & Company, Australia
30–52 Smidmore Street
Marrickville, NSW 2204, Australia

Harcourt Brace & Company, Japan
Ichibancho Central Building, 22-1 Ichibancho
Chiyoda-ku, Tokyo 102, Japan

A catalogue record for this book is available from the British Library

ISBN 0-7020-2141-5

Typeset by Florencetype Ltd, Stoodleigh, Devon
Printed in Great Britain by The Bath Press, Bath

Contents

Contributors   vii

Foreword   ix

Preface   xi

Acknowledgements   xiii

1 **Pathology of malignant and premalignant oesophageal and gastric cancers**   1
Mark K. Bennett

2 **Epidemiology and screening for oesophageal and gastric cancer**   35
William H. Allum

3 **Preoperative assessment and staging of oesophageal and gastric cancer**   59
John R. Anderson

4 **Anaesthetic aspects of oesophageal and gastric cancer surgery**   89
Ian H. Shaw

5 **Surgery for cancer of the oesophagus**   111
S. Michael Griffin

6 **Surgery for cancer of the stomach**   145
Simon A. Raimes

7 **Radiotherapy and chemotherapy in the treatment of oesophageal and gastric cancer**   191
Thomas N. Walsh

8 **Palliative treatments of carcinoma of the oesophagus and stomach**   213
Jane M. Blazeby, Derek Alderson

9 **Management of other oesophageal and gastric neoplasms**   245
Deirdre M. O'Hanlon, S. Michael Griffin

10 **Pathophysiology and investigation of GORD and motility disorders**   267
David F. Evans, Charles S. Robertson

11 **Treatment and complications of GORD**   299
Stephen E. A. Attwood, John Bancewicz

CONTENTS

12 Benign ulceration of the stomach and duodenum   **325**
John Wayman, Simon A. Raimes

13 The treatment of non-variceal upper gastrointestinal bleeding **361**
Robert J. C. Steele

14 Management and surgical treatment of morbid obesity   **391**
Peter M. Sagar

Index   **411**

Contributors

Derek Alderson *MD FRCS*
Reader in Surgery, University Department of Surgery, Bristol Royal Infirmary, Bristol, UK

William H. Allum *BSc MD FRCS*
Consultant Surgeon, Dorking Road, Epsom General Hospital, Epsom, Surrey; Honorary Consultant Surgeon, Gastrointestinal Unit, Royal Marsden Hospital, London, UK

John R. Anderson *BSc MB ChB FRCS(Ed & Glas)*
Consultant Surgeon, Southern General Hospital NHS Trust, Glasgow, UK

Stephen E. A. Attwood *MCh FRCS*
Consultant Surgeon, Hope Hospital, Salford, Greater Manchester, UK

John Bancewicz *MCh FRCS*
Reader in Surgery, Hope Hospital, Salford, Greater Manchester, UK

Mark K. Bennett *FRCPath*
Consultant Histopathologist, Freeman Hospital, Newcastle Upon Tyne, UK

Jane M. Blazeby *BSc FRCS*
Lecturer in Surgery, University Department of Surgery, Bristol Royal Infirmary, Bristol, UK

David F. Evans *BA, PhD*
Senior Lecturer in GI Science, St Bartholomew's & Royal London School of Medicine, Whitechapel, London, UK

S. Michael Griffin *MD FRCS FRCS(Ed) FCSHK*
Consultant Surgeon, Oesophago-Gastric Cancer Unit, Newcastle General Hospital, Newcastle Upon Tyne, UK

Deirdre O'Hanlon *FRCS*
Registrar in Surgery, St James Hospital, Dublin, Eire, UK

Simon A. Raimes *MD FRCS*
Consultant Surgical Gastroenterologist, Department of General Surgery, Cumberland Infirmary, Carlisle, UK

Charles S. Robertson *DM FRCS*
Consultant Surgeon, Worcester Royal Infirmary NHS Trust, Worcester, UK

Peter M. Sagar *BSc MD FRCS*
Consultant Surgeon, The General Infirmary at Leeds, Leeds, UK

Ian H. Shaw *BSc PhD MB BChir DA FRCA*
Consultant Anaesthetist, Department of Anaesthesia and Intensive Care, Newcastle General Hospital, Newcastle Upon Tyne, UK

Robert J. C. Steele *BSc MD FRCS*
Professor of Surgical Oncology, Department of Surgery, Ninewells Hospital, Dundee, UK

Thomas N. Walsh *MD MCh FRCSI*
Lecturer in Surgery, Department of Surgery, Royal College of Surgeons in Ireland, Beaumont Hospital, Dublin, Ireland

John Wayman *FRCS*
Research Fellow in the Oesophago-Gastric Cancer Unit, Newcastle General Hospital, Newcastle upon Tyne, UK

Foreword

General surgery defies easy definition Indeed, there are those who claim that it is dying, if not yet dead – a corpse being picked clean by the vulturine proclivities of the other specialties of surgery. Unfortunately for those who subscribe to this view, general surgery is not lying down, indeed it is rejoicing in a new enhanced vigour, as this new series demonstrates.

The general surgeon is the specialist who, along with his other colleagues, provides a 24-hour, 7-day, emergency surgical cover for his, or her, hospital. Also it is to general surgical clinics that patients are referred, unless their condition is manifestly related to one of the other surgical specialties e.g urology, cardiothoracic services, etc. Moreover trainees in these specialties must, during their training, receive experience in general surgery, whose techniques underpin the whole of surgery. General surgery occupies a pivotal position in surgical training. The number of general surgeons required to serve a community, outstrips that required by any other surgical specialty.

General surgery is a specialty in its own right. Inevitably, there are those who wish to practise exclusively one of the sub-specialties of general surgery, e.g. vascular or colorectal surgery. This arrangement may be possible in a few large tertiary referral centres. Although the contribution of these surgeons to patient care and to advances in their discipline will be significant, their numbers are necessarily low. The bulk of surgical practice will be undertaken by the general surgeon who has developed a sub-specialty interest, so that, with his other colleagues in the hospital, comprehensive surgery services can be provided.

There is therefore a great need for a text which will provide comprehensively the theoretical knowledge of the entire specialty and act as a guide for the acquisition of the diagnostic and therapeutic skills required by the general surgeon. The unique contribution of this companion is that it comes as a series, each chapter fresh from the pen of a practising clinician and active surgeon. Each volume is right up to date and this is evidenced by the fact that the first volumes of the series are being published within 12 months from the start of the project. This is a series which has been tightly edited by a team from one of the foremost teaching hospitals in the United Kingdom.

Quite properly the series begins with a volume on emergency surgery and critical care – two of the greatest challenges confronting the practising surgeon. These are the areas that the examination candidate finds the greatest difficulty in acquiring theoretical knowledge and practical experience. Moreover, these are the areas in which advances are at present so rapid that they constantly test the experienced consultant surgeon.

This series not only provides both types of reader with the necessary up-to-date detail but also demonstrates that general surgery remains as challenging and vigorous as it ever has been.

Sir Robert Shields *DL, MD, DSc, FRCS(Ed, Eng, Glas, Ire),*
FRCPEd, FACS
President, Royal College of Surgeons of Edinburgh

Preface

A Companion to Specialist Surgical Practice was designed to meet the needs of the higher surgeon in training and busy practising surgeon who need access to up-to-date information on recent developments, research and data in the context of accepted surgical practice.

Many of the major surgery text books either cover the whole of what is termed 'general surgery' and therefore contain much which is not of interest to the specialist surgeon, or are very high level specialist texts which are outwith the reach of the trainee's finances, and though comprehensive are often out of date due to the lengthy writing and production times of such major works.

Each volume in this series therefore provides succinct summaries of all key topics within a specialty and concentrates on the most recent developments and current data. They are carefully constructed to be easily readable and provide key references.

A specialist surgeon, whether in training or in practice, need only purchase the volume relevant to his or her chosen specialist field plus the emergency surgery and critical care volume, if involved in emergency care.

The volumes have been written in a very short time frame, and produced equally quickly so that information is as up to date as possible. Each volume will be updated and published as a new edition at frequent intervals, to ensure that current information is always available.

We hope that our aim – of providing affordable up-to-date specialist texts – has been met and that all surgeons, in training or in practice will find the volumes to be a valuable resource.

Sir David C. Carter *MD, FRCS(Ed), FRCS(Glas), FRCS(Eng), Hon FRCS(Ire), Hon FACS, FRCP(Ed), FRS(Ed)*
Chief Medical Officer in Scotland
Formerly Regius Professor of Clinical Surgery, University
Department of Surgery, Royal Infirmary, Edinburgh

O. James Garden *BSc, MB, ChB, MD, FRCS(Glas), FRCS(Ed)*
Professor of Hepatobiliary Surgery of the Royal Infirmary; Director of Organ Transplantation, University Department of Surgery, Royal Infirmary, Edinburgh

Simon Paterson-Brown *MS, MPhil, FRCS(Ed), FRCS(Eng), FCSHK*
Consultant General and Upper Gastrointestinal Surgeon, University Department of Surgery, Royal Infirmary, Edinburgh

Acknowledgements

We are indebted to all the authors who have contributed to this volume for their perseverance and expertise. We are grateful to our fellow editors for assistance and advice in the initial planning of this book. The series editors give special thanks to Rachael Stock and Linda Clark from W. B. Saunders for their initial persuasion, continuing enthusiasm and ongoing support.

S. M. GRIFFIN
S. A. RAIMES

I wish to thank my wife, Alison, my mother and my late father without whom I could not have completed this onerous but fulfilling project. I dedicate my efforts into this enterprise to my late father, whose inspiration and great surgical talents have always provided me with the enthusiasm to take on and complete yet more academic and clinical projects.

S. M. GRIFFIN

I am grateful to my wife, Theresa, for putting up with my endeavours and absences from family duties during the preparation of the book.

S. A. RAIMES

1 Pathology of malignant and premalignant oesophageal and gastric cancers

Mark K. Bennett

Introduction

Malignant tumours of the upper gastrointestinal tract appear as irregular mucosal ulcers, polypoid masses or diffuse thickenings of the bowel wall. In some, the adjacent mucosa shows the precursor changes, though in the majority these lesions are destroyed by the infiltrative edge of the tumour. Dysplasia which is regarded as the tumour precursor is defined in terms of both cytological (individual cell) as well as architectural (gland or mucosal) atypia. Other mucosal changes which predispose to the development of dysplasia may be present and these will include histopathological as well as 'molecular' abnormalities.

The commonest carcinoma of the oesophagus, the squamous carcinoma, is derived from the lining epithelium. Other tumours are thought to arise from the basal cells of the mucosa or from the submucosal glands and are seen especially at the oesophagogastric junction. Carcinoma *in situ* is potentially irreversible and is regarded as the precursor for squamous carcinoma as it shows cytological atypia throughout the full thickness of the epithelium. Lesser degrees of atypia are more difficult to define and are sometimes confused with regenerative changes. Metaplasia, which is the change from squamous to a glandular mucosa (Barrett's oesophagus) occurs as a result of reflux of gastric contents. The premalignant potential of this change and the subsequent malignant transformation to adenocarcinoma is at present hotly debated. The possibility that screening of high risk population groups and identification of individuals with precursor lesions is at present under intense investigation.

Gastric adenocarcinoma is a tumour derived from the lining mucosa which in the UK presents late in its natural history. This advanced cancer is the sixth most common and causes approximately 7600 deaths per annum[1] although the incidence has inexplicably been falling for several decades. As with oesophageal cancers, the precursor lesion is regarded as an area of dysplasia. The differentiation between what is regarded as carcinoma *in situ* and that of an intramucosal carcinoma is often impossible. Problems in interpreting the degree of cellular atypia in biopsy material and to distinguish lesser degrees of dysplasia is often difficult, especially in low risk areas. There are several predisposing conditions which are associated with or precede the development of dysplasia (see Table 1.3). One of the most important changes in the last 20 years is the recognition of early gastric cancer, with its potential to improve patient survival (from 17% to > 90%). In countries with a low incidence of gastric cancer, such as the UK, the proportion of early tumours still remains disappointingly low (10–12%).

Gastric carcinoma

Advanced gastric cancer

Approximately 90% of all malignant tumours of the stomach are adenocarcinomas. The majority of the remaining tumours are either malignant lymphomas or smooth muscle tumours. There are in addition a wide variety of other primary tumours arising from the stomach which reflect the tissue present within the mucosa and deeper structures. These include squamous and oat cell carcinomas, carcinoid tumours, benign and malignant mesodermally derived tumours (i.e. those coming from blood vessels, fat-cells and neural elements) and an assortment of rare tumours more often associated with extragastrointestinal sites such as the malignant fibrous histiocytoma, glomus tumours, teratoma and choriocarcinoma.

Advanced gastric cancer has shown significant changes over the recent decades. First, there has been a recognition that the histological type known as diffuse cancer (see below) has been increasing and now represents up to 30% of all gastric neoplasms.[2] The second change is the apparent epidemic increase in tumours confined to the oesophagogastric junction, which have a predilection to white male patients and represent in the USA up to 50% of gastric cancers.[3] These tumours show an aggressive behaviour with a worse prognosis than cancers in the rest of the stomach. There are several factors which might explain this including large size (> 5 cm) at presentation, early submucosal invasion, extension into the oesophagus, and because of their large size the more frequent involvement of the serosa and the finding of lymph node metastasis. Unlike the more distal tumours they are not associated with atrophic gastritis or intestinal metaplasia suggesting that there are demographic and pathological features similar to the adenocarcinoma found in Barrett's oesophagus.

Macroscopic features

The macroscopic appearances of an advanced gastric cancer can be divided into four types[4] (Figs 1.1 and 1.2 and Table 1.1). Though the

Figure 1.1 *The macroscopic appearances of an advanced gastric cancer. Borrman type I (a) and III (b).*

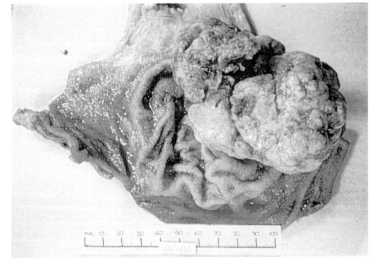

(a)

(b)

classification shown in Table 1.1 is commonly used in Germany and Japan it has never gained acceptance throughout the English-speaking world though as with all classifications it allows succinct categorisation of tumour appearances for comparative studies.

Histological features

The most widely accepted histological classification of gastric carcinoma is that by Lauren[5] who divided the tumours into two main types. Those which formed glandular structures were known as intestinal (53%) whereas those without any structure and secreting mucin were known as diffuse type carcinomas (33%) (Table 1.2; Figs 1.3 and 1.4). The remaining 14% had a mixed appearance with elements from both types and were regarded as unclassified. The macroscopic appearances

Table 1.1 *Macroscopic appearances of advanced gastric carcinoma (Borrman)*

Type 1 or fungating. A polypoid protrusion with a broad base, often soft, red in colour and may be slightly ulcerated.

Type 2. An excavated carcinoma which is dominated by the crater with slightly elevated margins. There is no definite infiltration of the adjacent mucosa.

Type 3. This is also ulcerative with mildly elevated (and infiltrated) margins.

Type 4. A diffusely thickened (schirrous type), also know as linitis plastica.

---

of these tumours depends on the relative proportions of collagen and mucus produced. One of the greatest problems with any pathological classification is that of reproducibility though this is minimised by having this simple division into two main histological types. From epidemiological evidence, it has become apparent that there is a wide variation in incidence between the intestinal and diffuse tumours, suggesting differences in the underlying aetiology. In an attempt to assess the prognostic value of the histological typing Goseki *et al.*[6] expanded this classification further and suggested that some types of tumour have a propensity to spread to the bone marrow, liver or directly to the peritoneum. However, in the other typing schemes such as those suggested by Ming[7] in which the tumours are split into expanding and infiltrating types or that proposed by the WHO where the tumours are organised into several different histological types (well/moderate and poorly differentiated, mucoid, signet ring and undifferentiated)[8] have not been shown to be independent factors in the prognosis of gastric cancer.

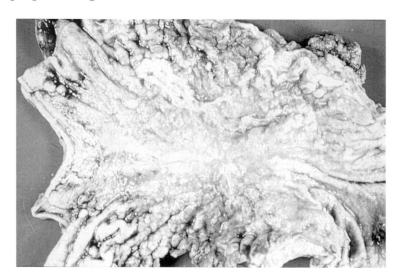

Figure 1.2 *A linitis plastica (Borrman type IV) in which there is diffuse infiltration of the wall of the stomach by tumour and apparent thickening of the rugal folds.*

Table 1.2 *Comparative histological features of advanced gastric carcinoma*

Features	Intestinal	Diffuse
Sex ratio M:F	2:1	Approximately 1:1
Mean age of detection in years	55	48
Decreasing incidence in western countries	Yes	No
5-year survival rate (all cases)	20%	Less than 10%
Major gross appearances	Intraluminal growth, fungating	Ulcerative infiltrating
Microscopic features differentiation	Well differentiated, glandular, papillary, solid	Poorly differentiated ring cells
Growth pattern	Expansile	Non-cohesive diffuse
Mucin production	Confined to gland lumen	Extensive often prominent in stroma around glands
Associated intestinal metaplasia	Almost 100%	Less frequent
Aetiological factors	Diet, environmental, *H. pylori*	Unknown, ? genetic factors associated with blood group A, *H. pylori*

Prognostic pathological features

Careful assessment of gastrectomy specimens have shown several prognostic features in advanced gastric cancer. The most important being the depth of invasion, involvement by tumour of the resection margin and the presence of lymph node metastasis.[9]

Serosal involvement is an ominous feature with a 5-year survival of just 7% whereas that for tumour infiltration restricted to the subserosa is about 29%. Penetration of the serosal surface may be the

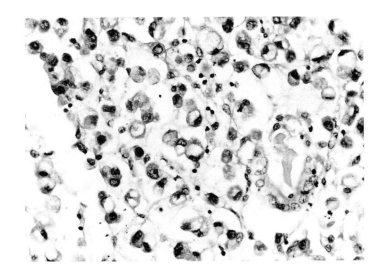

Figure 1.3 *A diffuse adenocarcinoma in which the tumour cells are widely dispersed and separated by a variable amount of stroma. Occasional cells show that their nuclei are displaced by the intracytoplasmic secretory vacuole (signet ring).*

Figure 1.4 *An intestinal adeno-carcinoma is composed of irregular glands which are lined by attenuated cuboidal epithelium showing there is invasion of the muscle layer (arrow head) and a mixed inflammatory infiltrate between the tumourous glands.*

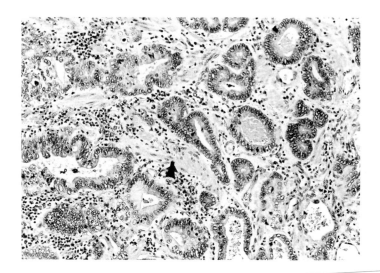

means by which transcoloemic dissemination occurs and the area of the serosal involvement has been looked at by several authors. Most have taken less than 2 cm in diameter as the limit indicating a better prognosis. Abe *et al.*[10] showed that less than 3 cm area of serosal involvement had a five-year survival 59.6% compared with 11.5% with tumours more than 3 cm. They also have suggested that if both the serosa and lymph nodes were involved then the diameter of serosal involvement is the more important factor in predicting the ultimate survival. It should be relatively easy at surgery to identify serosal involvement, but in nearly 10% of cases histological involvement was found where no macroscopic disease was thought to be present.[11] These tumours tended to be of large size to be undifferentiated histological type and with an infiltrative pattern.

The survival is also dependent on the number of nodes involved, the extension of metastasis through the capsule of nodes and involvement of the adjacent fibrovascular and fatty tissue, and whether the metastases were judged to be present macroscopically.[12] The depth of tumour penetration and the presence of nodal metastasis is the basis of the TMN staging of gastric tumours and this allows comparative data for prognosis and treatment.

Involvement of the duodenum in tumours of the distal stomach has been reported from 9 to 69% of the resections.[13,14] When present, it is regarded as a poor prognostic sign with a significant reduction in the 5-year survival rate to 8%, in comparison with those tumours restricted to the stomach. It should, however, be realised that in these tumours there is also an increased involvement of the serosa, with evidence of lymphatic and vascular invasion.

There have been other independent factors investigated which have shown positive predictive values, these have included blood and lymphatic invasion, patients who have had a total gastrectomy, or who are over 70 years of age, those with tumours with a diffuse infiltrating pattern, involvement of the entire stomach or measure more than 10 cm in diameter.[14] The only histological tumour type showing a worse prognosis is the adenosquamous carcinoma, an uncommon tumour, which is composed of both glandular and squamous elements. Those tumours which macroscopically appear as early gastric carcinoma but histologically are advanced cancers have a prognosis which is intermediate between the two groups.

Early gastric cancer

This is defined as a malignant tumour limited to the mucosa or submucosa and is independent of any lymph node metastasis. The penetration of the muscularis mucosae allows subdivision of the tumours into those that are intramucosal or submucosal types. A macroscopic classification was introduced by the Japanese Endoscopic Society where the tumour were grouped into predominately the protuberant type (type I), a superficial type where the mucosal changes are minimal (type II) or where there is a significant ulcerating lesion (type III).[15] Type I protruding polypoid tumours appear as a sessile smooth hemispherical nodule with a broad stalk, less than 3 cm in diameter and are often paler than the adjacent mucosa. Type II tumours are subdivided into three subsets (indicated by the suffix a, b or c), the slightly elevated (with a height no greater than that of the thickness of the adjacent mucosa), those which are 'flat' with little mucosal elevation and a third group in which there is mucosal erosion but not deep ulceration – the so called depressed lesions. More than one appearance can be found, especially if the tumours cover a large area when they are classified by the main type followed by the subsidiary types e.g. IIa + IIc (Fig. 1.5).

Early gastric cancers are found predominantly within the lower two-thirds of the stomach and vary in size from 3–5 mm to more than 8 cm. Mori et al.[16] have reported a small series of 21 patients with early carcinoma of the cardia. The ulcerating tumours (types III and IIc) are the most frequent accounting for 64% of the neoplasms followed by the exophytic lesions. The entirely flat IIb lesion is the least common and represents 14% of the tumours. Histologically the exophytic tumours tend to have a better differentiated intestinal type whereas the ulcerating tumours are more frequently associated with the signet ring or poorly differentiated histology. The flat lesions have a mixed histological pattern.

The prognosis for EGC is excellent with reported 5-year survival of 95%.[17] If the depth of invasion is taken into consideration then the survival at 15 years for those tumours confined to the mucosa is 87% and only slightly less when there is infiltration into the submucosa (75%).[18] Reports from Japan indicate that recurrence is due either to residual tumour in the gastric remnant or metastatic disease in the liver.[19,20] The features which are associated with haematogenous

Figure 1.5 *An early gastric carcinoma of the antrum showing areas of both a raised plaque and superficial mucosal erosions (type II a+c).*

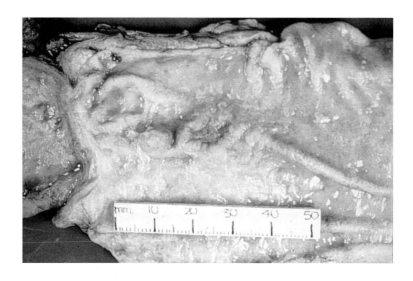

metastasis are intestinal tumours, submucosal invasion and involvement of the epigastric lymph nodes. Intramucosal EGC rarely have perigastric nodal metastasis (less than 5%) due to the paucity of intramucosal lymphatics and this is reflected in a 5-year survival rate of 100%. Invasion of the submucosa is associated with 10–20% nodal metastasis and a slightly reduced 5-year survival (between 90 and 95%).[21,22] Reports from the UK have suggested even higher rates of nodal metastases in EGC.[22] It is noteworthy that DNA analysis shows that aneuploid changes are more frequent in types I and IIa tumours though the ploidy status and nodal metastasis have not been shown to be consistently correlated.[23]

Precursors of gastric carcinoma

Chronic gastritis and intestinal metaplasia

The pathogenesis of gastric carcinoma is complex and multifactorial with several potential precursor lesions (Table 1.3). The most widely supported pathway from normal mucosa to cancer was suggested by Correa[24] and this is discussed in detail in Chapter 2. This has subsequently been added to as a result of the detailed examination of the mucosa by molecular techniques. Continuing inflammatory damage to the mucosa is considered one of the initiating insults which can lead to a chronic atrophic gastritis (Fig. 1.6) and intestinal metaplasia. The proliferative zone of the gastric mucosa produces not only cells for the surface but also the mucous and specialised glands which are found in the deeper parts of the mucosa. The pit epithelium responds to the loss of the surface cells by increasing its turnover by between three and four times. With the cell production redirected to the surface as a result of the inflammatory damage there is a loss of the cells maturing to form the deeper glands resulting in the apparent

Table 1.3 *Precursors of gastric carcinoma*

Chronic gastritis
Intestinal metaplasia of gastric mucosa
Gastric polyps
Gastric remnants (postgastrectomy state)
Ménétrièr's disease
Chronic peptic ulcer
Gastric epithelial dysplasia

'atrophy'.[25] On reviewing gastrectomies for carcinomas it has been noted that there is an increased incidence of chronic atrophic gastritis and gastric atrophy associated with intestinal type carcinomas. However, biopsies of the patients older than 60 years show that up to 40% have a similar atrophic gastritis, indicating that other factors must be implicated in carcinogenesis. In the past, environmental factors such as high dietary intake of salt, dried or pickled food were thought to enhance the development of the gastritis and would explain the geographical variation in the disease prevalence. The immune-mediated gastritis found in pernicious anaemia has a reported increased risk of developing carcinoma with a prevalence estimated at 1–3%.[26] It is, however, unclear whether the increased cancer risk is as a result of the pernicious anaemia or from dietary and/or environmental factors.

In addition to the inflammatory damage, the cells of the pits may undergo metaplasia towards intestinal epithelium.[27,28] This is seen as a change from the production of neutral to acid mucins, a change in function from a secretory to an absorptive cell type and the production of paneth cells (which are usually found in the small bowel). The initial

Figure 1.6 *The pyloric mucosa showing a quiescent atrophic gastritis with complete intestinal metaplasia. This has an irregular surface with elongation of the pits in which there are goblet cells. The normal serous glands are not present and in the lamina propria there is a mild mononuclear cell inflammatory infiltrate.*

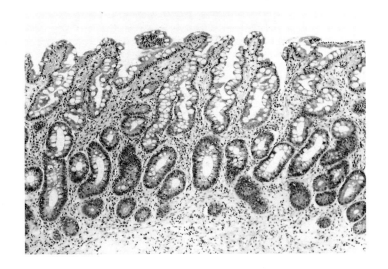

Figure 1.7
Intestinal metaplasia (type III). The superficial pits show both large solitary and multiple smaller secretory vacuoles within the apical portions of the cells. (Stained with alcian blue and PAS.)

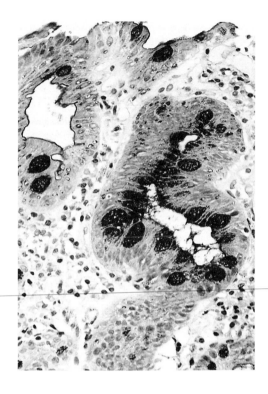

production of sialo acid mucins is usually found in the presence of paneth cells and is referred to as complete intestinal metaplasia (type II). With continuing damage, the pit cells change their morphology, produce a sulpha acid mucin which is more characteristic of colonic mucosa and there is loss of the paneth cells. These appearances are known as incomplete intestinal metaplasia (type III) (Fig. 1.7) and is a precursor of gastric atrophy. There is continuing controversy as to the value of identifying this colonic type mucin and its predictive value in identifying patients at risk of developing cancer.[29] There are significant differences in the expression of the sulpha mucins between the intestinal and diffuse type of carcinomas (80% and 20%, respectively) which has suggested differences in the underlying aetiology. It should be noted that intestinal metaplasia increases in prevalence and extent with age and is not infrequently associated with non-malignant disease, e.g. benign peptic ulceration. In these situations as well as those associated with the cancers, there are abnormalities of the mucin genes and cell kinetics.[30,31]

Any damage to the genome which occurs and is left unrepaired would be perpetuated in this hyperproliferative state and give rise to genomic instability.[32] Although it is possible to reverse the inflammatory changes, atrophy and more especially the colonic type intestinal metaplasia are regarded as irreversible. With the loss of fundic glands and the resulting hypochlorhydria the possibility exists for nitrosating bacteria to proliferate within the mucosa.[33–35] These bacteria are able

Figure 1.8
Helicobacter pylori, *the bacterium are found at the surface and in the mucus of the pits; in this silver stain they appear as black rods often curved at the apex of the cell.*

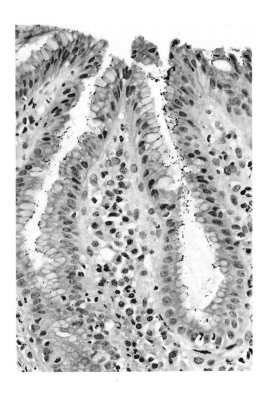

to convert nitrates into nitrites, as well as creating N-nitroso compounds by catalysing reactions between amines and amides and the nitrites. Ascorbic acid, the reduced form of vitamin C, appears to protect against neoplasia, possibly by scavenging both nitrites and reactive oxygen metabolites.

Recently *Helicobacter pylori* (Fig. 1.8) has been linked with gastric carcinogenesis.[36–39] There are several epidemiological studies showing a greater incidence of previous infection with *H. pylori* in gastric cancer patients than in controls, though the study designs have been questioned. This bacterium uses a variety of strategies to survive within the gastric mucus and may induce damage by several mechanisms. These include the production of a vacuolating toxin possibly associated with the *cag A* gene, the production of urease and ammonia, acetaldehyde and mucolytic factors. The other possibility is that of host response inducing the genomic change. *H. pylori* has a strong chemotactic effect for polymorphs and other inflammatory cells, which can produce both reactive oxygen metabolites, as well as plasma membrane-associated NADPH oxidase. Another potential mutagenic pathway is the production of nitrogen oxides and potent N-nitrosating agents from nitric oxide. Both of these latter pathways have been shown to cause mutations in p53 with its secondary effects on uncontrolled cell proliferation. The damage caused by *H. pylori* is not regarded as sufficient to induce gastric carcinoma but cofactors, possibly dietary, are presumed to be present and together initiate the steps required to convert a normal into a dysplastic mucosa. Lately it has also been noted that the immunological responses may play a part in perpetuating tumour growth in that antibodies which come from gastric cancer patients and react with *H. pylori* have been found to stimulate gastric cancer cells *in vitro*.[40]

Gastric mucosal polyps

Gastric polyps are found with increasing incidence with age; in some series they are present in up to 7% of patients over 80 years. The classification is important as it indicates whether or not they are premalignant or are just incidental and sometimes associated with tumours.[41,42] Gastric mucosal polyps fall into three main groups; the hyperplastic polyps, fundic gland polyps or neoplastic polyps (adenomas).

Hyperplastic polyps are the most frequently found usually with an equal sex distribution and occurring in later life with a mean age within the seventh decade. They represent 80–85% of all gastric polyps, are found in the antrum more than in the corpus, are often multiple and usually less than 1 cm in diameter. Histologically they are composed of disorganised and often hyperplastic glandular elements which are lined by regular epithelium and have an adjacent chronic gastritis. The risk of malignant transformation overall is approximately 0.5% and with rare exceptions this occurred in polyps greater than 2 cm in diameter.[43] The risk of detecting coexistent cancer in prospective studies varied from 4.5 to 13.5%.

Fundic gland polyps are present in up to 3% of endoscopies and form multiple sessile lesions confined to the body of the stomach. They were originally described in association with familial adenomatous polyposis,[44] but are now more frequently sporadic and are regarded as hamartomatous lesions. There is no evidence for an increased risk of gastric cancer.

Neoplastic polyps are also referred to as adenomas and histologically have a tubular configuration. They occur predominantly in the antrum, with no sex preference and more frequently in the elderly. Most are smaller than 2 cm. The risk of malignant transformation has been reported to occur in up to 40% of those adenomas greater than 2 cm. Although often found in isolation, coexistent cancers have been found in 3–25% though the malignant change is generally reported in the range 5–10%.[45] Histologically the polypoid epithelium shows dysplastic features with hyperchromasia, irregularity of maturation and abnormally situated mitoses; there is no evidence to suggest infiltration through the basement membrane.

Gastroduodenal polyps are found with familial adenomatous polyposis (FAP) with approximately a quarter of the patients having fundic gland or hyperplastic polyps. Often more than 50 fundic gland polyps are present and these develop at an earlier age than the sporadic cases. Of more concern is that 35–100% of cases are associated with adenomas and though they are less frequent in the stomach than duodenum they occur at a younger age (mean 37 years) than in the sporadic adenoma. The lesions are usually small and multiple; with time they increase in number and exhibit frequent malignant transformation.[46] Except in Japan the risk of gastric carcinoma is not increased in patients when compared with controls though the relative risk of duodenal and periampullary carcinoma is markedly increased.

The flat adenomas similar to those found in the colon are another form of tubular adenoma with variable degrees of dysplasia.[47] Macroscopically they appear as irregular impressions and occupy the full thickness of involved gastric glands. They may represent macroscopically a healing ulcer or depressed type of early gastric cancer. They occur in the distal two-thirds of the stomach, having similar demographic features to the commoner polypoid adenomas. A larger percentage of the adenomas are described as having high-grade dysplasia though the prevalence is unknown. In the Japanese literature, these lesions may represent up to 10% of all neoplastic polyps.

Gastric remnant

The risk of developing cancer following distal gastrectomy with gastroenteric anastomosis for treatment of benign peptic ulcer disease is controversial. By definition the cancer must be diagnosed 5 or more years after the original surgery so as to exclude small or early gastric neoplasms. There are a variety of benign histological changes associated with gastric remnants which include chronic gastritis and atrophy, fundic gland polyps, xanthomas, associated surface/foveolar hyperplasia and hyperplastic polyps with gastritis cystica profunda. There is, however, an increased risk of developing severe epithelial dysplasia although the malignant potential of the dysplasia is controversial.[48] The majority of the tumours are found at or close to the stoma site, rarely extend into the intestinal side of the anastomosis and show equal proportions of intestinal and diffuse cancers. The tumour in 40% of cases is restricted to the submucosa, i.e. an early gastric cancer. The risk of developing cancer is thought to be approximately twice that of the control population. Those who are at most risk have been identified as patients who have undergone surgery before the age of 40 and who have had a postsurgery interval of 15–20 years. The risk of this type of cancer is increased in countries with a high intrinsic rate of gastric cancer but apparently not in those with a lower rate. It has been suggested that selective surveillance should be considered for those patients who are symptomatic, who underwent surgery at a young age, those who are 20 years or more after surgery and for those who have high-grade dysplasia on endoscopy. In addition, cases of lymphoma of the stomach are now being described in the gastric stump.[49] A variety of non-gastric malignancies have been identified in follow-up series, and these have been predominantly lung, pancreatic ductal and colorectal cancers.

Ménétrièr's disease (hypertrophic gastropathy)

This is a rare cause of rugal hypertrophy characterised by hyperplasia of the surface cells, hypochlorhydria and a protein losing enteropathy. A review of the cases shows that approximately 10% are associated with cancer, diagnosed either simultaneously or within 12 months. However, follow-up in a total of 16 cases shows the risk of malignancy to be low or negligible.[50] A few cases however have been associated with gastric dysplasia.

Chronic peptic ulcer disease

The possibility of malignant transformation of gastric ulcers is controversial. Few long-term studies of peptic ulcers are available and these have shown a relative risk of developing cancer no more than twice that of the normal population.[51] The natural history of early gastric carcinoma is one of episodes of mucosal ulceration followed by repair, some of which may be related to active medical therapy. It is essential, therefore, to ensure that any mucosal ulcer is adequately sampled before making a diagnosis of a benign ulcer. At the present time it is thought that less than 1% of ulcers will have undergone malignant transformation. The epidemiological evidence would suggest that ulcers do not have a significant role in gastric carcinogenesis.

Gastric epithelial dysplasia

Dysplasia may occur in an epithelium which shows intestinal metaplasia and may be flat, depressed or polypoid.[52] It is generally classified into three grades: mild, moderate or severe. There is great interobservational variation between the mild and moderate grades. From retrospective studies high-grade dysplasia is closely associated with gastric carcinoma in the adjacent mucosa. Between 40 and 100% of early gastric cancers and 5 and 80% of advanced tumours show dysplasia. Although only 1–3% of gastric ulcers with an atrophic gastritis are associated with dysplasia. There are several problems associated with histological interpretation which include distinguishing regenerative atypia from true dysplasia, the ability to differentiate high-grade dysplasia from intramucosal carcinoma, a lack of experience due to the rarity of dysplasia (especially in low incidence areas) and the problem of sampling identical areas in the gastric mucosa on follow-up endoscopy. The natural history of dysplasia also compounds the potential 'premalignant' problem with regression reported in 60–70% in mild and moderate dysplasia. Severe dysplasia can also regress but this is less common (30–45%) with the majority of patients progressing to carcinoma (20–80%).[53] A diagnosis of severe dysplasia is a frequent marker of coexistent cancer with 50% of the tumours being diagnosed within 3 months of the initial finding of dysplasia on biopsy which is accompanied by a gross endoscopic lesion by erosion ulcer or polyp. The natural history of severe dysplasia without mucosal abnormality is unknown. The following protocol[34] has been suggested for surveillance of patients with dysplasia.

1. Mild dysplasia   Perform no or limited surveillance.
2. Moderate dysplasia   Similar to mild dysplasia but in addition a rapid follow-up endoscopy to detect any other abnormality which should be biopsied. Further management is defined as a result of the second evaluation.
3. Severe dysplasia   Immediate re-evaluation indicated if no cancer is detected and then regular surveying should be undertaken. Persistent severe dysplasia associated with gross lesion may be an indication for resection.

Gastrointestinal stromal tumours (GIST)

The stomach is the most frequent site within the gastrointestinal tract for these tumours, although the incidence and distribution varies depending on whether the data have been collected from post mortem or surgically resected specimens (and whether or not they were total or partial gastrectomies). They have been found in up to 0.18–46% of stomachs and up to 60% have been reported within the middle third by several authors. They range in size from under 1 cm where they are clinically asymptomatic to bulky 20 cm masses. Approximately three quarters are benign. The nomenclature of those tumours which were previously referred to as leiomyoma or leiomyosarcomas is undergoing a significant change.[54] They were thought to be derived from the mesoderm and are composed of spindle cells (Fig. 1.9) with a variable amount of extracellular collagen. Electron microscopy shows few features to suggest smooth muscle differentiation and in some a suggestion of neural differentiation is recognised. There is a variable expression of the putative markers of muscle, desmin (up to 20%), actin (up to 70%) whereas the marker of neural differentiation S100, is expressed in up to 15% of these tumours. Recently CD34 which is expressed in a variety of tissue including the spindle cells adjacent to smooth muscle bundles in the gastric stroma, has been found in 80–90% of tumours.[55] As a consequence these tumours are considered to be derived from undifferentiated stromal fibroblasts and hence have been termed gastrointestinal stromal tumours.

Apart from the histogenesis of the tumours, predicting clinical behaviour is also problematical. Because of the bland cytological features clinical information such as the presence of metastases or local invasion are important in indicating clinical malignancy. The most important histological feature after multivariant analysis has been the mitotic index, malignant behaviour being most likely when there are more than five mitotic figures per ten high power fields. Although

Figure 1.9
Gastrointestinal stromal tumours (GIST); the spindle cells have irregular nuclei with rounded ends and form loosely associated bundles separated by a collagenous matrix.

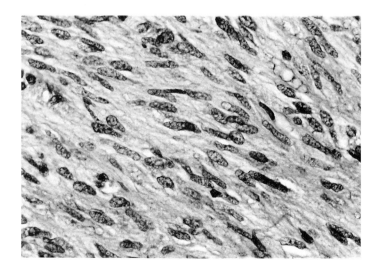

size is important, with 60% of the tumours more than 10 cm in diameter showing metastatic spread within five years, benign tumours of a similar size have been described. It is also important to recognise that these tumours may be part of a clinical syndrome such as Carney's triad. This consists of extra-adrenal paraganglioma together with pulmonary chondroma and stromal tumours of the stomach; the triad may be diagnosed if two of the three features are present. The stromal tumours are often multiple, as are the paragangliomas, and are more frequent in women who at presentation are on average only 15 years old.

Gastrointestinal lymphoma

The stomach is the most common site for gastrointestinal lymphomas in the United Kingdom whereas in the oesophagus this tumour is very rare. This is rather surprising since the stomach does not normally have any lymphoid tissue from which a lymphoid malignancy could arise. As nodal lymphomas often involve the gastrointestinal tract the diagnosis of a primary lymphoma requires strict criteria which were suggested in 1961.[56] For the diagnosis of a primary lymphoma, the tumour must be limited to the gastrointestinal tract and its contiguous lymph nodes. The present classification of the lymphomas[57] is shown in Table 1.4.

B-cell lymphomas of MALT type
Low-grade lymphomas occur in the elderly and present suggesting a diagnosis of gastritis or peptic ulcer disease.[58] They appear macroscopically as an ill-defined thickening of the mucosa with erosions, sometimes ulcerated (Fig. 1.10) and frequently multifocal. The mucosa contains lymphoid follicles which have a similar appearance to Peyer's

Table 1.4 *Primary gastrointestinal non-Hodgkin's lymphomas*

B-cell
1. MALT type
   (a) Low grade
   (b) High grade with or without low-grade component
   (c) Immunoproliferative small intestinal disease (low and high grade)
2. Mantle cell (lymphomatous polyposis)
3. Burkitt's and Burkitt-like
4. Other types of low or high-grade lymphoma corresponding to lymph node equivalents

T-cell
1. Enteropathy-associated T-cell lymphoma
2. Other types not associated with enteropathy
3. Rare types (including conditions that may simulate lymphoma)

patches, i.e. they simulate the Mucosa Associated Lymphoid Tissue (MALT). The characteristic lesion of a lymphoepithelial lesion (Fig. 1.11) is composed of small- to medium-sized tumour cells with irregular nuclei which infiltrate the pit epithelium. Pathologists have in the past referred to these as centrocyte-like cells though they have a variable appearance from small lymphocytes to monocytoid B cells. The lymphoepithelial lesion, is not pathognomonic of a lymphoma as it can also be demonstrated in an *H. pylori*-associated gastritis, Sjögren's syndrome and Hashimoto's thyroiditis. Plasma cells are not infrequently found and are regarded as reactive in nature. In recent studies up to 90% of the gastric MALT lymphoma were associated with *H. pylori* infection.[37] This has suggested a possible

Figure 1.10 *Non-Hodgkins lymphoma which shows superficial ulceration of the antrum with fibrous scarring of the adjacent mucosa.*

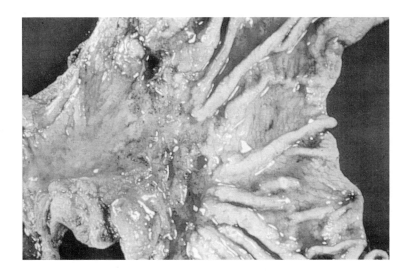

Figure 1.11
Lymphoepithelial lesion. An intense cellular cell infiltrate is present in the pits which are partially destroyed (arrow head).

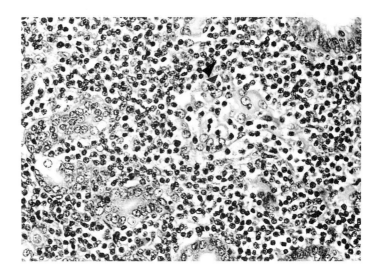

role not only in the initiation of the gastritis but also that the bacterial antigens could perpetuate the immunological drive from which the lymphomatous process develops. Initially the tumour effaces the lymphoid tissue of the adjacent mucosa then spreads to the contiguous lymph nodes. The subsequent development of a monoclonal proliferation requires accumulation of genetic abnormalities.[59] Both phenotypic and genotypic changes are noted in the lymphoid cells. This includes the expression of surface immunoglobulin, light chain restriction and monoclonal immunoglobulin gene rearrangement. Unlike the nodal lymphoma which has similar cytological features the genotypic investigations do not show rearrangement of the *bCL-2* gene, this and other aspects suggests that they do not share common features with nodal lymphomas.[60]

The high-grade lymphoma is thought to be a transformation from the low-grade tumour to a more aggressive cytological type and is the more frequent tumour. Unlike the low-grade lymphoma this type of tumour can be rarely distinguished from other high-grade nodal lymphomas and as the clinical behaviour is similar between the two, there is probably no reason to separate them in any pathological classification.

Most low-grade MALT lymphomas are associated with localised disease confined to the site of origin (stage IE or IIE) with slow dissemination. The favourable clinical behaviour may reflect the partial dependence on the *H. pylori* antigenic drive. Wotherspoon *et al.*[61] showed regression of the lymphoma following eradication of *H. pylori*. Generally there are excellent survival rates with reported 5- and 10-year survival rates of 91% and 75%, unlike the low-grade nodal lymphomas which are essentially incurable, most patients succumbing to their disease within 7–10 years. Some of the high-grade lymphomas have been reported as having a more favourable prognosis than their equivalent nodal disease though this is not as good as the low-grade tumours (75% at 5 years).

Other lymphomas

The majority of the remaining gastrointestinal lymphomas are restricted to the distal bowel with differences not only in the epidemiology but also the nature of the tumours. Immunoproliferative small intestinal disease is almost exclusively found in the Middle East and characterised by a diffuse lymphoplasmacytic infiltrate which synthesises abnormal α heavy chains giving a paraprotein without light chains. Lymphomatous polyposis can affect any part of the gastrointestinal tract but is predominantly found at the ileocaecal valve. The polyps characteristic of the condition range in size from 0.5 cm to 2 cm in diameter and are sometimes associated with diffuse or nodular lymphoid infiltrates within the bowel wall. Unlike the preceding forms of gastrointestinal lymphoma there is early involvement of the liver, spleen, bone marrow and peripheral nodes. The other forms of lymphoma, Burkitt's, Burkitt-like and the enteropathy associated T-cell lymphomas are nearly always confined to the distal small bowel.

Gastric carcinoids

Gastric carcinoids are derived from endocrine cells which have a characteristic distribution, staining pattern and electron microscopic appearance.[62] Proliferation of the endocrine cell population is brought about by hypergastrinaemia, atrophy of the corpus, genetic factors and possibly as a consequence of *H. pylori* infection. Endocrine cell proliferation can be found as a simple hyperplasia, a dysplasia or as a neuroendocrine (carcinoid) tumour. The simple hyperplasia may take on a variety of patterns and may lead eventually to nodule formation. A presumed multistep progression as a result of continuing proliferation results in dysplastic nodules with associated atypical cells and these are considered to be the precursor for the carcinoid tumour. Recently it has been found that there is an increased incidence of gastric carcinoids though at present this still represents only 0.3% of all malignant tumours.

Neuroendocrine tumours can be subdivided into four groups with different underlying clinical conditions, associated changes in the mucosa and behaviour patterns. Multiple well-differentiated tumours affecting predominantly middle-aged females (average age 51 years) are associated with pernicious anaemia and a hypergastrinaemia in one third. Where the tumours are invasive they tend to be limited to the submucosa and metastases are usually confined to the local lymph nodes (7–12%). No reported deaths are associated with these tumours. The possibility of reversibility, by antrectomy (to reduce the hypergastrinaemia) or with octreotide have demonstrated a reduction in the endocrine cell numbers at one month though there tends to be a rebound phenomenon at three months after stopping treatment.

The carcinoid tumours associated with the Zollinger–Ellison syndrome or those patients with MEN type 1 also have hypergastrinaemia and a predominance of middle-aged females (average 48 years). The tumours tend to be multicentric with a minimal gastritis but both hyperplasia and endocrine cell dysplasia are present. These tumours often extend into deep muscle and have lymph node metastasis.

More aggressive behaviour is seen in those solitary tumours occurring in men which have similar mucosal changes as those with Zollinger–Ellison syndrome. These patients present at about the same age (49 years), the mucosa shows a minimal non-specific gastritis and only focal hyperplasia but no dysplasia of the endocrine cells. The tumours tend to be larger (median 2 cm) and serosal infiltration with lymphatic and vascular invasion is recognised. Liver metastasis and an accompanying carcinoid syndrome have been reported. Metastases are present in 52% and approximately one-third of the patients will have died in a median of 51 months.

The fourth type of tumour showing neuroendrocrine differentiation is the poorly differentiated carcinoid. These also tend to be solitary and affect the acidopeptic mucosa with an accompanying chronic active gastritis. At presentation these tend to be slightly older than the other groups, median 65 years (range 41–76 years) and again males predominate. This is sometimes associated with a hypergastrinaemia or G-cell hyperplasia. The lesions tend to be large, deeply invasive and as a consequence the median survival is short (6.5 months with a range of 1–12 months) death frequently being tumour related.

Carcinoma of the oesophagus

Squamous carcinoma

There is a strong association between squamous cancer, alcohol intake and smoking in different parts of the world. Up to 80% of the male cases in USA, Latin America and Japan have a history of either one or the other factor, whereas in Iran and China these are not considered to be major causative agents.[63] Restricted diets with micronutritional deficiencies of vitamins A, C and riboflavin may potentiate dietary carcinogens. There is some evidence to suggest the human papilloma virus may be important in some tumours.

Several predisposing factors have been reported (Table 1.5). Achalasia has a reported risk of cancer development of between 0 and 33 times that of the normal population and a prevalence of approximately 3.7%.[64] Chemical strictures which have developed following mucosal damage from various ingested insults include lye.[65] The progression from a benign fibrous stricture to tumour occurs in 0.8–7.2% of patients, with a latent period of up to 40 years. Tylosis, a condition of abnormal keratinisation affecting the palms and soles of the feet, has been associated with a few cases of oesophageal cancer.[66] Postcricoid dysphagia with hypochromatic (iron deficiency) anaemia frequently with mucosal webs is known as Plummer Vinson or Patterson Brown Kelly syndromes. The webs consist of thin mucosal

Table 1.5 *Predisposing factors for oesophageal carcinoma*

Achalasia
Chemical strictures
Tylosis
Plummer Vinson or Patterson Brown Kelly syndrome
Oesophageal diverticulae
Barrett's oesophagus
Irradiation treatment

folds. Some epithelial changes extend into the oral mucosa these consist of epithelial atrophy or hyperkeratinization and could account for the high incidence (up to 16%) of these patients having aerodigestive cancers.[67] The pharyngo-oesophageal (Zenker's) diverticulum found at the border of the cricopharyngeus and the inferior constrictor muscles have a reported incidence of cancer of 0.3–0.8%.[68] The tumours tend to be at the apex of the diverticulum and by the time of diagnosis are usually in an advanced stage with extension through the wall. Barrett's oesophagus can occasionally be associated with a squamous carcinoma though an adenocarcinoma is more usual.[69] There is a slight increased incidence of squamous cancer in patients with coeliac disease though more frequently this condition has been complicated by small bowel lymphoma.[70] The least frequent possible aetiology is that of irradiation treatment as only 13 cases have so far been reported.[71]

The appearances of squamous carcinoma are usually in an advanced stage when resected and tend to have a fungating, ulcerating or infiltrating configuration, though occasional verrucous, polypoid or multifocal types are seen. Ulcerating lesions (Fig. 1.12) have raised rolled edges with necrotic centres whereas the stenosing variety shows a diffuse full circumferential infiltrating mass often with a grey white fibrous cut surface. The endoscopic appearances of early tumours may be better appreciated by use of the vital stains, toluidine blue or iodine. They have been reported as showing either a mosaic or hypervascular pattern or may remain occult.[72] The pathological findings are similar to the advanced stages with erosions, plaques or polypoid masses within the lumen.[73] If previous chemotherapy has been given then the tumour appearance changes as a consequence of tumour shrinkage and scarring.

Tumour infiltration and spread will depend on the site of the primary.[74] Approximately three-quarters of the tumours at presentation will extend through the submucosa and deep muscle layers into adventitial tissue and lymph nodes. Approximately 40% of tumours within the upper third of the oesophagus will spread to the abdominal nodes whereas approximately similar numbers from the lower third will extend into the cervical lymph node chains. Metastatic

Figure 1.12
Oesophageal carcinoma with a central ulceration and an irregular margin. To one side there is a smaller nodule which represents intramucosal spread.

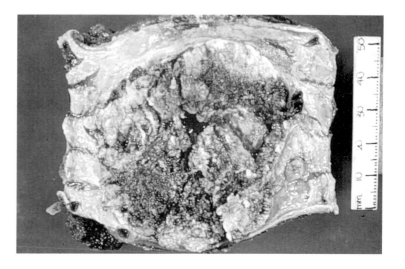

tumour to visceral organs, most frequently liver and lung, has been demonstrated in 40–75% whereas lymph nodes are involved in 70%.[75] The more undifferentiated the malignancy the greater the metastatic potential. An incidental second tumour of the aerodigestive tract can be found in one in ten patients and this may also be related to the use of tobacco and alcohol.

Depending on the degree of keratinisation, keratin whorl formation and the cytological atypia present, the histological appearances can be described as well, moderate or poorly differentiated (Fig. 1.13). Two variations are occasionally seen. These are the verrucous carcinoma which is similar to that found at other sites such as the penis or head and neck with a predominantly exophytic papillary and warty appearance which form an intraluminal fungating mass. Histopathological

Figure 1.13
Squamous carcinoma of the oesophagus which is formed from lobulated islands of prickle cells (arrow head).

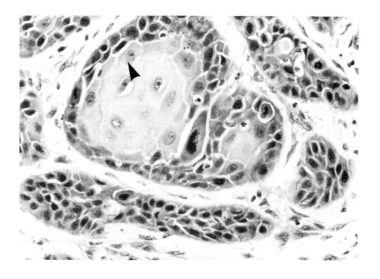

interpretation of these tumours is sometimes difficult especially when superficial biopsies have been taken. The two main differential diagnoses of this indolent malignant tumour are pseudoepitheliomatous hyperplasia which is a benign reactive change and a squamous papilloma which is very uncommon in humans and could be virally induced. The second variant is the carcinosarcoma,[76] which also appears as an exophytic mass and is composed of a mixture of both squamous and spindle cells. The latter are thought to be keratinocytes showing differentiation towards spindle cells and so giving rise to the appearance of a 'sarcoma'. Although the microscopic features are worrying the tumours behave in a less aggressive manner than the pure squamous carcinoma.

Precancerous conditions: dysplasia

Dysplasia and carcinoma *in situ* are regarded as precancerous conditions of the oesophagus and the atypia is similar to that found in other squamous epithelia such as the cervix or bronchial epithelium. There is irregular maturation of the keratinocytes with abnormally situated mitotic figures accompanied by nuclear enlargement and variation in size. If there is evidence that the squamous cells show some maturation this is regarded as dysplasia whereas the full thickness abnormality is classified as carcinoma *in situ*. The suggestion that these two conditions are premalignant has come from the finding of dysplasia in up to 8% of the population in high risk areas and the abnormalities of DNA within the mucosa.[77]

The finding of dysplasia is sufficiently worrying for surveillance to be contemplated as the risk of developing carcinoma is increased.[78] In screened high risk populations the finding of dysplasia predates the development of carcinoma by approximately five years. Carcinoma *in situ* can also be found at a distance from the primary tumour in up to 14% of resections. This is associated with the development of the secondary oesophageal malignancy or other tumours in the aerodigestive tract. The precursor lesion for development of dysplasia is not well identified though in areas of high risk there is an increased instance of moderate to severe chronic oesophagitis suggesting luminal damage may in part be responsible for this preneoplastic change.

Adenocarcinoma in Barrett's oesophagus

First described in 1950[79] Barrett's oesophagus is defined as the replacement of the squamous epithelium by a columnar-lined mucosa in the lower oesophagus (Fig. 1.14). This is usually regarded as a consequence of chronic gastro-oesophageal reflux and the metaplastic change can be towards either gastric fundal or cardiac type of mucosa as well as the more characteristic intestinal type.[80] The first paper describing a carcinoma associated with the metaplastic change was reported three years after the original paper. The incidence of these tumours has been the subject of many reviews and now accounts for 7–35% of tumours

Figure 1.14
Barrett's oesophagus in which the squamous epithelium is displaced uniformly away from the oesophago-gastric junction and the mucosa takes on the macroscopic appearances of that of the gastric mucosa.

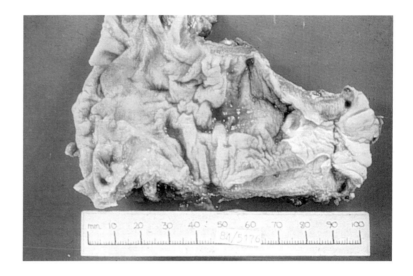

of the oesophagus.[81] The incidence of malignancy in cases of Barrett's has been estimated to vary between 1 in 80 and 1 in 440 cases, but is increasing at an alarming rate. From these figures it has been suggested that the risk of developing an adenocarcinoma is between 30 and 40 times that of the general population.

The predisposing factors to developing cancer in Barrett's oesophagus at the present time are unknown. The development of metaplasia is thought to be irreversible though some regression has been identified following antireflux surgery and recently with laser ablation. Despite the possibility of reversal, tumours may however develop after surgery.[82] The area of involvement and duration of the metaplasia appear insufficient to identify those patients at risk of developing malignancy.[83] From epidemiological studies Barrett's oesophagus is uncommon in the black population of America, whereas alcohol and smoking may predispose the conversion of Barrett's to a malignant process. This suggests that the population at risk are white males who smoke and use alcohol[84] and who possibly may benefit from a screening programme, although this risk is questioned by some authors.[85]

Macroscopically the tumours appear as exophytic masses, ulcers (Fig. 1.15) or endophytic irregular masses. Histologically the majority are adenocarcinoma with features similar to the intestinal type of gastric carcinoma though other variants including neoplasms showing additional neuroendrocrine features and even squamous carcinoma have been reported. To confirm that the tumour has arisen from a Barrett's oesophagus, the metaplastic change should be present in the adjacent mucosa though this has only been demonstrated pre-operatively in 35% of biopsy material.[86] In short segment Barrett's oesophagus, where the metaplastic epithelium is less than 2 cm in length, it may be difficult to demonstrate after resection due to the distortion of the mucosa by the tumour.

Figure 1.15
Barrett's oesophagus with an adeno-carcinoma showing an irregular ulcer-ating tumour which is encroaching upon the metaplastic mucosa. The residual squamous epithelium has been left as grey white mucosal islands separated by the bands of meta-plastic mucosa.

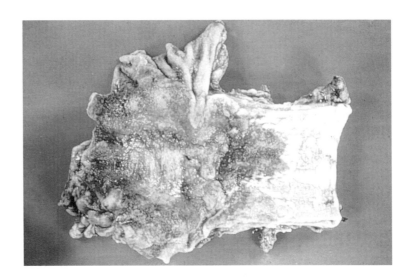

Dysplasia in Barrett's

The premalignant change in Barrett's has been given a variety of descriptive terms which have included carcinoma *in situ*, dysplastic change, adenomatous neoplasms, adenomatous hyperplasia, adeno-matous change, adenoma and oesophageal columnar intraepithelial neoplasia.[87] The latter may be preferable since it follows similar termi-nology being applied to other organs. As with other glandular mucosa, dysplasia can be categorised by its architectural disorganisation, changes in the epithelial morphology and cytology of the individual cells (Fig. 1.16).[88] Regenerative changes are often accompanied by significant atypia, within the base of the glands, a diagnosis of intra-epithelial neoplasia requires involvement of the entire mucosal thickness or the luminal portions of the mucosa. Three grades of dysplasia (mild, moderate and severe) have been suggested, though significant intra- and interobservational variation make this grading difficult to use. A scheme of reporting columnar intraepithelial neoplasia similar to that used in ulcerative colitis has also been suggested (Table 1.6). This is used to indicate the degree of confidence of the pathologist as to the diagnosis and the severity of the pre-malignant change. It has been recommended that the high-grade dysplasia should be confirmed by a second pathologist before treat-ment is started and a further four quadrant biopsies using jumbo forceps at 2 cm intervals to map the dysplasia[89] and detect possible synchronous cancers. At the present time the natural sequence is thought to be the progression from the intestinal type of metaplastic change through dysplasia to invasive cancer. The time interval between each of these phases is unknown but it is assumed to be a matter of years. Progression from high-grade dysplasia to cancer, however, can be as short as several months. The management of these lesions will be discussed in later chapters.

Figure 1.16
Dysplasia in a Barrett's mucosa. The glands are irregular and lined by an epithelium which is pseudostratified (arrowheads) and thickened in comparison with the normal columnar cells of the metaplastic mucosa.

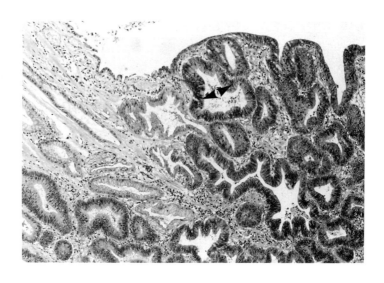

Other oesophageal tumours

In addition to the squamous and adenocarcinoma of the oesophagus there are two other malignant tumours which although uncommon should be considered in the differential diagnosis. The adenoid cystic carcinoma[90] is an uncommon tumour usually found in males over 60 years. Most have been reported in small series and represent 0.75–5% of oesophageal cancers. They are thought to arise from the ducts or acini of submucosal glands and present as ulcerating or fungating masses in the distal oesophagus. Microscopically they are similar to those found in the salivary gland and composed of islands of basophilic cells with thickening of the basement membrane and microcystic structures. These tumours are also reported in the trachea, breast, skin and cervix with variable survival though in the oesophagus most patients die within two years. These tumours are further discussed in Chapter 9.

Table 1.6 *Reporting classification of dysplasia in Barrett's oesophagus*

Negative for dysplasia
Indefinite for dysplasia
Probably negative
Unknown significance
Probably positive
Positive for dysplasia
Low-grade
Intermediate-grade
High-grade

Figure 1.17 *Oat cell carcinoma of oesophagus which is composed of sheets of undifferentiated cells with little cytoplasm showing streaming of the cells within the tumour. The appearances are similar to the more common bronchial oat cell and from which they must be differentiated.*

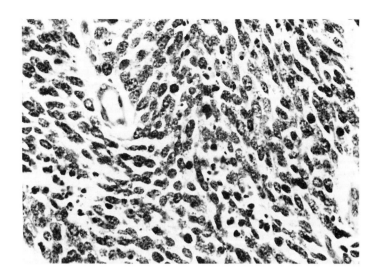

A similarly infrequent tumour is the small cell carcinoma which represents 0.05–18% of oesophageal cancers; approximately half of reported cases have come from Japan.[8,91] They present in the lower and middle third and are more usually found in males in the fifth to sixth decade. Exophytic or ulcerative growths measure on average 6 cm at presentation. It is unclear whether they arise from totipotential reserve cells at the base of the squamous epithelium or from oesophageal/tracheobronchial mucosa in the embryonic foregut (Fig. 1.17). As with lung equivalents ectopic hormone secretion (ACTH, calcitonin, somatostatin or gastrin) has been reported. These tumours are further discussed in Chapter 9.

The future: molecular aspects

Epithelial tumours result from the accumulation of multiple genetic defects which leads to uncontrolled growth.[92] Modification of the tumour growth occurs as a result of the local effects of cytokines, growth factors and the interaction with the stromal components. A stepwise progression has been suggested, from the possible precursor lesions to cancer although the initiating events are unknown. The most plausible pathway for gastric cancer is shown (Fig. 1.18) and indicates that the underlying mechanisms may be different for the diffuse and intestinal types of tumour.

There has been a massive explosion in the knowledge of the genetic abnormalities in both gastric and oesophageal cancer and these have been well reviewed.[93–95] The changes present can be classified as consisting of abnormalities in DNA content, in the karyotype (including allele loss), oncogene and tumour suppressant gene expression (or deletion), of cell cycle regulation and finally of DNA repair genes.

Figure 1.18
Genetic pathway for gastric carcinoma.

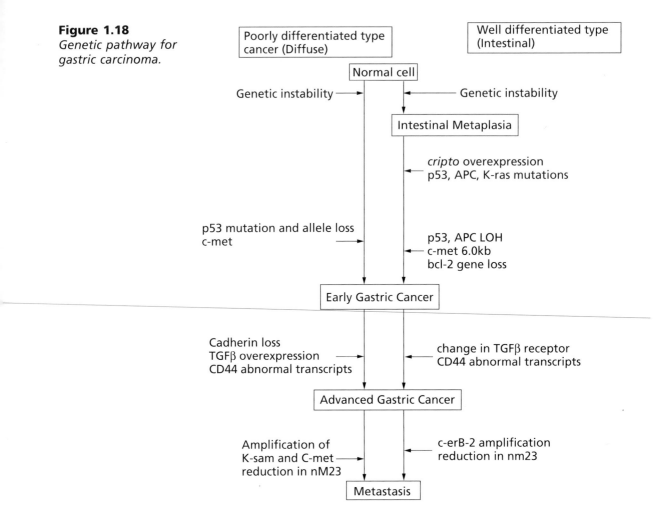

Gastric carcinoma

Heterogeneity of tumours is not only expressed in the morphological picture but also in its DNA content as up to 30% of tumours show a mixed diploid and aneuploid pattern. There are significant differences in the DNA content of tumours, for instance tumours of the cardia are nearly all aneuploid and have a poor prognosis.[96] Despite this, diffuse cancers with their poorer prognosis in general, tend to be less aneuploid than the intestinal type malignancies. The tumour suppressor gene p53, which is found on the short arm of chromosome 17, is thought to play a pivotal role in cell regulation and tumorigenesis. Its normal function is to put a brake on DNA replication and to act as a trigger for apoptosis, in response to significant DNA damage. Point mutations are the most frequent abnormality found and these and other defects are noted in up to 60% of tumours.

Abnormalities of the proto-oncogenes are now being described[97] which suggest that they are early events in carcinogenesis. Loss of heterozygosity (LOH) in the proto-oncogene C-met continues to be present in up to 30% of intestinal cancers and correlates with peritonal dissemination.[93] A member of the fibroblastic growth factor receptor family, K-sam is amplified in both diffuse and scirrhous carcinomas but not other types of tumours.[98] The finding of overexpression of c-erB-2 is controversial. In some tumours it has been associated with more rapid metastasis to the liver though in other reports overexpression had the reverse effect with patients having a longer survival.[97] Amplification and overexpression of *c-myc* is found in both intestinal metaplasia, in some cases of dysplasia and advanced gastric cancer but not in early gastric cancer.

The growth factors tumour growth factor-α (TGFα), epithelial growth factor (EGF), amphiregulin and interleukin 1α, which modulate interactions between tumour cells and stroma, are overexpressed in tumours. A new oncogene, *cripto*, a member of the EGF family is associated both with the intestinal metaplasia and carcinoma and so far there is good correlation between the tumour stage and the prognosis when expressing this oncogene. Deletions of the *cripto* gene occur both in intestinal metaplasia and well-differentiated adenocarcinoma although overexpression has been reported.

Abnormalities in the mismatch repair genes[99] have been found in significant numbers of diffuse (64%) adenocarcinoma whereas in comparison 7% of the intestinal type malignancies have similar defects. At the present time it is unclear whether this abnormality causes the accumulation of the genetic changes, of oncogenes or tumour suppressor genes in the same cancer.

The metastasis-related gene *CD44*[100] is a linking protein between the extracellular matrix and the cell surface. In cancers, this protein is defective and shows a significant difference in expression between intestinal and diffuse cancers. Another is *nM23* which is thought to be a suppressor gene for metastasis and encodes for nucleotide diphosphate kinase and the c-myc transcription factor. Overexpression of this gene in a primary tumour is found to be related to the reduced risk of developing metastasis.

Oesophageal carcinoma

Although the histological progression from normal to invasive squamous carcinoma is readily identified, the molecular basis is still unclear and is actively being researched.[98] In up to half the cases of squamous carcinoma, the *p53* gene has been found to be abnormal, either with point mutations or loss of heterozygosity. This genetic damage results in the loss of some of the regulatory mechanisms of proliferation and leads to uncontrolled cellular growth. In addition *p53* is often accompanied by abnormalities of several other tumour suppressor genes, including deletions or loss of heterozygosity of the retinoblastoma

(Rb, 48%), mutated in colorectal carcinoma (MCC, 63%), adenomatous polyposis coli (APC, 67%), deleted in colorectal cancer (DCC, 24%) genes. In nearly all cases one of these tumour suppressor genes is defective, and nearly three quarters of the squamous carcinomas have two abnormalities. As *p53* expression is found in normal and dysplastic epithelium, it has been suggested that this occurs early in the pathway leading to malignancy.

In Barrett's metaplasia, abnormalities of the *p53* increase with the progression from the intestinal type metaplastic mucosa through the grades of dysplasia to adenocarcinoma. In comparison with squamous carcinoma, it has been reported that there is preferential mutation of exon 5 whereas in the adenocarcinoma exon 8 is more frequently damaged. Mapping studies have shown similar defects of p53 throughout different parts of the tumour, suggesting a clonal origin and that this precedes losses in chromosome 17p unlike colorectal cancers.

Overexpression and amplification of oncogenes has also been found frequently in squamous carcinoma. In up to 70% of tumours epidermal growth factor receptor (EGFR) has been found overexpressed or abnormal. This has correlated well with the degree of dysplasia in the precursor lesions and with the frequency of lymph node metastases in resected tumours. The ligands for the receptor, EGF and TGFα as well as the messenger RNA, have been demonstrated both in tumours and in cell lines derived from squamous carcinoma. Recent interest has focused on the relationship between the tumour and the stroma, as these growth factors are produced by both components. The ras oncogene family, unlike other gastrointestinal tract cancers, appears not to have an important role in the genesis of squamous carcinoma.

Few studies have looked at the oncogenes and growth factors in adenocarcinoma, EGFR is amplified and there is overexpression of TGFα, h-ras and erb-B2. These factors are expressed in greater amounts with progression from normal to the malignant tumour.

As the pathways for tumour development are further understood, the function of 'molecular pathology' will be better defined in the future. This will enable the present diagnostic problems to be resolved. This includes the differentiation between regenerative hyperplasia and dysplasia, in order to provide more prognostic information and possibly recognised high risk groups in any surveillance programmes undertaken.

References

1. Smans M, Muir CS, Boyle P (eds). Atlas of cancer mortality in the European Economic Community. IARC Scientific Publication 107. 1992; 62–7 and 918–21.
2. Ideda Y, Mori M, Kamakura T, Haraguchi Y, Saku M, Sugimachi K. Improvements in diagnosis have changed the incidence of histological types in advanced gastric cancer. Br J Cancer 1995; 72: 424.
3. Blot WJ, Devesa SS, Kneller RW *et al.* Rising

incidence of adenocarcinoma of the esophagus and gastric cardia. JAMA 1991; 265: 1287–9.

4. Borrmann R. Makroskopische Formen des vorgeschritteten Magenkrebses. In: Henke F, Lubarach O (eds). Handbuch der speziellen pathologischen Anatomie und Histologie Vol 4/1. Berlin: Springer, 1926.

5. Lauren P. The two histological main types of gastric carcinoma: diffuse and so called intestinal-type carcinoma. Acta Pathol Microbiol Scand 1965; 64: 31–49.

6. Goseki N, Maruyama M, Takisawa T, Koike M. Morphological changes in gastric carcinoma with progression. J Gastroenterol 1995; 30: 287.

7. Ming S-C. Gastric carcinoma. A pathobiological classification. Cancer 1977; 39: 2475–85.

8. Watanabe H, Jass JR, Sobin LH. Histological typing of gastric and oesophageal tumours. WHO International Histological Classification of Tumours 2nd edn, Berlin: Springer-Verlag, 1990.

9. Boku T, Nakane Y, Minoura T et al. Prognostic significance of serosal invasion and free intraperitoneal cancer cells in gastric cancer. Br J Surg 1990; 77: 436.

10. Abe S, Shiraishi M, Nagaoka S, Yoshimura H, Dhar DK, Nakamura T. Serosal invasion as the single prognostic indicator in stage IIIA (T3N1M0) gastric cancer. Surgery 1991; 109: 582.

11. Ichiyoshi Y, Maehara Y, Tomisaki S et al. Macroscopic intraoperative diagnosis of serosal invasion and clinical outcome of gastric cancer: risk of underestimation. J Surg Oncol 1995; 59: 255.

12. Di Giorgio A, Botti C, Sammartino P, Mingazzini P, Flammia M, Stipa V. Extracapsular lymphnode metastases in the staging and prognosis of gastric cancer. Int Surg 1991; 76: 218.

13. Kakeji Y, Korenaga D, Baba H et al. Surgical treatment of patients with gastric carcinoma and duodenal invasion. J Surg Oncol 1995; 59: 215.

14. Nakamura K, Ueyama T, Yao T et al. Pathology and prognosis of gastric carcinoma. Findings in 10,000 patients who underwent primary gastrectomy. Cancer 1992; 70: 1030.

15. Murakami T. Pathomorphological diagnosis.

16. Mori M, Sakaguchi H, Akazawa K, Tsuneyoshi M, Sueishi K, Sugimachi K. Correlation between metastatic site, histological type, and serum tumor markers of gastric carcinoma. Hum Pathol 1995; 26: 504.

17. Farley DR, Donohue JH. Early gastric cancer. Surg Clin North Am 1992, 72: 401.

18. Tsuchiya A, Kikuchi Y, Ando Y, Yoshida T, Abe R. Lymph node metastases in gastric cancer invading the submucosal layer. Eur J Surg Oncol 1995; 21: 248.

19. Sano T, Sasako M, Kinoshita T, Maruyama K. Recurrence of early gastric cancer. Follow-up of 1475 patients and review of the Japanese literature. Cancer 1993; 72: 3174.

20. Kitamura K, Yamaguchi T, Okamoto K et al. Total gastrectomy for early gastric cancer. J Surg Oncol 1995; 60: 83.

21. Kim JP, Hur YS, Yang HK. Lymph node metastasis as a significant prognostic factor in early gastric cancer: analysis of 1,136 early gastric cancers. Ann Surg Oncol 1995; 2: 308.

22. Hayes N, Karat D, Scott D, Raimes S, Griffin SM. Radical lymphadenectomy for early gastric carcinoma. Br J Surg 1996; 83: 1421–3.

23. Brito MJ, Filipe MI, Williams GT et al. DNA ploidy in early gastric carcinoma (T1). A flow cytometric study of 100 European cases. Gut 1993; 34: 230–4.

24. Correa P, Chen VW. Gastric cancer. Cancer Surv 1994; 20: 55.

25. Wyatt JL. Gastritis and its relation to gastritic carcinogenesis. Semin Diagn Pathol 1991; 8: 137–48.

26. Sjoblom SM, Sipponen P, Jarvinen H. Gastroscopic follow-up of pernicious anemia patients. Gut 1993; 24: 28–32.

27. Silva S, Filipe MI. Intestinal metaplasia and its variants in the gastric mucosa of Portuguese subjects. A comparative analysis of biopsy and gastrectomy material. Hum Pathol 1986; 17: 988–95.

28. Sipponen P, Kimura K. Intestinal metaplasia, atrophic gastritis and stomach cancer: trends over time. Eur J Gastroenterol Hepatol 1994; 6: S79.

29. Stemmermann GN. Intestinal metaplasia of the stomach. A status report. Cancer 1994; 74: 556.

30. Ho SB, Shekels LL, Toribara NW et al. Mucin

gene expression in normal, preneoplastic, and neoplastic human gastric epithelium. Cancer Res 1995; 55: 2681.

31. Saegusa M, Takano Y, Okayasu I. Bcl-2 expression and its association with cell kinetics in human gastric carcinomas and intestinal metaplasia. J Cancer Res Clin Oncol 1995; 121: 357.

32. Correa P, Fox J, Fontham E *et al. Helicobacter pylori* and gastric carcinoma: serum antibody prevalence in populations with contrasting cancer risks. Cancer 1990; 66: 2569–74.

33. Sipponen P, Hyvarinen H. Role of *Helicobacter pylori* in the pathogenesis of gastritis, peptic ulcer and gastric cancer. Scand J Gastroenterol Suppl. 1993; 196: 3.

34. Antonioli DA. Precursors of gastric carcinoma: a critical review with a brief description of early (curable) gastric cancer. Hum Pathol 1994; 25: 994.

35. Hill MJ. Bacterial N-nitrosation and gastric carcinogenesis in humans. Ital J Gastroenterol 1991; 23: 17.

36. Correa P, Shiao YH. Phenotypic and genotypic events in gastric carcinogenesis. Cancer Res 1994; 54 (7 Suppl): 1941.

37. Eidt S, Stolte M. The significance of *Helicobacter pylori* in relation to gastric cancer and lymphoma. Eur J Gastroenterol Hepatol 1995; 7: 318.

38. Genta RM, Graham DY. *Helicobacter pylori*: the new bug on the (paraffin) block. Virchows Arch 1994; 425: 339.

39. Parsonnet J, Freidman CD, Vandersteen DP *et al. Helicobacter* infection and the risk of gastric carcinoma. N Engl J Med 1991; 325: 1127–31.

40. Vollmers HP, Dammrich J, Ribbert H *et al.* Human monoclonal antibodies from stomach carcinoma patients react with *Helicobacter pylori* and stimulate stomach cancer cells in vitro. Cancer 1994; 74: 1525–32.

41. Ming S-C. Malignant potential of epithelial polyps of the stomach. In Ming S-C (ed) Precursors of gastric cancer. New York: Praeger, 1984, pp. 219–31.

42. Nakamura T, Nakano GI. Histopathological classification, and malignant change in gastric polyps. J Clin Pathol 1985; 38: 754–64.

43. Hattori T. Morphological range of hyperplastic polyps and carcinomas arising in hyperplastic polyps of the stomach. J Clin Pathol 1985; 38: 622–30.

44. Iida M, Yao T, Watanabe H *et al.* Fundic gland polyposis in patients without familial adenomatotis coli: its incidence and clinical features. Gastroenterology 1984; 86: 1437–42.

45. Kolodziejczyk P, Yao T, Oya M *et al.* Long-term follow-up study of patients with gastric adenomas with malignant transformation. An immunohistochemical and histochemical analysis. Cancer 1994; 74: 2896.

46. Sarre RG, Frost AG, Jagelman DG *et al.* Gastric and duodenal polyps in familial adenomatous polyposis. A prospective study of the nature and prevalence of upper gastrointestinal polyps. Gut 1987; 28: 306–14.

47. Xaun ZX, Ambe K, Enjoji M. Depressed adenoma of the stomach revisited: histologic, histochemical and immunohistochemical profiles. Cancer 1991; 67: 2382–9.

48. Domellof L, Eriksson S, Janunger K-G. Carcinoma and possible precancerous changes of the gastric stump after Billroth II resection. Gastroenterology 1977; 73: 462–8.

49. Sebagh M, Flejou JF, Potet F. Lymphoma of the gastric stump. Report of two cases and review of the literature. J Clin Gastroenterol 1995; 20: 147.

50. Johnson MI, Spark JI, Ambrose NS, Wyatt JI. Early gastric cancer in a patient with Ménétrièr's disease, lymphocytic gastritis and *Helicobacter pylori*. Eur J Gastroenterol Hepatol 1995; 7: 187.

51. Lee S, Iida M, Yao T *et al.* Long-term follow-up of 2529 patients reveals gastric ulcers rarely become malignant. Dig Dis Sci 1990; 35: 763–8.

52. Morson BC, Sobin LH, Grundmann E, Johansen A, Nagayo T, Serck-Hanssen A. Precancerous conditions and epithelial dysplasia in the stomach. J Clin Pathol 1980; 33: 711–21.

53. Coma del Corral MJ, Pardo-Mindan FJ, Razquin S *et al.* Risk of cancer in patients with gastric dysplasia: follow-up study of 67 patients. Cancer 1990; 65: 2078–85.

54. Appelman H. Smooth muscle tumours of the gastrointestinal tract. What we know now that Stout didn't know. Am J Surg Pathol 1986; 10 (Suppl 1): 83–99.

55. van de Rijn M, Hendrickson MR, Rouse RV. CD34 expression by gastrointestinal tract stromal tumours. Hum Pathol 1994; 25: 766–71.

56. Dawson IMP, Cornes JS, Morson BC. Primary malignant lymphoid tumours of the intestinal tract. Report of 37 cases with a study of factors influencing prognosis. Br J Surg 1961; 49: 80–9.

57. Isaacson PG. Gastrointestinal lymphoma. Hum Pathol 1994; 25: 1020–9.

58. Montalban C, Castrillo JM, Abraira V et al. Gastric B-cell mucosa-associated lymphoid tissue (MALT) lymphoma. Clinicopathological study and evaluation of the prognostic factors in 143 patients. Ann Oncol 1995; 6: 355.

59. Inagaki H, Nonaka M, Nagaya S, Tateyama H, Sasaki M, Eimoto T. Monoclonality in gastric lymphoma detected in formalin-fixed, paraffin-embedded endoscopic biopsy specimens using immunohistochemistry, in situ hybridization, and polymerase chain reaction. Diagn Mol Pathol 1995; 4: 32.

60. Dierlamm J, Pittaluga S, Wlodarska I et al. Marginal zone B-cell lymphomas of different sites share similar cytogenetic and morphologic features. Blood 1996; 87: 299.

61. Wotherspoon AC, Doglioni C, Diss TC et al. Regression of primary low-grade B-cell gastric lymphoma of mucosa associated lymphoid tissue type after eradication of *Helicobacter pylori*. Lancet 1993; 342: 575–7.

62. Solcia E, Fiocca R, Villani L, Luinetti O, Capella C. Hyperplastic, dysplastic, and neoplastic enterochromaffin-like-cell proliferations of the gastric mucosa. Classification and histogenesis. Am J Surg Pathol 1995; 19: S1–7.

63. Munoz N, Crespi M, Grassi A, Wang Guo Qing, Shen Qiong, Li Zhang Cai. Precursor lesions of oesophageal cancer in high-risk populations in Iran and China. Lancet 1982; i: 876–9.

64. Streitz J Jr, Ellis F Jr, Gibb SP, Heatley GM. Achalasia and squamous cell carcinoma of the esophagus: analysis of 241 patients. Ann Thorac Surg 1995; 59: 1604.

65. Applequist P, Salmo M. Lye corrosion carcinoma of the esophagus. A review of 63 cases. Cancer 1980; 45: 2655–8.

66. O'Mahoney MY, Ellis JP, Hellier M, Mann R, Huddy P. Familial tylosis and carcinoma of the oesophagus. J R Soc Med 1984; 77: 514–517.

67. Chisholm M. The association between webs iron and post-cricoid carcinoma. Postgrad Med J 1974; 50: 215.

68. Huang B-S, Unni KK, Payne WS. Long term survival following diverticulectomy for cancer in pharyngooesophageal (Zenker's) diverticulum. Ann Thorac Surg 1984; 38: 207–10.

69. Tamura H, Schulman SA. Barrett-type esophagus associated with squamous carcinoma. Chest 1971; 59: 330–3.

70. Swinson C, Slavin G, Coles EC, Booth CC. Coeliac disease and malignancy. Lancet 1983; i: 111–15.

71. Sherrill DJ, Grishkin BA, Galal FS, Zajtchuk R, Graeber GM. Radiation induced associated malignancies of the oesophagus. Cancer 1984; 54: 726–8.

72. Contini S, Consigli GF, Di Lecee F, Chiapasco M, Ferri T, Orsi P. Vital staining of oesophagus in patients with head and neck cancer: still a worthwhile procedure. Ital J Gastroenterol 1991; 23: 5–8.

73. Bogomoletz WT, Molas G, Gayet B, Potet F. Superficial squamous cell carcinoma of the esophagus. A report of 76 cases and review of the literature. Am J Surg Pathol 1989; 13: 535–46.

74. Jaskiemdcz K, Banach L, Mafungo V, Knobel GJ. Oesophageal mucosa in a population at risk of oesophageal cancer: postmortem 72 studies. Int J Cancer 1992; 50: 32–5.

75. Sugimachi K, Matsuoka H, Ohno S, Mori M, Kuwano H. Multivariate approach for assessing the prognosis of clinical oesophageal carcinoma. Br J Surg 1988; 75: 1115–18.

76. Enrile FT, De Jesus PO, Bakst AA, Baluyot R. Pseudosarcoma of the esophagus (polypoid carcinoma of the esophagus with pseudosarcomatous features). Cancer 1975; 31: 1197–202.

77. Matsuura H, Kuwano H, Morita M et al. Predicting recurrence time of esophageal carcinoma through assessment of histological factors and DNA ploidy. Cancer 1991; 67: 1406–11.

78. Muir CS, McKinney PA. Cancer of the oesophagus: a global overview. Eur J Cancer Prev 1992; 1: 259.

79. Barrett NR. Chronic peptic ulcer of the oesophagus and 'oesophagitis'. Br J Surg 1950; 38: 175–82.

80. Womack C, Harvey L. Columnar epithelial line oesophagus (CELO) or Barrett's oesophagus: mucin chemistry, dysplasia, and invasive adenocarcinoma. J Clin Pathol 1985; 38: 477–8.

81. Cameron AJ, Ott BJ, Payne WS. The incidence of adenocarcinoma in columnar-lined (Barrett's) esophagus. N Engl J Med 1985; 313: 857–9.

82. Hamilton SR, Hutcheon DF, Ravich WJ, Cameron JL, Paulson M. Adenocarcinoma in Barrett's esophagus after elimination of gastro-esophageal reflux. Gastroenterology 1984; 86: 356–60.

83. Iftikhar SY, James PD, Steele RJ, Hardcastle JD, Atkinson MI. Length of Barrett's oesophagus: an important factor in the development of dysplasia and adenocarcinoma. Gut 1992; 33: 1155–8.

84. Rogers EL, Goldkind SF, Iseri OA et al. Adenocarcinoma of the lower esophagus: a disease primarily of white males with Barrett's esophagus. J Clin Gastroenterol 1986; 8: 613–18.

85. van der Burgh A, Dees J, Hop WCJ, van Blankenstein M. Oesophageal cancer is an uncommon cause of death in patient with Barrett's oesophagus. Gut 1996; 39: 5–8.

86. Haggitt RC. Barrett's esophagus, dysplasia, and adenocarcinoma. Hum Pathol 1994; 25: 982.

87. Lee GR. Dysplasia in Barrett's esophagus: a clinical pathologic study of six patients. Am J Surg Pathol 1985; 9: 845–52.

88. Miros M, Kerlin P, Walker N. Only patients with dysplasia progress to adenocarcinoma in Barrett's oesophagus. Gut 1991; 32: 1441–6.

89. Riddell RH. Dysplasia and regression in Barrett's epithelium. In: Spechler SJ, Goyal RK (eds) Barrett's esophagus: pathophysiology, diagnosis, and management. New York: Elsevier, 1985, pp. 143–52.

90. Cerar A, Jutersek A, Vidmar S. Adenoid cystic carcinoma of the esophagus. A clinicopathological study of three cases. Cancer 1991; 67: 2159–64.

91. Mori M, Matsukuma A, Adachi Y et al. Small cell carcinoma of the esophagus. Cancer 1989; 63: 564–73.

92. Correa P. Human gastric carcinogenesis: a multistep and multifactorial process – First American Cancer Society Award Lecture on Cancer Epidemiology and prevention. Cancer Res 1992; 52: 6735.

93. Tahara E. Genetic alterations in human gastrointestinal cancers. The application to molecular diagnosis. Cancer 1995; 75: 1410–17.

94. Wright PA, Quirke P, Attanoos R, Williams GT. Molecular pathology of gastric carcinoma: progress and prospects. Hum Pathol 1992; 23: 848–59.

95. Yonemura Y, Matsumoto H, Ninomiya I et al. Heterogeneity of DNA ploidy in gastric cancer. Anal Cell Pathol 1992; 4: 61.

96. Wright PA, Williams GT. Gastric carcinoma. In: Quirke P (ed) Molecular biology of digestive disease, 1st edn. London: BMJ Publishing Group, 1994, pp. 44–51.

97. Noguchi Y, Tsuburaya A, Makino T et al. Predictive value of c-erbB-2 and DNA ploidy patterns in gastric carcinoma recurrence. Int Surg 1993; 78: 107.

98. Stemmermann G, Heffelfinger C, Noffsinger A, Zhong Y, Miller MA, Fenoglio-Preiser CM. The molecular biology of esophageal and gastric cancer and their precursors: oncogenes, tumour suppressor genes and growth factors. Hum Pathol 1994; 25: 968–87.

99. Tamura G, Sakata K, Maesawa C et al. Microsatellite alterations in adenoma and differentiated adenocarcinoma of the stomach. Cancer Res 1995; 55: 1933.

100. Harn HJ, Ho LI, Chang JY et al. Differential expression of the human metastasis adhesion molecule CD44V in normal and carcinomatous stomach mucosa of Chinese subjects. Cancer 1995; 75: 1065.

2 Epidemiology and screening for oesophageal and gastric cancer

William H. Allum

Introduction

During the past century there have been remarkable changes in cancer of the oesophagus and stomach. World-wide both are major health problems and much effort has been directed to better understanding of the aetiology and to detecting disease at an early and treatable stage.

Oesophageal cancer is considerably less common than gastric cancer, although it is highly prevalent in parts of the world with high population density, such as China. Incidence in more developed countries has shown increases in the latter part of the century. The tumour type has shown corresponding changes with increased numbers of adenocarcinoma compared with squamous cell cancers and particularly affecting the lower third of the oesophagus.

Gastric cancer has shown an overall world-wide decrease in incidence, but has only recently been overtaken by lung cancer as the commonest world-wide malignancy. Developing countries have tended to predominate in incidence in the latter years although 50 years ago gastric cancer was very common in more socially advanced populations. Dietary and hygiene changes are likely to have been responsible. Nevertheless in more developed countries gastric cancer remains a significant health problem largely because of the plateau in age-standardised incidence reflecting the increase in the ageing population. The incidence of proximal tumours has markedly increased. Indeed the downward migration of oesophageal cancer and a proximal shift in gastric tumours suggests a common aetiology. Furthermore, this has resulted in tumours of the gastric cardia being considered as separate entities.

The overall poor results of treatment have reflected the advanced stage of most cases at presentation. Those parts of the world with high incidence have developed and pursued active mass screening programmes. These have certainly identified precursor lesions and premalignant conditions. Indeed, application of these programmes has produced a significant improvement in survival rates for gastric cancer, particularly in Japan. The knowledge of these changes and underlying conditions has enabled areas of lower incidence to pursue examination of those at estimated high risk. Not only has this begun to increase the number of earlier stage cancers but has also suggested ways in which primary and secondary prevention can begin to reduce overall disease incidence.

Oesophageal cancer

Incidence

In 1985, carcinoma of the oesophagus (ICD Code 150) was the ninth commonest form of malignancy world-wide comprising 4.0% of all cancers.[1] This report from the International Agency for Research in Cancer evaluated cancer incidence by type of country. In developed countries 61 000 cases were registered contrasting with developing countries where 243 000 cases were recorded, representing the fourth most common cancer in these countries. Males predominated with a male to female ratio of approximately 2:1. The highest rates were recorded in China such that 47% of all new cases occurred there. Incidence was not uniform. In Western Europe (France, West Germany, the Benelux Countries; population 155.0 million) there were approximately 9000 new cases contrasting with Northern Europe (UK, Scandinavia; population 83.2 million) where 6100 new cases were registered. The sex incidence was significantly different with a male to female ratio in Western Europe of 4.3:1 compared with 1.3:1 in Northern Europe. Subsequent studies have shown a steady increase in European incidence. Cheng and Day[2] have reported a 60% increase in age-standardised mortality for men in England and Wales between 1956–60 and 1986–90 with a corresponding increase of 35% for women. (Although mortality rates do not precisely correspond to incidence rates the overall poor survival justifies this method of estimation.)

Similarly in a 25-year review of oesophageal cancer in the West Midlands, UK, Matthews et al.[3] reported a rising incidence. The crude incidence over the whole period of study (1957–81) was 5.01 per 100 000 with an age-standardised rate of 3.31. Increasing incidence is apparent for the figures documented for 1957–61 (crude rate 3.63; age-standardised 2.74) compared to those for 1977–81 (crude rate 6.65; age-standardised 4.11). The increases occurred in both sexes with a trend towards a greater increase in women. Factors influencing this increase were partly improvements in registration efficiency but also the effect of the increasing age of the population and an overall increase in the incidence of the disease itself.

Changes in incidence and the actual burden of new cases over time are the result of changes in the size and composition of population and in the actual risk for a specific cancer. The influence of age has already been identified. In the Birmingham study the population was divided into groups (cohorts) according to their year of birth. There is a tendency in both sexes for those born more recently to have higher incidence rates. This implies that the risk in younger people is greater

Figure 2.1
Incidence changes for squamous cell carcinoma and adenocarcinoma of the oesophagus, 1962–1986.

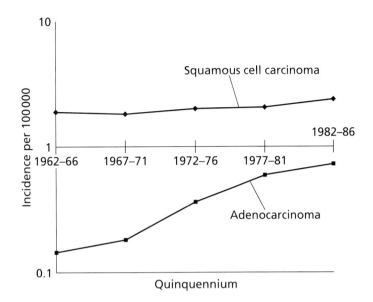

at each age than it was for their elders when they were at the same age. This trend together with the greater longevity of the population has significant implications for both clinical workload as well as the needs for general, social and health care with a predicted increased number of cases of oesophageal cancer.

The increase in incidence in the UK of oesophageal cancer has occurred in both histological subtypes. However, the rate of increase has been greatest for adenocarcinoma (Fig. 2.1).[4] Within the oesophagus there have been corresponding increases in each of the principal subsites. However, the greatest increase by approximately a factor of 5 has occurred in the lower third. When analysed by sex these changes are generally equally distributed although the rate of rise in the lower third has been greater in men.[3]

Demography of oesophageal cancer

Oesophageal cancer shows a remarkable preponderance for variation in prevalence and incidence. Differences between countries have already been described. However, enormous variations are seen between provinces or even districts within certain countries. In the West the incidence in France is three times greater than in Spain. Within France the national average of 10 per 100 000 rises to 30 per 100 000 in Burgundy and Normandy. These rates are dwarfed by the rates in Iran and China. In Linxian county of Northern China the age-adjusted incidence for men is 151 per 100 000 and 115 per 100 000 for women. In parts of Iran the highest world incidence rates have been recorded of 195 cases per 100 000 for females and 165 per 100 000 for males. These rates have tended to be stable for most of this century. However, in South Africa there have been significant increases in the last 40 years. This has particularly occurred in black people where incidence rates of 28.4 per 100 000 men and 17.8 per 100 000 women have been recorded. Furthermore, Yang and Davis[5] reported an increase in incidence in black men and women in the USA. This was most marked for squamous cell carcinoma which was 4–5-fold more common, yet the incidence of adenocarcinoma in the black population was 30% that of the white population. The incidence of squamous cell carcinoma in the black population increased by 30% between 1973 and 1982 with a parallel increase of 74% for adenocarcinoma in white men.

Although traditionally oesophageal cancer has occurred in the seventh and eighth decades, in those parts of the world where the disease is becoming more prevalent, the age at diagnosis is decreasing. McGlashan[6] reviewed death certification in South Africa and found very few cases of oesophageal cancer under 40 years of age for 1980–1982. However, during 1986–1988 8.8% of oesophageal cancer deaths occurred in the third and fourth decade.

These striking variations in incidence and the age of onset which occur in geographically related parts of the world have led to extensive studies searching for common aetiological factors which have resulted in the identification of several premalignant conditions.

Premalignant conditions

Squamous cell carcinoma

Overall squamous cell carcinoma is the commonest histological subtype. It is found predominantly in the areas of highest incidence. These areas are in those countries of low socioeconomic level where poverty and malnutrition predominate. Aetiological studies in Iran and China have evaluated the identification of oesophagitis as a premalignant lesion. It is a different type of oesophagitis from that found in the West and is not associated with gastro-oesophageal reflux (see below).[7] It is characterised by irregular friable mucosa with a varying extent of oedema, leucoplakia and hyperaemia yet without ulceration. There is clear cell acanthosis which manifests itself endoscopically as white patches of mucosa. It is usually found in the middle and lower third of the oesophagus. Frequently this type of oesophagitis is asymptomatic.

In a comparative study of high incidence areas in China and Iran, Munoz et al.[8] found similar changes in the different populations. In addition to the oesophagitis, these authors identified atrophy and dysplasia as common associated changes. From natural history studies over approximately 10 years they postulated a sequence of changes for chronic oesophagitis through atrophy and dysplasia to squamous carcinoma.

Others have reported similar evidence for this hypothesis. Guanrei and Songliang[9] compared endoscopic findings in high and low risk populations. Although chronic oesophagitis incidence was similar, changes of basal cell hyperplasia and dysplasia were more common in the high risk population. In 62 cases from a total of 186 in the high risk area, with dysplasia, 21 (33.8%) developed oesophageal cancer contrasting with five out of 124 with oesophagitis alone or simple hyperplasia (follow-up range 30–78 months). Crespi *et al.*[7] also reported a lower incidence of chronic oesophagitis and no cases of dysplasia in a low risk area of China compared with a high risk area.

In an attempt to identify the underlying cause of these histological changes Chang-Claude *et al.*[10] investigated a population of 15–26-year olds in a high risk area. Using a multivariate case-control analysis they compared a series of factors in those with mild and moderate oesophagitis with those with very mild oesophagitis and normal subjects. Significant changes were associated with ingestion of very hot beverages, a family history of oesophageal cancer, prevalence of oesophagitis among siblings and a low intake of fresh fruits and wheat flour products. Cigarette smoking and the use of cotton seed oil for cooking were usually observed in those with oesophagitis but there was not a striking difference according to level of risk.

Other similar studies have identified riboflavin deficiency[7] and vitamin A and C deficiency[11] as risk factors which are particularly important at a young age. Conversely vitamin C intake confers a protective benefit; Hu *et al.*[12] in a case-control study found that 100 mg vitamin C per day decreased risk by 39%. Overall, those with a nutritionally deficient diet have a higher incidence of oesophageal cancer in the high risk areas.[13]

Dietary habits and customs are additionally important to nutritional content. Hot drinks and coarse foods have been implicated. In both Iran and China wheat contains silica fibres and millet bran contains silica plates. Furthermore, nitrosamine precursors associated with mouldy or pickled foods are commonly ingested in areas of high risk. Not only do nitrosamines come from foodstuffs but also some other ingested substances. In France, apple brandy, in Northern Italy heavy tar-coated cigarettes and in Iran opium smoke are potent sources. The significance of nitrosamines is supported by work in animal models in which ingestion of nitrosamine induces similar lesions to those found in patients in Iran and China.[8]

It has thus been postulated that chronic oesophagitis is the common pathway towards oesophageal cancer. This may be induced directly by mechanical irritation, thermal injury or vitamin deficiencies. Alternatively the inflammatory injury producing oesophagitis increases the sensitivity of the oesophageal mucosa to carcinogens and hence malignant transformation.

Squamous cell carcinoma is also associated with a variety of uncommon conditions which can equally be explained by this hypothesis, relating to some form of inflammatory injury. Oesophageal strictures developing after ingestion of corrosive agents particularly in childhood are associated with a 1000-fold increase in the risk of carcinoma. There is a time delay of 20–40 years after ingestion of the corrosive and as a result tumours are seen at a younger age than normal.

Achalasia is associated but the magnitude of the risk is unclear. Again the risk appears to relate to retention oesophagitis secondary to stasis and exposure to possible carcinogens in fermenting food residue. There is a lead time of approximately 15–20 years and these cases warrant long-term surveillance. Treatment of the achalasia does not seem to reduce the risk.

The Plummer Vinson syndrome of dysplasia, iron-deficiency anaemia, koilonychia and oropharyngeal mucosal atrophy is associated with an increased risk of cervical oesophageal cancer. There are associated vitamin deficiencies including riboflavin that predispose to the carcinogenic tendencies already described.

Finally there is a familial tendency suggesting a genetic predisposition. Tylosis palmarum is a rare inherited autosomal dominant condition in which there is a very high incidence of squamous cell cancer. Perhaps of greater significance is the finding of the increased risk in low risk areas for offspring of parents with oesophageal cancer.[14] There are numerical and structural chromosomal aberrations in patients with a family history not seen in those without a family history.

Adenocarcinoma of the oesophagus

The different populations affected by adenocarcinoma of the oesophagus and the changes in disease pattern over recent years suggest a different aetiology to squamous carcinoma. It can arise from oesophageal mucosal glands, ectopic islands of gastric mucosa or from metaplastic columnar lined epithelium (Barrett's metaplasia). Incidence and aetiology are difficult to define precisely because of the potential for tumours of the gastric cardia to spread to the oesophagus. However, gastro-oesophageal reflux is responsible for typical reflux oesophagitis which although not a premalignant condition is complicated by Barrett's columnar lined oesophagus and reflux-induced stricture which are premalignant conditions.

Oesophageal glands are normally found throughout the oesophagus, ectopic gastric mucosa is most frequent in the upper thoracic and lower cervical oesophagus and by implication from incidence data both are relatively uncommon precursors. Barrett's metaplasia, however, affects the lower third and the increase in cancer incidence reflects increases in the occurrence of this change. In one study 86% of cases of adenocarcinoma revealed Barrett's metaplasia in the surrounding mucosa.[15]

Transformation of Barrett's metaplasia appears to resemble progress of intestinal metaplasia in the stomach (see below). There may be gastric cardia or body type epithelium of intestinal type and it is this latter type which may progress from atrophy to dysplasia and carcinoma. Identification of at-risk patients can be difficult. Although 10% of those with reflux oesophagitis have Barrett's metaplasia as many as 40% may be asymptomatic. Equally the risk of malignant transformation is difficult to determine. Survival data for patients with Barrett's metaplasia have shown little difference from the general population. However, the

Mayo Clinic have reported a 15% prevalence of malignancy which represents a 30-fold increase above the expected rate.

Predisposing factors to malignant transformation include male gender, race (more common in whites), tobacco smoking, length of the columnar lined segment, and previous gastric surgery with associated alkaline reflux. Alkaline reflux appears to discriminate between those at risk of progressing from metaplasia and those not progressing.[16] Furthermore antireflux surgery may actually arrest the progression of Barrett's metaplasia and in principle this should reduce the risk of progression to cancer.

Reflux stricture has been associated with an increased risk. However, most cases also have Barrett's metaplasia and it is thus likely that the latter is more important as a premalignant factor.

Gastric cancer

Incidence

Gastric cancer (ICD Code No 151) has shown a dramatic decrease in incidence over the past 100 years. In 1980 the IARC survey documented it as the commonest form of malignancy world-wide accounting for 10.5% of all registered cancers, a total of almost 670 000 cases per year world-wide. The follow-up survey from 1985 showed it to have fallen to second place behind lung cancer yet still accounts for 755 000 new cases of cancer world-wide each year.[1] Comparison with incidence data shows a decrease from 36 per 100 000 to 20 per 100 000 for men and from 31 to 11 per 100 000 for women between 1920 and 1985[17] in England and Wales. These rates of decline have been similarly documented in other Western series.[18] However, the incidence according to type of country relative to socioeconomic status shows little difference. In 1980 for developed countries, gastric cancer was fourth commonest and for developing countries second commonest with both having similar numbers of new cases (approximately 330 000 in each type of country). This is largely explained by the high incidence in Japan and East Asia as well as in China and Latin America. On an overall basis the number of new cases fell between 1975 and 1980 by 1.9% despite a world population increase of 9.4% which corresponds to an annual rate of decline in crude incidence rate of 2.2%.[19]

In the UK there have been a number of studies assessing in greater detail the nature of this decrease in incidence. In a 25-year review, Fielding et al.[20] reported an overall crude incidence of 24.8 in 100 000 (age adjusted 17.2 per 100 000). The figures for 1957–1961 were 23.4 and 17.40, respectively, falling to 24.8 and 15.3 for 1972–81. The decreases were most marked in women such that the age-standardised male to female ratio rose from 2.02 to 2.34. Analysis by date of birth has shown that those born in more recent years have a generally lower risk than their forebears.

Retrospective registry series are limited by the very nature of case collection. However, during the period 1957–81 Fielding et al.[20] found an increase in the numbers of specific subsites registered, this being

Figure 2.2
*Changes in incidence
by site of gastric
cancer, 1957–1981.*

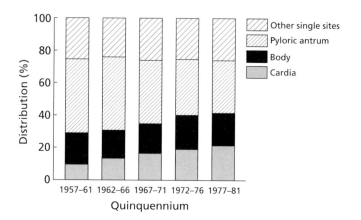

largely due to an improved quality of data recording. A steady rate of decrease in incidence is apparent for distal tumours. However, there is a significant rise in the incidence of carcinoma of the cardia (Fig. 2.2).[21] Others have found similar patterns. Antonioli and Goldman[22] compared a series of consecutive cases from 1938 to 1942 with a series from 1975 to 1978. In the older series there were no cases of cardia cancer contrasting with 27% of the total cases for the more recent period. Patterson *et al.*[23] reported a similar finding. However, the increase in proximal tumours was associated with a decrease in more distal lesions suggesting that the increase in proximal tumours was relative rather than absolute.

Despite an apparent decrease in incidence in Western series the actual effect in numbers of cases appears to be small. Sedgwick *et al.*[24] reviewed trends in incidence and mortality in Scotland and examined the associated surgical workload. It was apparent that although incidence had fallen marginally overall this was not the case for those aged over 65 and at most risk of developing the disease. As a result the number of surgical procedures slightly increased for 1988 when compared with 1979. Furthermore, with the increasing proportion of the population in the older age group the workload both clinically and socially is likely to increase.

The decline in gastric cancer suggests as with other cancers that its cause is largely environmental. Before reviewing the incidence for changes in environmental factors it is worth considering the principal pathological features as these reflect environmental influences.

Pathology of precursor lesions

The histological features of gastric adenocarcinoma are not homogeneous. Various subclassifications have been proposed based on cellular morphology. For epidemiological purposes, the classification by Lauren[25] has proved most useful. Essentially this proposed two major types: (1) intestinal in which features of intestinal mucosa were apparent and (2) diffuse in which cells were more randomly distributed.

The intestinal type has proved most interesting epidemiologically. It is more prevalent in the older age group contrasting with the diffuse type which has an equal sex incidence and occurs at a younger age. The intestinal type is more common in areas of high incidence whereas the diffuse type occurs equally irrespective of incidence rates. Furthermore, the excess incidence of intestinal type is associated with the high mortality seen in areas of high incidence.[26] Conversely the reduction in mortality in areas of decreasing incidence is associated with a reduction in incidence of the intestinal type.[27] Furthermore, this reduction is associated with the decrease in incidence in the distal stomach suggesting that the intestinal type is a disease of the gastric antrum.

It would thus seem that the two types represent different diseases and as a result have different aetiological factors. Correa and colleagues have proposed that there is a progression from normal gastric mucosa to carcinoma in high risk populations[28] (Fig. 2.3). The initial change is early onset superficial gastritis which, although reversible, is triggered by a variety of agents. Progression may occur to chronic gastritis which may be associated with varying degrees of atrophy. Within the areas of gastric atrophy intestinal metaplasia may occur and particularly in those areas where the metaplasia is similar to large bowel epithelium

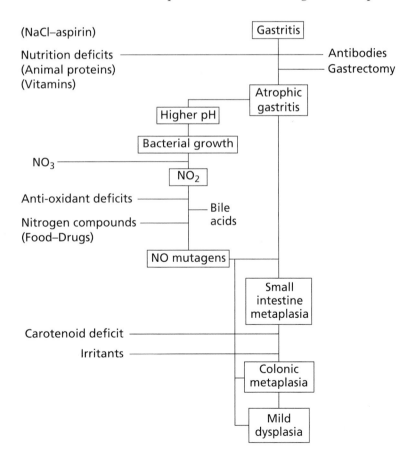

Figure 2.3 *Correa hypothesis for gastric carcinogenesis.*

(type III intestinal metaplasia), dysplasia may supervene and hence carcinoma of the intestinal type. The stages up to high-grade dysplasia are all spontaneously reversible. Cell kinetic studies suggest that the process may take up to 25 years to complete.

Evidence supporting the Correa hypothesis is available from high risk areas. Both intestinal metaplasia and chronic gastritis are found in association with intestinal type cancer. Intestinal metaplasia type III has been shown to increase the relative risk of gastric cancer by a factor of 4.58 when compared to type I.[29] Both precursor lesions are common in areas of high incidence. Intestinal metaplasia incidence in patients with the diffuse type of cancer is no different from the general population.

Other evidence comes from studies of chronic gastritis associated with autoimmune pernicious anaemia. Such patients are at risk from gastric cancer and the gastric mucosa from the early stage of the disease has similar features of intestinal metaplasia and gastric atrophy. Correa also defined an environmental type of gastritis which tends to be multifocal, has similar histological changes to those associated with intestinal metaplasia and has a prevalence which strongly correlates with population risk.

Demography of gastric cancer

Geography

Mortality rates for gastric cancer show wide variations which cannot reflect simple differences in diagnosis and treatment. Historically the decrease in incidence has tended to occur more recently in those areas with the highest incidence. Decreases in the USA were evident almost 70 years ago. Subsequent decreases in the UK began in the 1940s and it is only since 1960 that decreases in Japan have occurred.

Intercountry variations are well known between the Far East and the West. However, there are also significant intracountry variations. These largely reflect a north to south gradient which is particularly apparent in the northern hemisphere. Both in Japan and China mortality rates in the northern provinces are almost double those in the south. Similar differences are observed in the UK with higher standardised mortality rates in north and north western regions.

In the southern hemisphere, however, the gradient is the reverse. Indeed, the higher geographical latitude in both hemispheres have tended to be colder and more temperate and have a higher risk of gastric cancer, thus implicating environmental and particularly dietary factors in aetiology.

Socioeconomic influences

Gastric cancer appears to be a disease of lower socioeconomic groups. This reflects the persisting high incidence in poor areas such as Latin America and China considered as developing countries. However, evidence is not consistent. Comparison of urban and rural rates shows little difference although in areas of high incidence there is a trend for higher rates in rural areas possibly reflecting lower socioeconomic status.

An excess risk has been linked to certain occupations. Coal mining in the UK and the USA is associated as is the pottery industry in the North Midlands of the UK. The proposed mechanism involves swallowing dust-contaminated mucus cleared from the lungs and nasal passages. Evidence for such a relationship is circumstantial and certain occupations reflect social background and the risk may equally reflect life style, particularly dietary habits rather than actual occupational risk.

Exposure to potentially carcinogenic agents at an early age is clearly critical to the risk of developing both precursor lesions and subsequently gastric cancer. Evidence for this risk is available from migrant studies. Initial evidence from migrants to the USA from Japan showed that the high risk of the Japanese migrant was retained despite the lower incidence of the disease in the US. The longer the migrant lives in the area of lower incidence the more likely it is that the risk of gastric cancer reduces. However, it does not reach that of the host environment. For example, the US-born offspring of migrants show a similar risk to their country of birth. This would suggest that it is an environmental influence that is important rather than a genetic one. Interestingly, Correa et al.[30] have subsequently demonstrated that migrants developing gastric cancer are more likely to develop the diffuse type consistent with their new host country, further suggesting a relationship of intestinal type to environmental influences.

Aetiology of gastric cancer

Evidence from epidemiological studies is consistent with the Correa hypothesis for the development of intestinal type gastric cancer. Environmental influences are required to effect the multistage progression to malignant transformation. It would seem logical that the majority of environmental influences reflect what is ingested. However, definite evidence particularly from dietary influences is difficult to confirm as records for population dietary habits are incomplete and lack objectivity. Nevertheless, influences and trends can be drawn from dietary studies as long as their limitations are recognised.

Diet

The prevalence of gastric cancer in poor communities reflects both malnutrition and intake of poor quality diet. Foodstuffs that are cheap prevail as well as low cost methods of food preservations and preparation. Thus high carbohydrate intake has been implicated. Case-control studies have demonstrated consumption of cooked cereals, rice and starch to be higher in gastric cancer patients than controls. Other studies have shown no difference. It may, however, be an effect of the balance of carbohydrate in proportion to protein and fat. Areas with a high carbohydrate content have a low protein intake. Protein deficiency will impair gastric mucosal repair and indeed high carbohydrate/low protein may impair defence mechanisms against injurious agents.

In experimental models, N-nitroso compounds are well known to produce gastric cancers resembling the human form. Such compounds may be generated from interaction of nitrite with certain substances in foods. Nitrite is generated from nitrate by interaction with nitrate-reducing bacteria found when gastric juice is more alkaline than usual. This is particularly the case after gastrectomy and in pernicious anaemia, both conditions associated with a greater risk of gastric cancer. Sources of nitrate in the diet have been cured meat, fish and vegetables. Nitrate fertilisers may equally reach the human food chain. However, vegetables are often high sources of nitrate yet are considered protective. This may reflect the associated high content of vitamin C which may block *in vivo* nitrosation. Such conflicting epidemiological evidence mitigates against nitrate/nitrite as gastric carcinogens. However, in combination with other agents these may initiate progressive gastric epithelial change.

Salt preservation of food was practised during the early years of this century throughout the world. In some land-locked parts of the world this still occurs. In such areas and in those practising salt preservation there have been high rates of gastric cancer. In animal models, mice fed diets rich in salt had a high rate of gastritis. Increased absorption of polycyclic aromatic hydrocarbons occurred in the presence of high salt intake suggesting that salt acts as a promoter of carcinogenesis.

In human studies evidence of salt as a carcinogen is limited. In Japan where gastric cancer mortality is falling the intake of salt per capita has shown little change. However, the consumption of salted and pickled fish is high in Japanese and Columbians and correlates with their disease incidence. On the basis that salt induces injury to the gastric mucosa it may act like a high carbohydrate intake as an initiator to allow access for more potent carcinogens.

In contrast with the previous foodstuffs, fresh vegetables and fruit act to protect against gastric carcinogenesis. This effect may merely be a part of a more balanced diet or may reflect the content of anticarcinogens, such as vitamin A, C and E. Vitamin C in particular inhibits intragastric formation of nitrosamines from nitrite and amino precursors. Both vitamins A and E act as antioxidants within the cell as well as regulating cell differentiation and protecting the gastric mucosal barrier. However, dietary studies have failed to confirm these theoretical advantages.

Intercountry variations in fruit and vegetable intake has not paralleled differences in gastric cancer incidence. It is possible, however, that prolonged exposure is more relevant, again supporting the philosophy of a balanced diet rather than one supplemented with a potentially beneficial foodstuff. Indeed, secondary prevention studies are currently being assessed where the precursor changes in high risk areas can be reversed with supplemental vitamin C.[31]

Finally a practical innovation in this century seems to be most important. There has been the rapid and widespread use of refrigeration initially for storage and transportation and by the 1950s and

Figure 2.4 *Annual trends for proportion of households with electric refrigeration and age-adjusted death rates for stomach cancer in Japan, 1966–1985.[75]*

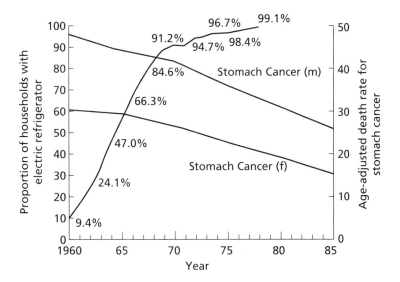

1960s for domestic use. Indeed, the reduction in mortality observed in Japan shows an inverse relationship with the increase in ownership of domestic refrigerators (Fig. 2.4). The effect of refrigerators is likely to be twofold, increasing the intake of fresh and frozen produce and altering the consumption of salted and pickled foods.

Helicobacter pylori

The Correa hypothesis implicates other factors which may induce gastric mucosa change. The identification and characterisation of the effect of *Helicobacter pylori* on gastric mucosa has raised the potential for a role in gastric carcinogenesis. The initial effect is acute inflammation. Since the infection does not resolve spontaneously, an effect is likely to persist for a long time and may proceed to chronic gastritis and associated mucosal atrophy. Furthermore *H. pylori* induces tissue monocytes to produce reactive oxygen intermediates which are potent carcinogens. In addition infection is associated with a significant reduction in gastric juice ascorbic acid further implicating antioxidant activity.[32]

Evidence for a relationship with gastric cancer comes from epidemiological studies. In South America in areas with a high incidence of gastric cancer, *H. pylori* is endemic particularly in the young.[33] In rural China there is a significant correlation between gastric cancer mortality and *H. pylori* infection.[34] Communities throughout the world selected for their gastric cancer rates have been randomly examined for *H. pylori* infections. A significant correlation was found between *H. pylori* infection and both incidence and mortality of gastric cancer.[35] These authors concluded that there was an approximately sixfold increased risk of gastric cancer in populations with 100% *H. pylori* infection compared with populations that have no infection. Furthermore, the presence of *H. pylori* in poor communities reflects the established associations between low socioeconomic groups and gastric cancer.

Although there is epidemiological evidence to associate gastric cancer with *H. pylori*,[36] it does not mean that the two are causally related. Indeed the odds ratios reported are not particularly high. Second, several at-risk populations do not have high *H. pylori* infection rates. Third, there is a significant difference in disease pattern from duodenal ulceration which is strongly associated with *H. pylori*.[37] Finally, there is an inverse relationship between the rate of *H. pylori* infection and the increasing severity of precancerous lesions; chronic gastritis (72% *H. pylori* positive), intestinal metaplasia (63%), dysplasia (44%) and carcinoma (35%).[38]

Nevertheless, there is sufficiently strong evidence to propose a role for *H. pylori* in gastric cancer development. Simple eradication of the infection may have a major impact on gastric cancer incidence. However, this has major methodological implications as *H. pylori* seropositivity is very common and many of those infected are unlikely to progress. As with other factors it is likely that *H. pylori* is an initiator for gastric carcinogenesis and acts in combination with other agents.

Oesophago-gastric and cardia cancers

The incidence data have shown that oesophagogastric cancer is slowly merging to principally occur at the cardia. These are all adenocarcinomas and many authorities are beginning to consider them as separate tumours from more proximal oesophageal cancers and more distal gastric cancers.

Mass surveys have demonstrated cardia adenocarcinoma has a high incidence in areas where oesophageal cancer is common.[39] The natural history of the two sites appears to be similar. Guanrei *et al.*[40] reported on a group of patients with early oesophageal squamous carcinoma and early adenocarcinoma of the cardia who refused any treatment. Progression to advanced disease was similar at 4–5 years. Survival from diagnosis was also similar with a median of 74 months.

Proximal gastric tumours are more likely to occur in men and this parallels the male predominance in the increasing incidence of lower third adenocarcinoma. Aetiologically there may also be a difference in *Helicobactor* infection which is less likely in cardia tumours. Equally life style may be relevant. Powell and McConkey[4] demonstrated that the increase of adenocarcinoma of the lower third of the oesophagus and the cardia was mainly in social classes I and II, i.e. professional and managerial occupations.

Such evidence could, therefore, suggest that the tumours are similar. This has a significant implication for management as each site should be considered in a similar manner. Furthermore, with the projected increases in incidence there are significant effects on workload and healthcare planning. Separation of management and treatment of oesophageal and gastric cancer should no longer occur, particularly if improvement in overall outcome is to occur. These cancers need to be assessed by the same multidisciplinary team.

Screening for oesophageal and gastric cancer

Screening programmes for any disease are dependent on a number of criteria. In the population to be screened the disease must be common. A reliable and accurate test which is as sensitive and specific as possible is required. The tests should be acceptable to the screened population. There should be an effective treatment for the screened abnormality with minimum morbidity and mortality. Finally not only does the treatment need to show an improvement in results but also implementation of the screening programme should result in an overall benefit for the screened population.

The world-wide differences in incidence of oesophageal and gastric cancer allow the implementation of screening programmes for asymptomatic populations only in those areas where the incidence is high. However, lessons from these programmes have increased knowledge of natural history and have allowed high-risk groups to be targeted in low-risk areas in order to detect disease at an earlier stage.

Oesophageal cancer screening

Asymptomatic screening

Evaluation of asymptomatic screening for carcinomas of the oesophagus has centred around those parts of China with highest incidence. The screening test involves swallowing a small deflated balloon which is then inflated at the lower end of the oesophagus. The balloon surface is covered with a fine mesh which on withdrawal from the oesophagus scrapes the mucosa to collect cells. A cytological smear is then made from the scrapings for microscopic examination. Those individuals found to have abnormalities are then subjected to endoscopy and appropriate biopsy. Radiology has very little place. In 132 subjects with early oesophageal cancer detected in this way, 26% had normal radiological appearances.[41]

The efficiency of this technique has had varying reports. Shu,[42] reviewing data based on 500 000 examinations, suggested an accuracy for the differentiation of benign for malignant of 90%. Mass surveys have shown that 73.8% of detected cancers were either *in situ* or minimally invasive. In a provincial review, Huang[43] reported on 17 000 examinations screened during a one-year period. Abnormalities were found in 68% of the population with low grade dysplasia in 37%, high grade in 26% and *in situ* cancer 2%. A group with high-grade dysplasia were followed for up to eight years. Regression to normal or low-grade change was observed in 40%, 20% remained as high grade, 20% fluctuated between high and low grade and 20% developed cancer. In the absence of dysplasia, 0.12% developed cancer. Progression from dysplasia to *in situ* cancer occurred over 3–12 years and for *in situ* cancer over 3–7 years. Tumour risk was consistent with a known distribution of middle third chronic oesophagitis in 76%. It would seem that the duration of severe dysplasia is the greatest risk for malignant transformation. Follow-up by endoscopy is, therefore, important and in order to ensure biopsy of the same site vital stains have been used.

Huang[44] reported that staining with toluidine blue was effective for identifying neoplastic epithelium; 84% of cancers were identified in positively staining areas.

The problem associated with this approach is the management of dysplasia. Oesophageal dysplasia is a dynamic process with both spontaneous regression and progression. Furthermore, even if *in situ* cancer develops, progress to advanced disease is often prolonged and may be associated with prolonged survival. In one series of 23 untreated patients, 11 developed late-stage disease at a mean of 55 months. In the remainder there was no change for over 6 years and the five-year survival of the group was 78%.[45] Five-year survival needs to be considered with caution as detection of asymptomatic slowly progressive disease introduces lead time bias and this can falsely give the impression that treatment results for screen-detected cases are better.

As a result a UICC recommendation has been to limit oesophageal cancer screening to areas of high risk.[46] The aim is to identify the natural history of dysplasia more completely; it would certainly not be justifiable to recommend oesophagectomy for those with dysplasia. Furthermore, common standards are required for the classification of dysplasia to identify those changes with greatest risk. Finally once the assessment is more reliable, control studies should be developed to determine whether screening intervention can reduce mortality for oesophageal cancer.

Symptomatic screening

Symptomatic screening is useful for those individuals considered at high risk for oesophageal cancer. The incidence in low risk areas is too low to justify a mass screening programme. The principal method of assessment is endoscopy with biopsy. Thus for tylosis, achalasia and corrosive stricture, regular endoscopies are recommended. This should start 10 years after diagnosis for achalasia and ingestion of the corrosive agent.

Barrett's metaplasia is usually combined with dysplasia prior to development of invasive malignancy. Again, endoscopy and biopsy are the most appropriate forms of assessment. Reid *et al.*[47] have recommended four quadrant biopsies to be taken at 2 cm intervals on an annual basis. Although a sensitive indicator for adenocarcinoma, since the changes are site specific, once dysplasia has been found, 40% have a co-existent adenocarcinoma.[48] Latterly more specific markers of disease activity have been sought involving molecular biopsy markers.[49] Random assessment, however, is relatively inefficient as the return is low. In practical terms, high-risk groups such as those with a long segment of columnar metaplasia and those with alkaline reflux should be targeted. Equally those considered fit enough for surgery should be included which raises the question of the age of surveillance intervention. Prophylactic resection has been suggested for high-grade dysplasia and early invasive cancer as results are better than those with more established disease.[50] It would seem appropriate to start at 50 years of age allowing for the considerations already described.

Gastric cancer screening

Asymptomatic

The size of gastric cancer as a public health problem in Japan led to the development during the 1960s of a mass screening programme for all over the age of 40 years. The programme has been based on double-contrast radiology with endoscopy assessment of any abnormalities.[51] Members of the public are invited to undergo radiology in mobile units at which seven films are taken after the ingestion of an effervescent contrast agent. Screening is undertaken annually or biannually depending on the area of Japan and the associated risk of disease. Governmental recommendations set a target of 30% for the annual examination rate. In 1985 over 5 million were examined representing 13% of the at-risk population. Therein lies one of the problems with any screening programme, namely the cooperation of the public. Despite recognition of gastric cancer as a public health problem, attendance for screening is low.

Screening in this way detects disease at an early stage. Approximately half the cases diagnosed are limited to the mucosa or submucosa (early gastric cancer). Interestingly half of those detected are symptomatic and an alternative approach could be envisaged. In keeping with the criteria for a screening programme there has been a highly significant decrease in mortality since mass screening was introduced. However, as already discussed there may be other reasons for the decline in mortality.

Oshima *et al.*[52] compared screened and unscreened populations to determine whether screening was important over and above the other influences on the decrease in mortality. In a case-controlled study they found that the risk of dying from gastric cancer among screened cases was at least 50% less than that for non-screened cases. Similar results have been reported by other Japanese groups.

However, the actual effect on mortality remains to be proven as none of the studies have been randomised or controlled. Again, as with oesophageal screening there is the risk of lead time bias. Nevertheless, as Hisamichi observes, the Japanese could not wait to see if their incidence would follow the decreases in trends of incidence observed in the West and wanted to speed up the decline in mortality.

As a result the UICC recommended that studies should be continued in Japan to resolve the problem, but screening in this way should not be adopted as public health programmes in other parts of the world.[46] Despite this recommendation other countries have developed similar programmes to cope with their high incidence. In Chile, for example, where incidence is 75% that of Japan, there has been an increase in early detection after the introduction of mass screening.[53] Furthermore, the Chileans have found that mass contrast radiology is efficient

Figure 2.5
Classification of macroscopic subtypes of early gastric cancer.

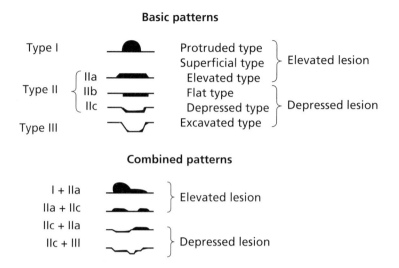

despite its critics. They would recommend its use as an inexpensive assessment particularly in poor countries with high risk.

As well as producing a significant influence on the way in which the disease is managed in Japan, the Japanese screening approach has enabled greater understanding of the endoscopic appearances of early gastric cancer and precursor lesions. Macroscopically EGC has been described as protruding (type I), superficial (type II) and excavated (type III).[54] Type II is further divided into elevated (IIa), flat (IIb) and depressed (IIc) (Fig. 2.5). A further subclassification of the type I/IIa (protruding lesion) has been designed; sessile (I), semi-spherical (II), spherical (III) and pedunculated (IV). Pedunculated lesions less than 20 mm are usually benign, but sessile and semi-spherical are usually malignant. Spherical lesions greater than 10 mm and all lesions greater than 20 mm are likely to be malignant.

Knowledge of the morphological appearances is useful in areas of high incidence where screening is active. However, for areas of low incidence where more often than not type IIc or III lesions are seen, more practical advice has been given by Sano *et al.*[55] An elevated lesion is likely to be limited to the mucosa if the surface is regular and not ulcerated. Small depressed lesions which are shallow with either no or slight gastric fold convergence are likely to be mucosal. However, more depressed lesions with a stiff base and irregular nodularity and fold convergence will penetrate at least to the submucosa. Finally, irregular ulcerating lesions are most likely to show full thickness wall penetration.

Screening assessment can be supplemented by endoluminal ultrasound (EUS). Experienced endoscopists with EUS can identify the four layers of the gastric wall.[56] Shallow lesions are usually straightforward to assess. However, limitations are inherent as fibrosis secondary to ulceration can be difficult to differentiate from penetration by tumour.

The identification and review of precursor lesions has equally been advanced by experience from screening. Areas of gastric atrophy, intestinal metaplasia and dysplasia need to be actively surveyed. Again, as with the oesophagus the changes are in a dynamic equilibrium and spontaneous regression can occur. However, in contra-distinction to the oesophagus once severe dysplasia has been identified on more than one biopsy on two separate occasions, surgery should be recommended as progression to cancer is inevitable.[57]

In order to ensure the same site is assessed vital dye sprays have been used during endoscopy. Intestinal metaplasia shows highly reproducible rates of positive staining after spraying with methylene blue.[58] The frequency of repeat endoscopy is contentious. However, the increased risk of intestinal metaplasia type III (colonic type) and dysplasia merits repeat endoscopy every 6–12 months.[59]

Symptomatic screening

In areas of low risk, asymptomatic screening is not justifiable. There is a small group who should be considered for regular assessment by virtue of their concurrent conditions. Pernicious anaemia imposes a three–fourfold risk over the normal population. However, screening of such individuals may be limited, as in one survey of gastric cancer 1.3% had pernicious anaemia. Patients who have undergone gastric resection for benign disease have been considered to have a greater risk possibly because of increased alkaline reflux. However, again this group provides only a small portion of gastric cancers detected in a screening programme.[60]

Since half of those that were detected in Japan through screening had symptoms, efforts have been made to further evaluate symptoms in low-risk populations. In the UK increased availability of endoscopy has been assessed as an influence on gastric cancer diagnosis.[61] However, large numbers of endoscopies in the population with dyspepsia have been performed without significant findings. Many of the diagnoses have been of functional disorders. Subsequently groups have assessed symptomatic scoring symptoms to form a profile of the at-risk patient.[62,63] Unfortunately these profiles have tended to identify only those with advanced disease or have proven too cumbersome for routine use.

Since EGC in the UK tends to peak in incidence approximately 10 years younger than advanced disease[64] and since dyspepsia as a new symptom is associated with early disease or dysplasia,[65] those over 40 with dyspepsia can be considered as a high-risk group. A recent study had evaluated endoscopic examination of such a group of patients before any treatment had been started. During a four-year period 2600 patients were examined from a 100 000 population. Gastric cancer was diagnosed in 57 (2%) with 12 (22%) being limited to the mucosa and submucosa. In a further 493 (19%) precursor lesions were identified in whom six were subsequently found to have early gastric cancer on follow-up endoscopy.[66] Those with gastric cancer proceeded to resection and comparison of this group with those diagnosed in the 5 years

Figure 2.6 *Survival after early detection of gastric cancer (study population) compared with historical control population (pre-study population).*

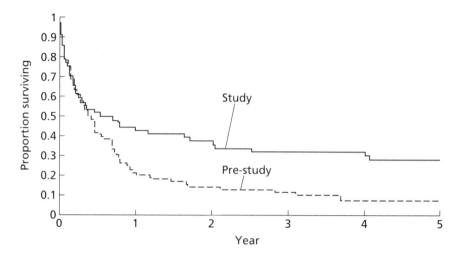

prior to the study shows an overall 20% survival advantage for the 'screened' population[67] (Fig. 2.6).

The problem with the approach in this study remains the large number of examinations for limited clinical benefit to the patient. Certainly a diagnosis can be achieved and management pursued appropriately. Indeed, this has significant health economic implications. However, as regards early diagnosis of cancer there are limitations. Nonetheless, the benefit for survival suggests application of similar schemes in other areas of low incidence. Experience of the endoscopist is critical. In the early phase a low threshold for biopsy of any abnormality is appropriate. Improvements in resolution with video endoscopy have aided diagnosis of small lesions as has the descriptive morphology from Japanese studies.

A variety of markers have been assessed to aid prediction of significant gastric mucosal change and so enable more specific use of endoscopy. Tumour markers such as the oncofetal antigens have been extensively assessed. However, none have the required sensitivity or specificity for either early or advanced disease. Serum levels of gastric hormones have been investigated as changes in pepsinogen and gastric levels appear to relate to mucosal change. Two types of pepsinogen have been identified as having a potential role: pepsinogen I arising from cells of the gastric body and pepsinogen II from cells of the body and antrum. Stemmerman *et al.*[68] found low pepsinogen I levels to be specific for extensive intestinal metaplasia. Furthermore, low serum pepsinogen I and raised gastric levels were found in pernicious anaemia complicated by gastric atrophy.[69] Kekki *et al.*[70] have suggested that low serum pepsinogen I is useful for screening as it is markedly reduced in atrophy of gastric body mucosa.

In gastric cancer low pepsinogen is found with a moderate elevation in pepsinogen II. A ratio of the two has been proposed as a screening test.[71,72] Farinati *et al.*[73] found similarly for pepsinogen levels but also found reduced gastrin concentrations. This equally has been assessed as a ratio with reasonable sensitivity and specificity. However, although there appears to be a relationship with prediction for precursor changes or malignancy, when these parameters have been assessed in an early detection programme, limitations were observed because of false positive values.[74]

The role of *H. pylori* as a marker for endoscopy is receiving considerable attention. Both serological estimation and breath tests depending on exhalation of urea have been investigated. Serology has been assessed for concordance with underlying histological presence of *H. pylori*. Farinati *et al.*[38] found 82% agreement between a measurable antibody response and the histological evidence of *H. pylori* infection. Urea breath tests are in routine use for *Helicobacter* eradication programmes for duodenal ulceration. Again the problem is one of specificity and sensitivity. *H. pylori* seropositivity does not necessarily imply active infection. Equally seropositivity is a common finding and may not be specific for the at-risk population. It increases with age and to a certain extent parallels gastric atrophy which is equally an age-related phenomenon and in the majority does not progress to cancer. However, evidence of infection at an early age does identify a group at risk and therefore worthy of consideration for endoscopic follow-up. Further investigation is required and longitudinal studies may resolve the issue of which patients with *H. pylori* seropositivity warrant close endoscopic follow-up.

Summary and future

Oesophageal cancer incidence is increasing with a particular change in adenocarcinoma. Although gastric cancer is decreasing, the workload is staying constant. Management principles of the two diseases particularly in the developed world are converging. Thus separation of the two diseases is becoming blurred and this has important implications for health planning.

In developing countries the results of primary and secondary prevention programmes are eagerly awaited to determine specifically if *H. pylori* eradication and improvements in diet can reduce incidence. In developed countries the role of *H. pylori* remains to be evaluated particularly as an indicator of early diagnosis. The concentration of disease at the oesophageal hiatus strongly implicates reflux as an important factor. However, which patients are at high risk and require careful assessment and review remains to be established.

The poor end results of the past remain as potent influences on the philosophy towards treatment of gastro-oesophageal cancer. Greater appreciation of the curability of early disease by both medical and public education must become a priority.

References

1. Parkin DM, Pisani P, Ferlay J. Estimates of the worldwide incidence of eighteen major cancers in 1985. Int J Cancer 1993; 54: 594–606.
2. Cheng KK, Day NE. Oesophageal cancer in Britain. BMJ 1992; 304: 711.
3. Matthews HR, Waterhouse JAH, Powell J, McConkey CC, Robertson JE. Cancer of the oesophagus. Clinical Cancer Monographs Vol. 1. London: Macmillan, 1987.
4. Powell J, McConkey CC. The rising trend in oesophagus adenocarcinoma and gastric cardia. Eur J Cancer Prevent 1992; 1: 265–9.
5. Yang PC, Davis S. Incidence of cancer of the oesophagus in the US by histologic type. Cancer 1988; 61: 612–7.
6. McGlashan WD. Oesophageal cancer in the black peoples of South Africa 1980–82. S Afr J Sci 1988; 84: 92–9.
7. Crespi M, Munoz N, Grassi A et al. Precursor lesions of oesophageal cancer in a low-risk population in China: comparison with a high-risk population. Int J Cancer 1984; 34: 599–602.
8. Munoz N, Crespi M, Grassi A, Qing S, Cai LZ. Precursor lesions of oesophageal cancer in high risk populations in Iran and China. Lancet 1982; i: 876–9.
9. Guanrei Y, Songliang Q. Endoscopic surveys in high and low risk populations for oesophageal cancer in China with special reference to precursors of oesophageal cancer. Endoscopy 1987; 19: 91–5.
10. Chang-Claude JC, Wahrendorf J, Liang QS et al. An epidemiological study of precursor lesions of oesophageal cancer among young persons in a high risk population in Huixian, China. Cancer Res 1990; 50: 2268–74.
11. Iran-IARC Study Group. Oesophageal cancer studies in the Caspian Littoral of Iran: results of population studies. A prodrome. J Natl Cancer Inst 1979; 59: 1127–38.
12. Hu J, Nyren O, Wolk A et al. Risk factors for oesophageal cancer in northeast China. Int J Cancer 1994; 57: 38–46.
13. Yang CS. Research on oesophageal cancer in China: a review. Cancer Res 1980; 40: 2633–44.
14. Li JY, Ershaw AG, Chen ZJ et al. A case-control study of cancer of the oesophagus and gastric cardia in Linxian. Int J Cancer 1989; 43: 755–61.
15. Haggitt RC, Tryzelaar J, Ellis FH. Adenocarcinoma complicating columnar epithelium-lined (Barrett's) oesophagus. Am J Clin Pathol 1978; 70: 1–5.
16. Attwood SEA, Ball CS, Barlow AP, Jenkinson L, Norris TL, Watson A. Role of intragastric and intraoesophageal alkalinisation in the genesis of complications in Barrett's columnar lined lower oesophagus. Gut 1993; 34: 11–15.
17. Davis DL, Hoel D, Fox J, Lopez A. International trends in cancer mortality in France, West Germany, Italy, Japan, England and Wales and the USA. Lancet 1990; 336: 474–81.
18. Howson CP, Hiyama T, Wynder EL. The decline in gastric cancer: epidemiology of an unplanned triumph. Epidemiol Rev 1986; 8: 1–27.
19. Parkin DM, Laara E, Muir CS. Estimates of the worldwide frequency of sixteen major cancers in 1980. Int J Cancer 1988; 41: 184–97.
20. Fielding JWL, Powell J, Allum WH, Waterhouse JAH, McConkey CC. Cancer of the stomach. Clinical Cancer Monographs Vol. 3. London: Macmillan, 1989.
21. Allum WH, Powell DJ, McConkey CC, Fielding JWL. Gastric cancer: a 25-year review. Br J Surg 1989; 76: 535–40.
22. Antonioli DA, Goldman H. Changes in the location and type of gastric adenocarcinoma. Cancer 1982; 50: 775–81.
23. Patterson ID, Easton DF, Corbishley CM, Gazet J-C. Changing distribution of adenocarcinoma of the stomach. Br J Surg 1987; 74: 481–2.
24. Sedgwick DM, Akoh JA, Macintyre IMC. Gastric cancer in Scotland: changing epidemiology, unchanging workload. BMJ 1991; 302: 1305–7.
25. Lauren P. The two histological main types of gastric carcinoma: diffuse and so-called intestinal-type carcinoma: an attempt at a histoclinical classification. Acta Pathol Microbiol Scand 1965; 64: 31–49.
26. Munoz N, Correa P, Cuello C et al. Histologic types of gastric carcinoma in high- and low-risk areas. Int J Cancer 1968; 3: 809–18.
27. Munoz N, Asvall J. Time trends of intestinal and diffuse types of gastric cancer in Norway. Int J Cancer 1971; 8: 144–57.

28. Correa P. A human model of gastric carcinogenesis. Cancer Res 1988; 48: 3554–60.

29. Filipe ML, Munoz N, Matko I *et al*. Intestinal metaplasia types and the risk of gastric cancer: a cohort study in Slovenia. Int J Cancer 1994; 57: 324–9.

30. Correa P, Sasano N, Stemmerman N *et al*. Pathology of gastric carcinoma in Japanese populations: comparisons between Miyagi prefecture, Japan and Hawaii. J Natl Cancer Inst 1973; 51: 1449–59.

31. Munoz N, Vivas J, Buiatta E *et al*. Chemoprevention trial of precancerous lesions of the stomach in Venezuela. Eur J Cancer Prevent 1993; 2 (Suppl 1): 5.

32. Sobala GM, Schorah CJ, Shires S. Gastric ascorbic acid concentration and acute *Helicobacter pylori* infection. Rev Esp Enf Digest 1990; 78 (Suppl 1): 63.

33. Correa P, Fox J, Fontham E *et al*. *Helicobacter pylori* and gastric carcinoma. Serum antibody prevalence in populations with contrasting cancer risks. Cancer 1990; 66: 2569–74.

34. Forman D, Sitas F, Newell DG *et al*. Geographic association of *Helicobacter pylori* antibody prevalence and gastric cancer mortality in rural China. Int J Cancer 1990; 46: 608–11.

35. Eurogast Study Group. An international association between *Helicobacter pylori* infection and gastric cancer. Lancet 1993; 341: 1359–62.

36. Forman D, Newell DG, Fullerton F *et al*. Association between infection with *Helicobacter pylori* and risk of gastric cancer: evidence from a prospective investigation. BMJ 1991; 302: 1302–5.

37. Forman D. *Helicobacter pylori* infection: a novel risk factor in the aetiology of gastric cancer. J Natl Cancer Inst 1991; 83: 1702–3.

38. Farinati F, Valiante F, Germania B *et al*. Prevalence of *Helicobacter pylori* infection in patients with precancerous changes and gastric cancer. Eur J Cancer Prevent 1993; 2: 321–6.

39. Guanrei Y, Sunglian Q. Incidence rate of adenocarcinoma of the gastric cardia and endoscopic classification of early cardial carcinoma in Henan province, the People's Republic of China. Endoscopy 1987; 19: 7–10.

40. Guanrei Y, Songliang Q, He H, Guizen F. Natural history of early oesophageal squamous carcinoma and early adenocarcinoma of the gastric cardia in the People's Republic of China. Endoscopy 1988; 20: 95–8.

41. Wang G-Q. Endoscopic diagnosis of early oesophageal carcinoma. J R Soc Med 1981; 74: 502–3.

42. Shu Y-J. Cytopathology of the oesophagus. Acta Cytol 1983; 27: 7–16.

43. Huang G-J. Recognition and treatment of the early lesion. In: Delarae NC, Wilkins EW, Wong J (eds) International trends: general thoracic surgery 4. Oesophageal cancer. St Louis: Mosby, 1988, pp. 149–52.

44. Huang GJ. Early detection and surgical treatment of oesophageal carcinoma. Jpn J Surg 1981; 11: 399–405.

45. Yanjun M, Li G, Xianzhi G, Weheng C. Detection and natural progression of early oesophageal carcinoma – preliminary communication. J R Soc Med 1981; 74: 884–6.

46. Chamberlain J, Day NE, Hakama M *et al*. UICC workshop of the project on evaluation of screening programmes for gastrointestinal cancer. Int J Cancer 1986; 37: 329–34.

47. Reid BJ, Weinstein WM, Lewin KJ *et al*. Endoscopic biopsy can detect high-grade dysplasia or early adenocarcinoma in Barrett's oesophagus without grossly recognisable neoplastic lesions. Gastroenterology 1988; 94: 81–90.

48. Skinner DB, Walther BC, Riddell RH *et al*. Barrett's oesophagus: comparison of benign and malignant cases. Ann Surg 1985; 198: 554–65.

49. Reid BJ, Bloung PL, Rubin CE, Levine DS, Haggitt RC, Rabinovitch PS. Flow-cytometric and histological progression to malignancy in Barrett's oesophagus: prospective endoscopic surveillance of a cohort. Gastroenterology 1992; 102: 1212–19.

50. Skinner DB. The columnar lined oesophagus and adenocarcinoma. Ann Thorac Surg 1985; 40: 321–2.

51. Hisamichi S. Screening for gastric cancer. World J Surg 1989; 13: 31–7.

52. Oshima A, Hirata N, Ubakata T, Umeda K, Fujimoto L. Evaluation of a mass screening programme for stomach cancer with a case-control study design. Int J Cancer 1986; 38: 829–34.

53. Llorens P. Gastric cancer mass survey in Chile. Semin Surg Oncol 1991; 7: 339–43.

54. Murakami T. Pathomorphological diagnosis.

Definition and gross classification of early gastric cancer. In: Murakami T (ed.) Early gastric cancer, Gann Monograph on Cancer Research 11. Tokyo: University of Tokyo Press, 1971, pp. 53–66.

55. Sano T, Okuyama Y, Kobori O, Shimuzu T, Morioka Y. Early gastric cancer: endoscopic diagnosis of depth of invasion. Dig Dis Sci 1990; 35: 1340–4.

56. Tio TL, Schowink MH, Cikot RJML, Tytgat GNJ. Preoperative TNM classification of gastric carcinoma by endosonography in comparison with the pathological TNM system: a prospective study of 72 cases. Hepatogastroenterology 1989; 36: 51–6.

57. Landsdown M, Quirke P, Dixon MF, Axon ATR, Johnston D. High grade dysplasia of the gastric mucosa: a marker for gastric carcinoma. Gut 1990; 31: 977–83.

58. Suzuki S, Suzuki H, Endo M, Takemoto T, Kondo T. Endoscopic dyeing method for diagnosis of early cancer and intestinal metaplasia of the stomach. Endoscopy 1973; 5: 124–9.

59. Rokkas T, Filipe MI, Sladen GE. Detection of an increased incidence of early gastric cancer in patients with intestinal metaplasia type III who are closely followed up. Gut 1991; 32: 1110–13.

60. Oshima A, Sakagami F, Hawai A, Fujimoto I. Evaluation of a mass screening programme for gastric cancer. In: Hirayama T (ed.) Epidemiology of stomach cancer (WHO-CC Monograph), Tokyo: WHO, 1977, pp. 35–45.

61. Gear MWL, Barnes RJ. Endoscopic studies of dyspepsia in a general practice. BMJ 1980; 280: 1136–7.

62. Mann J, Holdstock G, Herman M, Machin D, Loehry CA. Scoring system to improve cost-effectiveness of open access endoscopy. BMJ 1983; 287: 937–40.

63. Davenport PM, Morgan AG, Darkborough A, De Dombal FT. Can preliminary screening of dyspeptic patients allow more effective use of investigational techniques? BMJ 1985; 290: 217–20.

64. Fielding JWL, Ellis DJ, Jones BG et al. Natural history of 'early' gastric cancer. BMJ 1980; 281: 965–7

65. De Dombal FT, Price AB, Thompson H et al. The British Society of Gastroenterology early gastric cancer/dysplasia survey: an interim report. Gut 1990; 31: 115–20.

66 Hallissey MT, Allum WH, Jewkes AJ, Ellis DJ, Fielding JWL. Early detection of gastric cancer. British Medical Journal 1990; 301: 513–5.

67. Hallissey MT, Jewkes AJ, Allum WH, Harrison JD, Fielding JWL. The impact of the dyspepsia study on deaths from gastric cancer. In: Nishi M, Sugano H, Takahashi T (eds) International Gastric Cancer Congress, Bologna, 1995, Vol. 1.

68. Stemmerman GM, Ishidata T, Samloff IM et al. Intestinal metaplasia of the stomach in Hawaii and Japan. Am J Dig Dis 1978; 23: 815–20.

69. Varis K, Samloff IM, Ihamaki T, Siurala M. An appraisal of tests for severe atrophic gastritis in relatives of patients with pernicious anaemia. Dig Dis Sci 1979; 24: 187–91.

70. Kekki M, Samloff IM, Varis K, Ihamaki T. Serum pepsinogen I and serum gastrin in the screening of severe atrophic corpus gastritis. Scand J Gastroenterol 1991; 26 (Suppl 186): 109–16.

71. Nomura AMY, Stemmerman GM, Samloff IM. Serum pepsinogen I as a predictor of stomach cancer. Ann Intern Med 1980; 93: 537–40.

72. Huang SC, Miki K, Furihata C, Ichinose M, Shimuzu A, Oka H. Enzyme linked immunosorbent assays for serum pepsinogens I and II using monoclonal antibodies – with data on peptic ulcer and gastric cancer. Clin Chim Acta 1988; 175: 37–50.

73. Farinati F, Di Mario F, Plebani M et al. Pepsinogen A/pepsinogen C or pepsinogen A multiplied by gastrin in the diagnosis of gastric cancer? Ital J Gastroenterol 1991; 23: 194–6.

74. Hallissey MT, Allum WH, Fielding JWL. Serum screening tests for gastric cancer and high risk groups. Eur J Surg Oncol 1986; 12: 398.

75. Hirayama T. Actions suggested by gastric cancer epidemiological studies in Japan. In: Reed PI, Hill MJ (eds) Gastric carcinogenesis. Amsterdam: Excerpta Medica, 1988, pp. 209–28.

3 Preoperative assessment and staging of oesophageal and gastric cancer

John R. Anderson

Introduction

The pretreatment staging of oesophageal and gastric cancer is essential to guide the clinician in planning therapy. Preoperative staging will allow stratification for neoadjuvant or other treatment and will identify those patients who would not benefit from surgery. Radiotherapy (in oesophageal cancer) and surgery (for both oesophageal and gastric cancer) remain the only proven treatments to cure patients of these distressing conditions. Neoadjuvant therapy using combinations of chemotherapy and/or radiotherapy is being increasingly used in protocols for the multimodality management of both conditions.

There are now a variety of non-operative methods for palliating the symptoms of oesophageal and gastric cancer involving metallic stents, laser therapy, pulsion or traction intubation, brachytherapy and local injection of alcohol. These treatments may be used singly or in combination with each other or with other modalities such as chemotherapy and/or radiotherapy in an effort to improve the quality of life. Many patients, especially with gastric cancer, will still require surgery for palliation but careful and accurate staging should prevent unnecessary laparotomy/thoracotomy and ill-advised resection which carry a high operative risk. Full recovery from surgery may also significantly affect the quality of life in a patient whose life expectancy is limited.

Preoperative staging will inevitably understage the disease but will identify patients with distant metastases in whom surgical resection may be inappropriate. Postoperative staging taking into account findings at surgery and histopathological examination will allow for accurate comparisons between reported series and will also guide the clinician when discussing prognosis with the patient.

Preoperative assessment

Radiological investigations

Contrast examinations

In the endoscopic era barium radiology of the oesophagus and stomach is still a useful tool in the diagnosis of oesophageal and gastric cancer. The two methods of examination are complimentary. In Western countries contrast radiological investigation of the oesophagus and stomach has been less appreciated, mainly because panendoscopy has been considered to give better diagnostic yields. The Western literature suggests that X-ray is less accurate and misses more lesions than endoscopy. However, is should be borne in mind that most reports are written by gastroenterologists expressing the endoscopic point of view and that endoscopy is usually used as the final arbiter in any such comparisons. Most of these communications, however, do not deal with early oesophageal and gastric cancer.

Oesophagus

Double contrast barium radiology should initially be taken with the patient erect with at least one film including the pharynx and one including the open lower oesophageal sphincter. Further films should then be taken both supine and erect.

Carcinoma of the oesophagus usually starts as a flat intramucosal lesion, with advancement of growth either in an infiltrative or polypoidal manner with possible ulceration accompanying the former. The length of the tumour as seen on swallow examination provides good correlation with the depth of extension and with curability.[1] With oesophageal cancers under 5 cm in length, 40% are localised, 35% have evidence of distant metastases or are unresectable and 25% are locally advanced. When the oesophageal tumour is greater than 5 cm in length 75% have evidence of metastases or are unresectable, 25% are locally advanced and only 10% are localised. Another useful sign of local mediastinal invasion is deviation of the axis of the lumen of the oesophagus within the lesion in relation to the expected luminal axis of the oesophagus. Rosenberg et al.[1] have shown that when this criterion was used alone there was a false positive rate for mediastinal invasion of 10% and a false negative rate of 8%. When the barium flow through the stricture is completely outwith the projected axis of the oesophagus then the lesion is almost always unresectable.

Detection of early oesophageal cancer

Yang et al.[2] have described four macroscopic types of early oesophageal carcinoma, occurring in the high incidence area of China: congested, erosive, plaque-like and polypoidal. Erosive lesions are the commonest of all early lesions accounting for 45%. The earliest radiological abnormality is an area of mucosa that is a little flattened or nodular and rigid with incomplete distensibility. This is usually best seen tangentially. An 'en face' view will usually show an oesophageal fold stopping at the upper limit of the tumour associated with mucosal irregularity and nodularity. These areas usually persist as an area of incomplete collapse when a peristaltic wave passes down the oesophagus. The presence of a mound or plaque suggests submucosal invasion.[3] Minor surface irregularities should be reported in detail so that a careful endoscopic examination can be carried out with biopsy and/or cytology. In high risk areas such as China comparisons of balloon cytology, radiology and endoscopy show detection rates of 98%, 38% and 85%, respectively.[4] In these areas of high incidence concomitant oesophagitis is almost universal in the adult population and these figures may not be directly transferable to the situation in Western countries.

Stomach

Advanced carcinomas are characterised by malignant invasion into or beyond the muscularis propria and manifest radiologically as polypoidal, ulcerating or infiltrating lesions. This produces the characteristic fluoroscopic findings of rigidity and absent peristalsis at the site of the tumour. Polypoidal carcinomas on double contrast examination, produce striking luminal defects frequently with irregular advancing tumour margins. With ulcerating carcinomas the most common radiological feature is an irregular nodular tumour mass which is sharply demarcated from the surrounding normal mucosa. The associated irregular ulcer crater usually fails to penetrate beyond the normal gastric contour (Fig. 3.1). Diffuse infiltrating carcinomas or linitis plastica result in an abrupt circumferential narrowing of the gastric lumen with various abnormalities of the mucosal surface pattern. Mucosal folds will be absent, being replaced by a smooth featureless surface or one which exhibits nodularity due to submucosal tumour infiltration.

Detection of early gastric cancer

Advances in the diagnosis of gastric adenocarcinoma have resulted from extensive Japanese experience with double contrast barium

Figure 3.1
Ulcerated gastric carcinoma. Barium meal appearance – shaded area shows barium in stomach, non-shaded area shows projection of cancer into lumen.

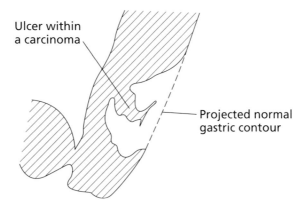

Ulcer within a carcinoma

Projected normal gastric contour

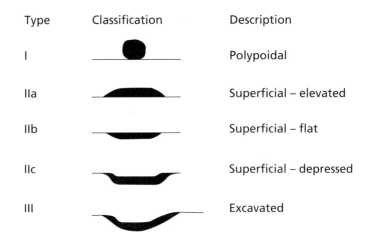

Figure 3.2 *Early gastric cancer.*

Type	Classification	Description
I		Polypoidal
IIa		Superficial – elevated
IIb		Superficial – flat
IIc		Superficial – depressed
III		Excavated

meals. This is especially true of early gastric cancer which accounts for approximately 35% of all cancers seen in Japan.[5] Classification of early gastric cancer (EGC) refers to the macroscopic appearance applicable to both radiology and endoscopy and is shown in Fig. 3.2. A common misconception is that early lesions are always small; they can be sizeable tumours with either extensive mucosal involvement or prominent intraluminal masses. Approximately 70% are of the superficial depressed type (IIc). Contrast radiological diagnosis is based on an analysis of the depression and the associated radiating folds. Depressions are irregular and uneven due to proliferation of the malignant tissue. Radiating folds extending to the malignant area reveal characteristic changes such as abrupt tapering, clubbing, interruption or fusion. Excavating (type III) cancers differ from the superficial depressed types by virtue of a greater depth of erosion. Early polypoidal carcinomas (type I) exhibit radiological features similar to those of benign tumours.

Computed tomography and magnetic resonance imaging

Computed tomography (CT) and more recently magnetic resonance imaging (MRI) have been promoted as effective preoperative decision making modalities for staging tumours of both the oesophagus and stomach. However, the ability of both imaging techniques to stage these tumours accurately has recently been questioned.

Oesophagus

Post-mortem studies have shown invasion of mediastinal structures to be present in almost 20% of cases, with 12% invading the trachea or bronchi and 2% invading the heart and aorta respectively.[6] The main sites of distant metastases are to liver, lung, bone and kidney, and occur respectively in 19%, 11%, 5% and 4% of patients. Many retrospective studies have reported that CT is accurate in the preoperative staging of oesophageal carcinoma, and in evaluating resectability.[7–12]

Table 3.1 *Incidence of local spread of oesophageal carcinoma (CT versus autopsy)*

		Incidence of invasion of		
		trachea/bronchus	aorta	heart
Retrospective studies[7–12]	286	35% (20–46)	27% (17–49)	13% (0–18)
Autopsy study[6]	2240	12%	2%	2%

However, many of these studies have lacked precise correlations to surgery and pathology (Table 3.1). Prospective studies have shown CT to be less accurate in pretreatment staging than had been suggested by the retrospective studies.[13–15] There are several explanations for the discrepancies in the reported results in the literature: the method of assessing a tumour as locally advanced, the lack of surgical correlation, and differences in the apparatus and scanning technique.

One area of great controversy is the loss of the perioesophageal fat plane. When present, invasion is highly unlikely but when absent, even in well nourished patients, it cannot be taken as absolute evidence of invasion. This may account for the overestimation of tracheal, bronchial, aortic and cardiac invasion in many studies. Extra-oesophageal tumour extension, in particular to the tracheobronchial tree, aorta and heart can be determined using the following signs: (a) the presence of an intraluminal bud; (b) obvious displacement and deformation of the tracheobronchial tree, aorta or pericardium; (c) increased thickness of the membranous trachea, bronchus, wall of the aorta or left atrium; (d) growth extending beyond the posterior wall of the trachea at the level of the aortic arch. Invasion of the aorta is more difficult to ascertain and although it occurs less commonly, it is obviously of importance to the surgeon. Picus *et al.*[10] have suggested that aortic invasion is considered indeterminate with contact of 45–90° between the aorta and tumour and that invasion can only be predicted with accuracy if there is 90° contact. This has been challenged by Fekete *et al.*[15] who found six patients with almost total circumferential tumour growth around the aortic circumference and in whom aortic invasion at surgery was not found. A recently introduced criterion for aortic invasion is based on the loss of the paravertebral fat space present in the triangle formed by the aorta, oesophagus and vertebral body.[16] If this fat space is completely obliterated by soft tissue in a patient with an oesophageal cancer, invasion of the aorta is usually present.

Owing to the variability of the normal anatomy at the gastro-oesophageal junction the findings on CT in patients with carcinoma of the gastro-oesophageal junction should be interpreted with caution.[17–19] A co-existing hiatus hernia may mimic or obscure both oesophageal or gastric invasion. CT is inaccurate in predicting diaphragmatic invasion although this in itself does not often preclude surgical resection. Diaphragmatic invasion can be considered present on CT when the crura are surrounded by a tumour mass. The close relationship of the oesophagus, gastro-oesophageal junction and diaphragm and the absence of an intervening fat plane are the main reasons for the difficulty in assessing diaphragmatic involvement. Preoperative staging of carcinoma of the cardia varies in accuracy from 68 to 86%. CT does not reliably detect the presence of lymph node metastases. It is impossible to differentiate abnormally enlarged nodes that contain tumour from those that are enlarged due to benign reactive hyperplasia. The use of size as a criterion for malignant involvement varies with different authors from 5 to 15 mm.[15] Lymph nodes of more than 1 cm in diameter can be seen within the mediastinum in healthy people.[20] It is also well known that nodes of normal size may contain metastatic deposits. The sensitivity for the detection of mediastinal lymph nodes is about 48% with a specificity of 90% and an accuracy of 70%.[17] Subdiaphragmatic lymphadenopathy can be detected with a sensitivity of 61%, a specificity of 94% and an accuracy of 82%, but lower figures are found in prospective studies.[18] Malignant cervical or supraclavicular lymphadenopathy occurs in about 60% of patients with upper third carcinomas. Overhagen et al.[21] have studied 100 patients with oesophageal carcinomas using transcutaneous sonography of the neck. Lymph nodes were considered abnormal if greater than 5 mm in diameter along the short axis. Ultrasonography detected enlarged supraclavicular lymph nodes in 22 patients whereas CT (obtained in 90 of the 100 patients) detected enlarged nodes in only 15. A total of 23 patients underwent fine needle aspiration biopsy under ultrasound guidance, 16 of whom had proven metastases histologically. In only three of these 16 patients were the lymph nodes palpable. Further studies are required to confirm these results.

CT scanning is, however, of value in the detection of distant metastases. With regard to the liver, several studies have demonstrated the overall accuracy in detecting liver metastases of the order of 80–98%.[17,18,22] Smith et al.[22] compared the accuracy of scintiscan, ultrasound and CT in patients with a variety of primary tumours with potential hepatic involvement and found little difference in the accuracy of the three techniques. Scintigraphy and ultrasound had an accuracy of 80% and CT 84%. They concluded that lesions less than 3 cm in diameter were liable to be missed by all three techniques. Advances in technique and the evolution of newer CT scanners has brought the size of lesions easily seen down to about 1 cm. The results of isotope scanning for detecting liver metastases are conflicting. Lamb and Taylor[23] found that both liver scintigraphy using technetium sulphur colloid and ultrasound were 97% accurate in determining the presence or absence of liver metastases in 100 patients with colorectal cancer. Most authors, however, have reported accuracies of the order of 64–80% for the detection of hepatic scintiscans.[22,24,25] Grey-scale ultrasound when used to enhance the diagnostic accuracy of scintigraphy has been shown to have an accuracy of 93%.[26] Most authors have not been able to reproduce this level of accuracy and figures of 75–80% are reported in the literature.[22,27] Pulmonary metastases are shown more frequently on CT than on simple chest radiography. Peritoneal metastases are not usually recognised by CT.

Magnetic resonance imaging is an alternative to CT. Studies comparing these two imaging modalities in the staging of oesophageal carcinoma have found that MRI has approximately the same success rate in predicting mediastinal invasion as CT. The accuracy for CT and MRI in the detection of tracheal or bronchial invasion was 89% and 90%, respectively.[17] Accuracy rates of 75% for aortic invasion and 88% for pericardial invasion have been reported for MRI.[28] In general the sensitivity and specificity of MRI is comparable to CT. MRI is limited, however, in its ability to examine more than one organ system or one area of the body during a single examination. MRI is an acceptable substitute for CT in the detection of liver metastases but it is less useful in the evaluation of pulmonary metastases. It is difficult to obtain a high quality study of the entire mediastinum and the upper abdomen in one sitting. Because of this, the higher cost and more limited availability of MRI, CT will remain the primary investigation.

Stomach

Early hopes that CT would provide accurate staging for gastric carcinoma have not been substantiated. This is partly because of the problem of nodal status as mentioned in the section on oesophageal cancer.

The CT appearances of gastric carcinoma are variable. It usually presents with focal or diffuse wall thickening, frequently projecting into the lumen of the stomach with or without ulceration. The thickness of the stomach wall in the distended stomach with gastric carcinoma is greater than 5 mm and a thickness of over 2 cm usually correlates with transmural extension.[29] Assessment of contiguous adjacent organ extension is unreliable unless a large bulk of tumour is present in the adjacent structure. Peritoneal carcinomatosis is poorly diagnosed. In 1988 Sussman *et al.*[30] reported a series of 75 patients with adenocarcinoma of the stomach and showed that CT was a poor method of staging; 47% of patients were incorrectly staged by CT, 31% understaged and 16% overstaged. Understaging was due to the factors described above and overstaging was due to overdiagnosed malignant lymphadenopathy and invasion of contiguous organs as predicted by a loss of the fat plane. As has been described with oesophageal carcinoma this sign is unreliable for a number of reasons. The patients are often emaciated and the fat plane may also be lost due to inflammatory adhesions. Pancreatic invasion has been described when the fat plane is intact. The sensitivity of CT to detect invasion of the pancreas is abysmal – with a sensitivity of only 27%.[30]

Technical improvements in high resolution CT together with intravenous contrast and oral ingestion of water to distend the stomach have resulted in improvements in the diagnostic accuracy over conventional

CT. Cho et al.[31] studied 52 patients with pathologically proven gastric cancers with an overall detection rate for the primary tumour of 88% (46 of 52 cases). Five of the nine early gastric cancers and 41 of the 43 advanced cancers were diagnosed. The uninvolved gastric wall showed a two or three layer pattern on the dynamic CT scan. These layers corresponded to the inner mucosal layer showing marked enhancement, the outer submucosal layer with lower attenuation and another outer muscular–serosal layer showing moderate enhancement. The four early cancers were missed owing to their small size and a partial volume effect. The advanced cancers showed moderate to marked heterogenous enhancement in the early phase and homogenous enhancement of the entire lesion in the equilibrium phase of the dynamic CT. This is related to the neovascularity of gastric cancer. These workers were unable to differentiate between EGC involving the mucosa or submucosa and more advanced carcinoma involving the muscular or subserosal areas of the gastric wall. The overall accuracy of dynamic CT in determining the T category was 65% and the accuracy in determining the degree of serosal invasion was 83%. Similar figures have been reported by other workers.[32] A recent study assessing high resolution CT and adjacent organ invasion has shown that an absence of fat planes or an irregularity of the border between the tumour and the adjacent organ was not found to be significantly related to invasion.[33] This group of Japanese workers assessed the mean densities at the region of interest and found them to be significantly greater at invasion sites than at non-invasion sites. This allowed invasion of the pancreas, liver and colon to be assessed with an accuracy of 75%, 61% and 78%, respectively. They still found however that CT has limited value in differentiating inflammatory adhesions with fibrosis or oedema from true invasion.

Dynamic CT showed a sensitivity of 74%, a specificity of 65% and an accuracy of 70% in assessing metastases to regional lymph nodes.[31] The detection rate of lymph node metastases was low when perigastric nodes were close to the primary tumour. Peritumoral lymph node involvement often appears confluent with the primary tumour. The detection rate was much higher in N_2 nodes especially in nodes associated with the left gastric, splenic or coeliac arteries. N_2 nodal status is of more importance to the surgeon.

CT scanning to detect distant metastases produces accuracy figures similar to those seen in oesophageal cancer and the arguments relating to MRI are similar. Despite the increasing accuracy of CT it is still not sufficient to determine specific procedures for patients with gastric cancer prior to surgery.

Endoscopy

Upper gastrointestinal endoscopy with biopsy with or without cytological examination is the most important investigation in the diagnosis of oesophageal and gastric carcinoma and should be performed in any patient in whom the disease is suspected.

Oesophagus

The appearances of early squamous cell carcinoma at endoscopy vary widely. The most common appearance is that of a superficial erosive cancer consisting of a slightly depressed lesion with grey erosions in a reddish mucosa. Early squamous carcinomas have also been described as whitish elevated plaques, slight depressed erythematous areas or as erosions suggestive of gastro-oesophageal reflux disease. Superficial polypoidal lesions also occur and when present are more likely to be associated with symptoms than other macroscopic types. In a recent Japanese study it was shown that endoscopy permitted a correct diagnosis of early oesophageal carcinoma in 100% of patients but contrast radiology only detected 47% of lesions.[34] The majority of lesions missed were of the superficial type. Endoscopic biopsy and brush cytology are complementary investigations and if facilities are available both should be performed. Several factors influence the accuracy of endoscopic biopsy including the number of biopsy specimens taken. When six to ten specimens are obtained the diagnostic accuracy exceeds 80%.[35] With advanced carcinoma prebiopsy dilatation may be necessary to enable biopsies to be taken from the central portion of the tumour rather than from the proximal limit of the tumour which may reveal non-neoplastic mucosa due to submucosal tumour infiltration. This is especially true of adenocarcinoma at or close to the cardia. Dilatation should be performed in order to examine the distal limit of the tumour. The accuracy of endoscopy brush cytology or cytological examination using the balloon technique is reported to exceed 70%.[35,36] By combining the results of cytology and multiple endoscopic biopsies an accuracy approaching 100% can be obtained.[35]

In vitro dye staining is being used increasingly in some centres to facilitate detection of early oesophageal cancer.[37] The stains most commonly used are 1–2% Lugol's iodine, 1–2% toluidine blue and 1–2% methylene blue. Lugol's solution stains non-keratinised squamous epithelium in proportion to its intracellular glycogen content. Early oesophageal cancer consistently shows negative staining allowing more accurate biopsies to be undertaken. Lugol's solution is not useful for isolating dysplastic epithelium because about 50% of such areas are stained positively. Using toluidine blue, dysplastic epithelium usually stains blue. Methylene blue can be used to stain columnar epithelium as it is taken up by goblet cells but not by the squamous epithelium. Methylene blue may also accentuate mucosal relief making differentiation of columnar and squamous epithelium more obvious endoscopically.

Macroscopically advanced cancer is traditionally classified into three main types: (1) exophytic or polypoidal, (2) ulcerative and (3) diffusely infiltrative. Many forms may co-exist within any single tumour. Usually a major part of the circumference of the oesophageal lumen is covered by the tumour. A diffusely infiltrative carcinoma manifests itself as obvious thickening and rigidity of the oesophageal wall of variable length with fixation of the irregularly thickened, coarsely nodular, usually non-ulcerated mucosa to the deeper layers of the oesophageal wall. Luminal narrowing is usually present. A peculiar form of oesophageal cancer described as 'superficial spreading cancer' is defined as a lesion with intramucosal extension of the tumour of at least 2 cm from the main bulk of the tumour.[38] The boundary between involved and uninvolved mucosa may be indistinguishable. It is important to realise that oesophageal cancers have a tendency to spread submucosally and to establish satellite lesions at some distance from the obvious primary tumour. Small mucosal elevations especially proximal to the main lesion should be given special attention and accurate biopsies taken. Whether these lesions represent intramural metastases from the submucosal spread or primary intramucosal carcinomas (the so called 'field change') remains controversial.

In patients with a Barrett's oesophagus the goal of endoscopic surveillance is to detect neoplastic lesions that may not be apparent on gross endoscopic examination. A systematic series of endoscopic biopsies should be carried out as high-grade dysplasia and early adenocarcinoma can be detected in mucosa that is endoscopically unremarkable.[39] Early cancers are sometimes associated with friability of the mucosa, superficial erosions, ulcerations, nodularity, plaques, polyps or early strictures. Endoscopic cytology is considered a complement but not an alternative to biopsy.[40]

Stomach

With regard to gastric cancer it is possible endoscopically to define the nature of the cancer, its situation and its dimensions. From its size and cell type the possibility of spread can be predicted. All endoscopists should be acutely aware of various macroscopic appearances of early gastric cancer (Fig. 3.2) with multiple biopsies being taken from any mucosal gastric lesion. This is especially true of patients at risk of gastric carcinoma, i.e. those with pre-existing gastric ulcers, patients who have undergone previous gastric surgery for benign disease, those with a family history of carcinoma of the stomach, those with atrophic gastritis and patients with pernicious anaemia. Brush cytology of suspicious gastric lesions has recently been shown to have a sensitivity almost as high as that of oesophageal cytology. In a study of 903 patients with gastric carcinoma, cytology yielded positive results in 785 (sensitivity 87%) and biopsies were positive in 826 (sensitivity 92%). When the two techniques were combined a positive diagnosis was established in 886 patients (sensitivity 98%).[41] In 52 patients with negative biopsies cytology was positive and a further eight patients had positive cytology in whom biopsies had not been obtained. Cytology therefore added 60 positive results to the overall diagnostic yield (6.7%). In this study, brushings were done after the biopsy had been taken which may lead to difficulty in retrieving precise samples from the bleeding abraded surface and improvement in the accuracy of cytology might have been obtained if the cytological sampling had been done before the biopsy as has been advocated.[42] Better results are obtained if the brush used for cytology is immersed in saline and stirred vigorously, with centrifugation of the resulting fluid rather than directly smeared on to slides.[43] Cytology, however, does add to the expense and requires an experienced endoscopist and cytopathologist.

It is important for the surgeon to know which histological type of gastric carcinoma is present – diffuse or intestinal – as they possess different biological behaviours.[44] Patients with the diffuse type of tumour usually have a worse prognosis.

Endoscopic ultrasonography

Endosonography has become an established diagnostic tool for the local staging of oesophageal and gastric carcinomas. Endoscopic ultrasound (EUS) is superior to CT in the local staging of oesophageal and gastric tumours.

Using EUS at 7.5–12 MHz frequency, the wall of the oesophagus and stomach can be imaged as a five layer structure of alternating bright (hyperechoic) and dark (hypoechoic) bands. For clinical purposes the first two layers correspond to the superficial and deep mucosa, the third layer to the submucosa, the fourth layer to the muscularis propria and the fifth layer to the serosa/adventitia.

Japanese investigators using this modality have directed their attention to the detection of EGC corresponding to T_1 tumours. In this high incidence area extensive nodal dissection for EGC has been questioned for certain groups of patients with mucosal tumours and the endoscopic treatment of cancers with minimal chance of lymph node metastases has also been reported. The relative reluctance to clinically predict lymph node status by EUS reflects the fact that the Japanese definition of EGC does not require negative nodal status. In contrast Western investigators have directed their attention toward recognition of resectable from non-resectable cancers and between curative and non-curative disease. As a result emphasis has been placed on detection of invasion of neighbouring organs, as shown by the loss of the fifth layer and tumour mass confluent with the adjacent organ. However, the results from both Western and Japanese investigators show very similar results.

Unlike CT which can only assess lymph node size, EUS provides additional information regarding shape, border demarcation, echo intensity and echo texture. In general it is thought that rounded, sharply demarcated, homogenous, hypoechoic features indicate malignancy whereas elongated, heterogenous, hyperechoic, lymph nodes with indistinct borders are more likely to be benign or inflammatory. However, these endosonographic features may not be evident in cases of micrometastases and evaluation of these features is subjective and may vary between different observers and possibly between the same observer on different occasions. In a study of 100 patients with oesophageal carcinoma Catalano et al.[45] found an overall sensitivity in the detection of malignant lymph nodes of 89%. When EUS imaged

Table 3.2 *Accuracy of EUS in oesophageal carcinoma (T + N stage) (%)*

Histology	Catalano[50]	Rösch[51]	Grimm[52]	Dittler[53]
T_1	33	50	90	81
T_2	75	78	86	77
T_3	82	91	93	89
T_4	89	80	83	88
N_0	94	42	85	70
N_1	89	89	88	74

lymph nodes of any sort the likelihood of N_1 disease was 86% whereas when lymph nodes were not seen the chance of N_0 disease was 79%. When at least one predicted feature of malignancy was present specificity increased from 75% to 92%, but when all four features were present metastases were found histologically in 100% of cases. The features most sensitive for discriminating benign from malignant lymph node was the central echo pattern followed in order by border, shape and size.

Oesophageal carcinoma

The accuracy of EUS in assessing the depth of tumour invasion within the oesophageal wall and of assessing N_1 nodes is shown in Table 3.2.[46-49] The high accuracy rates in N staging predominate in the literature although there are reports which do not confirm these results. In a study of 16 surgically resected specimens EUS visualised only 30% of the lymph nodes.[50] This study also questioned the subjective appreciation of the echo structure within lymph nodes and found significant variation between two examiners when compared with the grey-scale values on computer analysis.

Tumour-induced stricture precluding passage of the endosonography probe is common and is usually associated with advanced tumour stage (T_3, T_4).[49] Attempts to dilate the tumour prior to EUS may be associated with a significant perforation rate.[46] Some authors have suggested that in patients with stenosis, tumour staging should be confined to the proximal edge of the tumour. This approach will understage patients who have coeliac lymphadenopathy but was found to be accurate in the T staging of impassable tumours in 88% of patients. This staging is in fact more accurate than in those patients who have a difficult carcinoma to transverse where the accuracy is reduced to 46%.[51] The low accuracy for moderate strictures is related to the reduced distance between the tumour and the transducer which hampers visualisation of the individual wall layers.

Gastric carcinoma

The overall T staging accuracy for gastric carcinoma is slightly less than that for oesophageal carcinoma.[48,52,53] Certain regions of the

Table 3.3 *Accuracy of EUS in gastric cancer (T + N stage) (%)*

Histology	Rösch[51]	Grimm[52]	Dittler[53]	Ziegler[56]
T_1	71	90	81	91
T_2	64	79	71	81
T_3	83	62	87	86
T_4	64	89	79	89
N_0	75	85	93	88
N_1	86	50	65	64

stomach are difficult to assess completely with endosonography and these include the lesser curve immediately distal to the cardia, segments of the fundus and the prepyloric regions. Concurrent ulceration may be associated with peritumour inflammation and may lead to overstaging. Distinguishing between T_2 (infiltration of the subserosa) and T_3 (invasion of the serosa) lesions may be technically difficult on EUS. The accuracy of T and N staging for gastric carcinoma is shown in Table 3.3.[47,48,52,53] Ziegler *et al.*[52] have shown that assessment of T and N stage by EUS is significantly more accurate than CT or intraoperative assessment. The T stage accuracy of EUS, CT and intraoperative assessment by the surgeon was 86, 43 and 56% and the N stage accuracy of EUS, CT and intraoperative assessment was 74, 51 and 54%, respectively. The linear extent of gastric carcinoma has important implications when planning surgical therapy. Maruta *et al.*[54] have shown that the horizontal length of the hypoechoic region in the gastric wall corresponds to neoplastic tissue on histological evaluation in the absence of ulceration. When ulceration is present this hypoechoic area corresponds more closely to the fibrosis associated with malignancy, the actual tumour being smaller than the endosonographic hypoechoic area.

Laparoscopy

Both hepatic and parietal peritoneal metastases associated with either oesophageal or gastric carcinoma are associated with a poor prognosis. Knowledge of their presence or absence should have a significant bearing on the therapeutic decisions made in patients where their presence is confirmed.

The increasing use of chemotherapy, radiotherapy, intubation, stent insertion and laser therapy or combinations of these treatment modalities means that patients with disease incurable by surgery can usually be adequately palliated until their death.

In a large study of 369 patients with carcinoma of the oesophagus and cardia, Dagnini *et al.*[55] found metastases to liver, peritoneum, omentum, stomach and intra-abdominal lymph nodes in 52 patients (14%). Laparoscopic false negative results in patients subjected to laparotomy was only 4.4% (2.8% to the liver, 1.2% to peritoneum and 0.4% to the omentum). They concluded that laparoscopy was an effective procedure to stage oesophageal carcinoma. In a comparative study of laparoscopy, ultrasound scanning and scintigraphy in patients with oesophageal and gastric carcinoma Shandall and Johnson[27] showed that laparoscopy was more accurate in detecting hepatic metastases and this obviated the need for surgery in 29 patients (58%). They concluded that laparoscopy was useful in patients with oesophageal carcinoma, but in gastric carcinoma the value was doubtful as they felt a high percentage of patients would require palliative surgery. Gross et al.[56] studied 46 consecutive patients and found 27 patients with incurable disease and in whom surgery was not undertaken. Our own studies comparing laparoscopy, CT and ultrasound in 90 patients with either carcinoma of the oesophagus or cardia and in a further 103 patients with gastric carcinoma have shown laparoscopy to be more sensitive and accurate in the detection of hepatic and peritoneal metastases (Tables 3.4 and 3.5).[18,57] Laparoscopy was significantly more sensitive and accurate than ultrasound at diagnosing nodal metastases from oesophageal carcinoma and although more accurate

Table 3.4 *Hepatic metastases*

	Laparoscopy	CT	US
Sensitivity (%)			
Oesophageal carcinoma	88	56	48
Gastric carcinoma	96	52	37
Specificity (%)			
Oesophageal carcinoma	100	97	97
Gastric carcinoma	100	92	95
Accuracy (%)			
Oesophageal carcinoma	96	85	83
Gastric carcinoma	99	79	76

Table 3.5 *Peritoneal metastases*

	Laparoscopy	CT	US
Sensitivity (%)			
Oesophageal carcinoma	89	0	22
Gastric carcinoma	69	8	24
Specificity (%)			
Oesophageal carcinoma	100	100	100
Gastric carcinoma	100	100	100
Accuracy (%)			
Oesophageal carcinoma	98	–	89
Gastric carcinoma	94	81	84

and sensitive than CT this did not reach statistical significance. The sensitivity of laparoscopy for nodal metastases was 51% with an accuracy of 72%. In gastric carcinoma laparoscopy is more sensitive and accurate then either CT or ultrasound in diagnosing nodal metastases with a sensitivity of 54% and an accuracy of 65%. One of the major benefits of laparoscopy is the opportunity to obtain tissue samples accurately under direct vision not only from the liver but also from nodal or peritoneal metastases often confirming or refuting the results of other non-invasive investigations.

The recent introduction of laparoscopic ultrasound has been shown to improve the overall accuracy of staging in patients with oesophageal and gastric cancer. It was significantly more accurate than conventional investigations for staging the primary tumour (T grade) and for the assessment of intra-abdominal malignant lymphadenopathy (N stage).[58] It seems likely that the addition of ultrasonography to laparoscopy should improve the N staging of patients with oesophageal and gastric cancers and may improve the accuracy of liver metastases but this needs to be tested in a prospective study. One additional value of the use of laparoscopy under general anaesthesia as a separate staging procedure is that it will occasionally show patients who display significant cardiovascular instability during anaesthesia or a very slow functional recovery and these patients may be precluded from major resectional surgery, being considered unfit.

Additional investigations

Plain chest radiography has a limited role in assessing patients but should probably be undertaken in all with oesophageal and gastric cancer. Radiological features of aspiration pneumonia may be the first evidence of an oesophageal or proximal gastric lesion. Occasionally evidence of pulmonary metastases may be present.

Rigid bronchoscopy should be carried out on all patients with upper and middle third lesions to assess the tracheobronchial tree. Direct invasion can be seen and, if appropriate, biopsied. Significant compression of the trachea or the carina as well as the fixity can be assessed. Further investigations should be carried out as deemed clinically appropriate. Isotope bone scanning is superior to skeletal radiology in the detection of bone metastases. CT scanning of the head or isotope brain scan are useful in those patients exhibiting cerebral symptoms who may have intracranial metastases.

Summary

The appropriate management of patients with oesophageal and gastric cancer depends on accurate preoperative staging of the disease. Conventional preoperative staging based on physical examination, barium swallow and meal, endoscopy, bronchoscopy and CT or MRI often understages the disease. The reasons for the inaccuracy are the inability to determine the depth of oesophageal or gastric wall involvement, the extent of infiltration to other organs and the underestimation of lymph node metastases.

Pretherapy staging is more accurate when combined with laparoscopy with or without ultrasound and EUS. However, if this additional information does not alter the selection of treatment modalities for patients with oesophageal and gastric cancer it remains but an intellectual exercise. Fok *et al.*[59] in a study of endosonography in patients with oesophageal carcinoma confirmed that EUS can provide more precise preoperative staging but when surgery is the preferred treatment for palliation even in advanced stages of the disease the additional information gained by EUS did not help in guiding the decision to operate, or in the type of operation used, both being determined by the more simple conventional preoperative investigations. The impact of EUS on treatment, especially non-resectional, has yet to be determined. Most authors using laparoscopy have shown that improved pretreatment staging will reduce the number of patients undergoing non-resectional surgery.[56,60] More accurate preoperative staging will allow stratification within clinical trials and the use of repeated endoscopic ultrasonography should be useful in patients undergoing non-resectional treatment, e.g. radiotherapy or laser recanalisation.

At the present time it would appear that a battery of tests is needed in patients with oesophageal and gastric carcinoma once the diagnosis has been confirmed by endoscopy and biopsy. CT is useful for the detection of pulmonary and hepatic metastases with a low false negative rate. In those patients in whom surgery is being considered as a curative procedure, laparoscopy with or without ultrasound increases the staging as far as intra-abdominal metastatic disease is concerned. Endoscopic ultrasonography gives valuable information regarding the depth of the tumour and nodal status. Further studies are required to assess the accuracy of laparoscopy with ultrasound, and to combine laparoscopy with EUS as complimentary staging procedures. As technology develops the role of the various investigations used to stage patients with oesophageal and gastric cancer will change.

Intraoperative assessment and staging

With modern preoperative staging techniques it should be possible to embark on a resection for oesophageal or gastric cancer with a definite plan for the extent and radicality of the procedure. However, the first step in the operation and prior to beginning the resection, is careful operative staging of the cancer. There are two basic aims in performing staging at this point.

1. Confirm preoperative staging and in particular ensure that the cancer has not been understaged. Evidence of distant metastases

must be sought as this is an obvious indication of incurability and radical resection is not worthwhile, indeed the benefit of any resection is questionable in many patients as it will only be for palliation of symptoms.

2. Accurately stage the cancer to determine the extent of the surgical resection and develop a therapeutic plan. At this stage it is important to decide whether localised direct spread can be completely resected, the extent of the nodal dissection and the need for resection of other organs.

The steps in intraoperative assessment are to detect the following:

1. The presence of hepatic metastases not detected on preoperative scanning or laparoscopy. If there is any doubt about abnormal areas in the liver then needle core biopsies should be sent for urgent frozen section histology.
2. The presence and extent of peritoneal deposits. These should have been detected by preoperative laparoscopy, though this may not have been deemed necessary in elderly patients with obstructing distal cancers.
3. The extent of the primary tumour and in particular the proximal and distal palpable margins. The lateral margin must also be carefully evaluated to stage the depth of invasion and the presence of fixity to adjacent structures. It is important to decide whether adherence to another organ is inflammatory or neoplastic although this is often difficult to determine with certainty.
4. The extent of lymph node involvement. If enlarged nodes are within the planned extent of the en bloc resection then it is not vital to decide whether they are malignant. Enlarged nodes that cannot be safely resected and lie outside the margins of the resection are regarded as distant metastases and should be sampled and sent for frozen section histology – if positive the resection should be regarded as palliative and so either reduced or abandoned for a different treatment modality.
5. Other intraoperative investigative techniques may be helpful and are described in the respective chapters.

Clinico-pathological staging

The final staging of oesophageal and gastric cancer is important as it allows an accurate prediction of prognosis and may also indicate the need for adjuvant therapy. Importantly staging allows comparison of results, not only of different treatment strategies but also between different centres.

The final staging of a cancer relies on a combination of the results of preoperative investigations, the intraoperative macroscopic findings and the pathological microscopic analysis if the cancer is resected. The staging systems for gastric and oesophageal cancer are different and there are several systems presently in use for each.

Gastric cancer

There are three main staging systems presently used in different countries, although since 1986 there has been an attempt to use an agreed unified TNM system. It is, however, important to be aware of the various systems.

Japanese Research Society for Gastric Cancer – PHNS System

This is the most systematised and detailed system for staging gastric cancer. There are rules for both the macroscopic intraoperative findings and the histological findings. The PHNS system is derived from the TNM system, but takes into account four factors.[61]

P factor – Grade of peritoneal dissemination (Table 3.6).
H factor – Presence of liver metastases (Table 3.6).
N factor – Extent of lymph node involvement (Table 3.7).
S factor – Extent of invasion of serosal surface of the stomach (Table 3.7).

Table 3.6 *Clinical staging of gastric cancer – PHNS system*

P factor

P_0	no evidence of peritoneal spread
P_1	peritoneal spread limited to supracolic area including greater omentum but not the diaphragm
P_2	small number of nodules on diaphragm and/or below mesocolon
P_3	numerous nodules on diaphragm or below mesocolon

H factor

H_0	no liver metastases
H_1	metastases in one lobe
H_2	small number of metastases in both lobes
H_3	multiple metastases in both lobes

Table 3.7 *Clinical staging of gastric cancer – PHNS system*

N factor

N_0	no lymph node involvement
N_1	group 1 nodes involved
N_2	group 2 nodes involved
N_3	group 3 nodes involved
N_4	nodes involved extending beyond group 3

S factor

S_0	no serosal invasion
S_1	suspected serosal invasion
S_2	definite serosal invasion
S_3	serosal invasion and invasion of contiguous structures

Figure 3.3
*Location of primary
gastric cancer.*

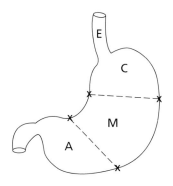

Anatomical description

The stomach is subdivided into three sections – upper (C), middle (M) and lower (A) (Fig. 3.3). When the carcinomatous infiltration is completely limited to one of the three sections this is expressed by indicating the appropriate letter. If the lesion extends across the dividing line the section primarily involved is listed first followed by the less involved section or sections. For example MCA indicates a tumour arising in the middle portion but extending into the upper third and to a lesser extent the lower third. In describing the site of the primary lesion the stomach is also separated into four parts looking at the cross section of the stomach.

Pathological description

It is with regard to the N factor that the Japanese have carried out considerable research and revision over that in the original TNM classification. Basically the lymph node drainage is divided into three tiers around each part of the stomach. Each lymph node group has been numbered and named (Fig. 3.4a and b). Table 3.8 lists the N_1, N_2 and N_3 node groups in relation to the site of the primary tumour. Any nodal metastases outside these groups are classed as N_4. Nodal involvement can be assessed intraoperatively, but only very detailed

Table 3.8 *Lymph node groups in relation to site of gastric cancer*

Lymph node group	Location of tumour			
	AMC, MAC, MCA, CMA	A, AM	M, MA, MC	C, CM
N_1	1,2,3,4,5,6	3,4,5,6	1,3,4,5,6(2MC)	1,2,3,4s
N_2	7,8,9,10,11	1,7,8,9	2,7,8,9,10,11	4d,5,6, 7,8,9,10,11
N_3	12,13,14, 110,111	2,10,11, 12,13,14	12,13,14	12,13,14, 110,111

Figure 3.4
(a) Perigastric lymph nodes; (b) extra-gastric lymph nodes.

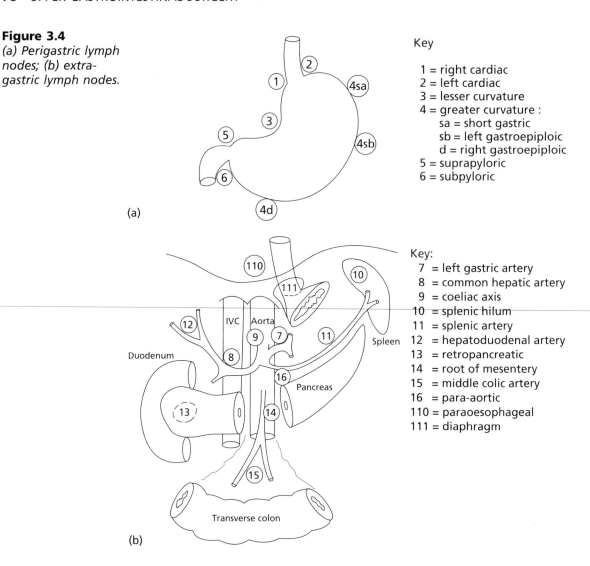

Key

1 = right cardiac
2 = left cardiac
3 = lesser curvature
4 = greater curvature :
    sa = short gastric
    sb = left gastroepiploic
    d = right gastroepiploic
5 = suprapyloric
6 = subpyloric

(a)

Key:
  7 = left gastric artery
  8 = common hepatic artery
  9 = coeliac axis
10 = splenic hilum
11 = splenic artery
12 = hepatoduodenal artery
13 = retropancreatic
14 = root of mesentery
15 = middle colic artery
16 = para-aortic
110 = paraoesophageal
111 = diaphragm

(b)

histological studies can accurately determine the N factor after which it is designated as pN.

Although serosal involvement and peritoneal dissemination can be assessed at operation, histology is still needed to confirm this aspect of staging. Serosal involvement is described on the basis of both the macroscopic findings (Table 3.7) and also on histological assessment. Depth of invasion of the cancer can only be determined accurately by histological analysis and is designated the symbol pT. There are five layers to the stomach wall – mucosa (m), submucosa (sm), muscularis propria (pm), subserosa (ss) and serosal (s). Early gastric cancer (m or sm) is pT_1, deeper invasion without breach of the serosa is pT_2 and confirmed serosal involvement is pT_3. Invasion of an adjacent structure is pT_4.

Table 3.9 *Stage classification based on gross findings in gastric cancer (PHNS system)*

Stage	Peritoneal metastases	Liver metastases	Nodal metastases	Serosal invasion
I	P_0	H_0	N_0	S_0
II	P_0	H_0	N_1	S_1
III	P_0	H_0	N_2	S_2
IV	P_1, P_2, P_3	H_1, H_2, H_3	N_3, N_4	S_3

Table 3.10 *Staging based on histopathology in gastric cancer (PHNS system)*

Stage	Macroscopic or histological			Histological
	Peritoneal metastases	Liver metastases	Nodal metastases	Depth of invasion
I	P_0	H_0	N_0	ps
II	P_0	H_0	N_1	ssy
III	P_0	H_0	N_2	se
IV	P_1, P_2, P_3	H_1, H_2, H_3	N_3, N_4	si,sei

ps, deepest layer invaded is muscularis mucosa, border distinct; ssy, deepest layer invaded is subserosa, border ill-defined; se, serosa involved; si, infiltration of neighbouring tissue; sei, coexistence of se and si.

The completed PHNS staging process allows each case to be allocated to a stage of the disease as shown in Table 3.9. The staging is refined on the basis of the microscopic findings (Table 3.10). It should be noted that the final staging also takes account of resection margins and if malignant cells are detected histologically within 10 mm of the proximal and distal margins then the cancer is down staged.

AJC and UICC modifications of the TNM system

These two systems are modifications of Kennedy's original description of the TNM system.[62] The American Joint Committee on Cancer Staging Systems and the UICC staging systems were widely adopted in the USA and Europe.[63,64] The AJC system has gained more popularity in the United Kingdom and is outlined in Table 3.11. In this system R is used to indicate whether there is evidence of residual cancer after the resection; R_0 indicates complete resection, R_1 microscopic evidence of residual cancer and R_2 is macroscopic residual cancer. This R factor should not be confused with the Japanese use of R for the level of nodal resection which has now been changed to D to avoid confusion.

Table 3.11 *Clinical staging of gastric cancer – AJC*

T factor	T_1	confined to the mucosa and submucosa
	T_2	involving the muscularis propria and the subserosa
	T_3	spread to involve the serosa
	T_4	spread to contiguous structures
N factor	N_0	no nodal metastases
	N_1	perigastric nodes within 3 cm of primary tumour
	N_2	nodes greater than 3 cm from tumour involved
	N_3	non-excised nodes involved
M factor	M_0	absence of metastatic disease
	M_1	presence of metastatic disease

Internationally Unified TNM System

The use of three different staging systems for gastric cancer, even though all are based on TNM, has led to considerable confusion. In order to try and eliminate this confusion and to introduce the most recent progress in diagnosis and treatment the Japanese have proposed an acceptable unified staging system. The concept is that of TNM, i.e. there are only three basic prognostic variables, with the proviso that in patients who are M_0 the pT and pN factors have almost equal significance. M_1 includes third and fourth tier nodes, peritoneal seedlings, liver and distant metastases. Stages 1 and 3 have been subdivided into A and B to allow tighter grouping of prognostic groups. The Unified TNM Staging System and approximate 5-year survival figures are shown in Table 3.12. This system was approved by the UICC and AJC in 1985 and in Japan in 1986. Use of this system is strongly recommended.

Oesophageal cancer

The TNM classification for oesophageal cancer has evolved since 1976. The Japanese Society for Esophageal Diseases system is used to define the anatomical location of the tumour.[65] The TNM staging system then classifies the primary tumour, nodal spread and distant metastases.

Anatomical description

This has not changed since the original description by the Japanese Society in 1976.[65] The oesophagus is divided into four parts.

1. *Cervical oesophagus* (Ce) – between the cricopharyngeus muscle and the upper border of the sternum.
2. *Intrathoracic oesophagus* – is further subdivided into three parts:
   (a) Upper intrathoracic (Iu) – extends from thoracic inlet to the level of the tracheal bifurcation, approximately 24 cm from the upper incisor teeth.

Table 3.12 *Internationally Unified TNM Staging System for gastric cancer*

T factor	T_1	Tumour limited to mucosa or submucosa
	T_2	Tumour involves muscularis propria or subserosa
	T_3	Tumour penetrates serosa
	T_4	Tumour involves contiguous structures
N factor	N_0	No node metastases
	N_1	Involvement of perigastric nodes within 3 cm of margin of primary
	N_2	Involvement of perigastric nodes greater than 3 cm from tumour margin or nodes along left gastric, common hepatic, splenic and coeliac arteries.
		Involvement of any other abdominal nodes is classed as distant metastases (M_1)
M factor	M_0	No evidence of distant metastases
	M_1	Evidence of distant metastases

Stage grouping				Approximate 5-year prognosis[a]
Stage IA	pT_1 pN_0 M_0			95+%
Stage IB	pT_1 pN_1 M_0	pT_2 pN_0 M_0		85–90%
Stage II	pT_1 pN_2 M_0	pT_2 pN_1 M_0	pT_3 pN_0 M_0	70–80%
Stage IIIA	pT_2 pN_2 M_0	pT_3 pN_1 M_0	pT_4 pN_0 M_0	45–50%
Stage IIIB	pT_3 pN_2 M_0	pT_4 pN_1 M_0	pT_4 pN_2 M_0	15–25%
Stage IV	Any case with M_1			0–10%

[a] Survival estimates based on Japanese and best results from Western studies

(b) Middle intrathoracic (Im) – proximal half of the oesophagus between the tracheal bifurcation and the oesophagogastric junction. The lower level is approximately 32 cm from the upper incisor teeth.

(c) Lower intra-thoracic (Ei) – This lower part of the oesophagus includes the abdominal oesophagus (Ea) and the distal half of the oesophagus between the tracheal bifurcation and the oesophagogastric junction. It is about 8 cm long and the lower level is about 40 cm from the upper incisor teeth.

The Japanese Society only classified squamous cell carcinomas. As a result the TNM classification, which was unified to include the UICC and AJC classifications, has included adenocarcinomas. Adenocarcinomas arising in the region of the oesophagogastric junction pose a problem for classification. They may arise in one of three ways.

1. Metaplasia columnar epithelium in the lower oesophagus.
2. Glandular epithelium of the cardia of the stomach.
3. Fundus of the stomach with proximal spread.

The tumour is described as Ec when the major portion is in the oesophagus, E = C where there are equal lengths in the oesophagus and stomach and Ce when the bulk of the tumour is in the proximal stomach. The major problem with this classification is the inability to identify the true oesophagogastric junction in patients with circumferential cancers in this area.

The anatomical sites of the regional lymph nodes that are involved in oesophageal cancer are listed according to the TNM classification:

Cervical oesophagus – scalene, internal jugular, upper cervical, paraoesophageal, supra-clavicular and cervical.
Intrathoracic oesophagus – internal jugular, tracheobronchial, superior mediastinal, paratracheal, perigastric (excluding coeliac), carinal, pulmonary hilar, perioesophageal, left gastric, paracardial, nodes of the lesser curve of the stomach and posterior mediastinal nodes.

These nodes differ slightly from the nomenclature as described by the Japanese Society in 1976 (see Fig. 3.5). However, the groups are broadly similar.

The most common metastatic sites are the liver, lungs, pleura and less commonly the kidneys and brain. Tumour may extend directly into mediastinal structures before distant spread is evident.

Figure 3.5 *Lymph node groups.*

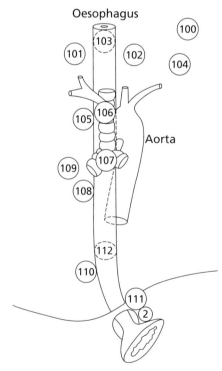

Key:
100 = lateral cervical
101 = cervical paraoesophageal
102 = deep cervical
103 = retropharyngeal
104 = supraclavicular
105 = upper thoracic paraoesophageal
106 = paratracheal
107 = tracheal bifurcation
108 = middle thoracic paraoesophageal
109 = pulmonary hilum
110 = lower thoracic paraoesophageal
111 = diaphragmatic
112 = posterior mediastinal
  2 = left cardiac

Rules for classification

Clinical staging

This depends on the anatomical extent of the tumour that can be determined prior to treatment. Assessment includes physical examination, endoscopic biopsies, laboratory studies and imaging as previously described. The location of the tumour, depth of invasion and evidence of nodal and distant spread should be described.

Histopathological staging

This is based on the findings at surgical exploration and on resection of the oesophagus and resected en bloc tissues and other tissue biopsies. Extension of the tumour into adjacent structures and evidence of distant spread should be carefully documented.

A single classification serves all regions of the oesophagus for both clinical and histopathological staging. The adjacent structures invaded depends on the location of the primary tumour. Involved structures should be specified in the description.

TNM definition

Primary tumour (T factor) – depth of invasion is shown in Table 3.13.
Regional lymph nodes (N factor) – the definition of regional node metastases has been revised since the original description by the Japanese Society. Any lymph node involved in the regions that have been described already are now classified as N_1 disease. Any nodes outwith the specific regional nodes are defined as distant metastases (M_1). (See the list above and Table 3.13 for further details.)
Distant metastases (M factor) – this is subdivided into M_0 where no distant metastases are detected and M_1 where there is evidence of distant metastases. Although the Japanese have added pleural dissemination as a separate category (PL), this is included in the M factor

Table 3.13 *Clincopathological staging of oesophageal cancer*

T factor	T_x	Primary tumour cannot be assessed
	T_0	No evidence of primary tumour
	T_{is}	Carcinoma *in situ*
	T_1	Tumour invades lamina propria or submucosa
	T_2	Tumour invades muscularis propria
	T_3	Tumour invades adventitia
	T_4	Tumour invades adjacent structures
N factor	N_x	Regional nodes cannot be assessed
	N	No regional node metastases
	N_1	Regional node metastases
M factor	M_x	Presence of distant metastases cannot be assessed
	M_0	No distant metastases
	M_1	Distant metastases

Table 3.14 *Staging based on clinical or operative findings in oesophageal carcinoma*

Stage	T	N	M
0	T_{is}	N_0	M_0
I	T_1	N_0	M_0
IIA	T_2, T_3	N_0	M_0
IIB	T_1, T_2	N_1	M_0
III	T_3, T_4	N_1	M_0
IV	any T	any N	M_1

in the unified TNM classification where pleural metastases are recorded as M_1.

Clinicopathological staging

The preoperative and intraoperative findings are refined after histological examination of the resected specimen to allow the cancer to be classified into one of four stages (Table 3.14). As with gastric cancer there are three staging systems currently in use. The Japanese PHNS system is again the most meticulous, but is not widely used outside Japan. It is important to use an agreed unified staging system so that results can be easily compared. The UICC and AJC system which is easier to use is shown in Table 3.14. These definitions are taken from the latest TNM classification (1996).[64]

It must be emphasised that the N factor in the staging system is not the same as the extent of lymphadenectomy. Three fields of lymphadenectomy are described and defined for lymph node clearance during oesophageal resection:

Field 1 – this refers to resection of nodes in the abdominal compartment.
Field 2 – thoracic lymphadenectomy
Field 3 – cervical area lymphadenectomy

This is covered in detail in Chapter 4.

Summary

The staging systems currently in use for oesophageal and gastric cancer are based on meticulous preoperative, intraoperative and histopathological assessment. Not all patients will proceed to surgical treatment and for those who do a proportion will not undergo a resection. Staging systems importantly still allow accurate staging of such cases. The most accurate staging relies on detailed histopathological analysis of the resected specimen and this information is then combined with the clinical information to allow clinicopathological staging. Adoption of recognised and preferably unified agreed systems allows comparison of results and accurate prediction of prognosis.

None of the staging systems to date place any emphasis on host defence mechanisms. Although some biological markers and acute phase proteins have shown promise with regard to predicting prognosis, none have gained clinical popularity.[66] The addition of information about host response may allow a more accurate prediction of prognosis when combined with conventional histopathological staging data. In the future this may be important in determining the most appropriate treatment modalities for each case.

References

1. Rosenberg JC, Roth JA, Lichter AS, Kelson DP. Cancer of the oesophagus. In: Devita VT, Hallman S, Rosenberg SA (eds) Cancer: principles and practice of oncology. London: JB Lippincott, 1985, pp. 621–57.
2. Yang G, Huang H, Sungliang Q, Yuming C. Endoscopic diagnosis of 115 cases of early oesophageal carcinoma. Endoscopy 1982; 14: 157.
3. Sata T, Sakai Y, Kajita A et al. Radiographic microstructures of early oesophageal carcinoma: correlation of specimen radiography with pathologic findings and clinical radiography. Gastrointest Radiol 1986; 11: 12–19.
4. Zhang DW. Fiberesophagoscopic diagnosis. In: Huang GJ, K'ai WY (eds) Carcinoma of the esophagus and gastric cardia. Berlin: Springer Verlag, 1984, pp. 217–36.
5. White RM, Levine MS, Enterline HT, Lanfer I. Early gastric cancer – recent experience. Radiology 1985; 155: 25–7.
6. Postlethwait RW. Surgery of the esophagus. New York: Appleton-Century-Crofts, 1979.
7. Daffner RH, Halber MD, Postlethwait RW, Korobkin M, Thompson WM. CT of the esophagus. II carcinoma. Am J Roentgenol 1979; 133: 1051–5.
8. Coulomb M, Lebas JF, Sarrazin R, Geindre M. L'apport de la tomodensitometric an bilan d'extension des cancers de l'oesophage. J Radiol 1981; 62: 475–87.
9. Moss AS, Schnyder P, Thoeni RF, Margulis AR. Esophageal carcinoma, pre-therapy staging by computed tomography. Am J Roentgenol 1981; 136: 1051–6.
10. Picus D, Balfe DM, Koelher RE, Roper CL, Owen JW. Computed tomography in the staging of esophageal carcinoma. Radiology 1983; 146: 433–8.
11. Thompson WM, Halvorsen RA, Foster WL, Williford ME, Postlethwait RW, Korobkin M. Computed tomography for staging esophageal and gastro-esophageal cancer: re-evaluation. Am J Roentgenol 1983; 141: 951–8.
12. Schneekloth G, Terrier F, Fuchs WA. Computed tomography in carcinoma of esophagus and cardia. Gastrointest Radiol 1983; 8: 193–206.
13. Samnelsson L, Hambraeus GM, Mercke CE, Tylen V. CT staging of oesophageal carcinoma. Acta Radiol (Diagn) 1984; 25: 7–11.
14. Quint LE, Glazier GM, Orringer MB, Gross BH. Esophageal carcinoma: CT findings. Radiology 1985; 155: 171–5.
15. Fekete F, Gayet B, Frija J. CT scanning in the diagnosis of oesophageal disease. In: Jamieson GG (ed) Surgery of the oesophagus. Edinburgh: Churchill Livingstone, 1988, pp. 85–9
16. Halvorsen RA, Thompson WM. Gastrointestinal cancer, diagnosis staging and the follow-up role of imaging. Semin Ultrasound, CT, MRI 1989; 10: 467–80.
17. Thompson WM, Halverson RA. Staging esophageal carcinoma II: CT and MRI. Semin Oncol 1994; 21: 447–52.
18. Watt I, Stewart I, Anderson D, Bell G, Anderson JR. Laparoscopy, ultrasound and computed tomography in cancer of the oesophagus and cardia: a prospective comparison for detecting intra-abdominal metastases. Br J Surg 1989; 76: 1036–9.
19. Halvorsen RA, Thompson W. Computed tomographic staging of gastrointestinal tract malignancies. Part I. Esophagus and stomach. Invest Radiol 1987; 22: 2–16.
20. Schnyder PA, Gamsu G. CT of the pre-tracheal-retrocaval space. Am J Roentgenol 1981; 136: 303–8.

21. Overhagen H, Lameris JS, Berger MY *et al*. Improved assessment of supraclavicular and abdominal metastases in oesophageal and gastro-oesophageal carcinoma with the combination of ultrasound and computed tomography. Br J Radiol 1993; 66: 203–8.

22. Smith TJ, Kemeny MM, Sugarbaker PH *et al*. A prospective study of hepatic imaging in the detection of metastatic disease. Ann Surg 1982; 195: 486–91.

23. Lamb G, Taylor I. An assessment of ultrasound scanning in the recognition of colorectal liver metastases. Ann R Coll Surg Engl 1982; 64: 391–3.

24. Castagna J, Benfield JR, Yamada H, Johnson DE. The reliability of liver scans and function tests in detecting metastases. Surg Gyencol Obstet 1972; 134: 463–6.

25. Lunia S, Parthasarathy KL, Bakshi S, Bender MA. An evaluation of 99mTc–sulfur colloid liver scintiscans and their usefulness in metastatic workup: a review of 1424 studies. J Nucl Med 1975; 16: 62–5.

26. Sullivan DC, Taylor KJW, Gattschalk A. The use of ultrasound to enhance the diagnostic utility of the equivocal liver scintigraph. Radiology 1978; 128: 727–52.

27. Shandall A, Johnson C. Laparoscopy or scanning in oesophageal and gastric cancer. Br J Surg 1985; 72: 449–51.

28. Quint LE, Glazier GM, Orringer MB, Esophageal imaging by MR and CT: study of normal anatomy and neoplasms. Radiology 1985; 156: 727–31.

29. Hada M, Hihara T, Kakishita M. Computed tomography in gastric carcinoma: thickness of gastric wall and infiltration to serosa surface. Radiat Med 1984; 2: 27–30.

30. Sussman SK, Halvorsen RA, Illescas FF *et al*. Gastric adenocarcinoma: CT versus surgical staging. Radiology 1988; 167: 335–40.

31. Cho JS, Kim JK, Rho SM, Lee HY, Jeong HY, Lee CS. Pre-operative assessment of gastric carcinoma: value of two-phase dynamic CT with mechanical iv injection of contrast material. Am J Roentgenol 1994; 163: 69–75.

32. Minami M, Kawawuchi N, Itai Y, Niki T, Sasaki Y. Gastric tumours: radiologic–pathologic correlation and accuracy of T staging with dynamic CT. Radiology 1992; 185: 173–8.

33. Tsuburaya A, Naguchi Y, Matsumoto A, Kobayashi S, Masukawa K, Horiguchi K. A preoperative assessment of adjacent organ invasion by stomach carcinoma with high resolution computed tomography. Jpn J Surg 1994; 24: 299–304.

34. Adachi Y, Kitamura K, Tsutsui S, Ikeda Y, Matsuda H, Sugimachi K. How to detect early carcinoma of the esophagus. Hepato-gastroenterol 1993; 40: 207–11.

35. Witzel L, Halter F, Gretillat PA *et al*. Evaluation of specific value of endoscopic biopsies and brush cytology for malignancies of the oesophagus and stomach. Gut 1976; 17: 375–7.

36. Hanson JT, Thoreson C, Morissey JF. Brush cytology in the diagnosis of upper gastrointestinal malignancy. Gastrointest Endosc 1980; 26: 33–5.

37. Kawai K, Takemoto T, Suziki S, Ida K. Proposed nomenclature and classification of the dye-spraying techniques in endoscopy. Endoscopy 1979; 11: 23–5.

38. Soga J, Tanaka O, Sasaki K *et al*. Superficial spreading carcinoma of the esophagus. Cancer 1981; 50: 1641–5.

39. Reid BJ, Weinstein WM, Lavin KJ *et al*. Endoscopic biopsy can defect high grade dysplasia or early adenocarcinoma in Barrett's oesophagus without grossly recognizable neoplastic lesions. Gastroenterology 1988; 94: 81–90.

40. Levine DS, Reid BJ. Endoscopic diagnosis of esophageal neoplasms. Gastrintest Endosc Clin North Am 1992; 2: 395–413.

41. Cusso X, Mones J, Ocana J, Mendez C, Vilardell F. Is endoscopic gastric cytology worthwhile? An evaluation of 903 cases of carcinoma. H Clin Gastroenterol 1993; 16: 336–9.

42. Chambers LA, Clark WE. The endoscopic diagnosis of gastroesophageal malignancy: a cytologic review. Acta Cytol 1986; 30: 110–14.

43. Waldron R, Kerrin M, Ali A *et al*. Evaluation of the role of endoscopic biopsies and cytology in the detection of gastric malignancy. Br J Surg 1990; 77: 62–3.

44. Miwa K. Cancer of the stomach in Japan. Gann Monogr Cancer Res 1979; 22: 61.

45. Catalano MF, Sivak MV, Rice T, Gragg LA, Van Dam J. Endosonographic features predictive of lymph node metastasis. Gastrointest Endosc 1994; 40: 442–6.

46. Catalano MF, Van Dam J, Sivak MV.

Malignant esophageal strictures: staging accuracy of endoscopic ultrasonography. Gastrointest Endosc 1995; 541: 535–9.

47. Rosch T, Lorenz R, Zehker K et al. Local staging and assessment of resectability in carcinoma of the esophagus, stomach and duodenum by endoscopic ultrasonography. Gastrointest Endosc 1992; 38: 460–7.

48. Grimm H, Binmoeller KF, Hamper K, Koch J, Henne-Bruns D, Soehendra N. Endosonography for preoperative locoregional staging of esophageal and gastric cancer. Endoscopy 1993; 25: 224–30.

49. Dittler HJ, Siewert JR. Role of endoscopic ultrasonography in esophageal carcinoma. Endoscopy 1993; 25: 156–61.

50. Heintz A, Mildenberger P, Georg M, Braunstein S, Junginger Th. Endoscopic ultrasonography in the diagnosis of regional lymph nodes in esophageal and gastric cancer – results of studies in vitro. Endoscopy 1993; 25: 231–5.

51. Hordijk ML, Zander H, van Blankenstein M, Tilanus HW. Influence of tumour stenosis on the accuracy of endosonography in preoperative T staging of oesophageal cancer. Endoscopy 1993; 25: 171–5.

52. Zeilger K, Sanft C, Zimmer T et al. Comparison of computed tomography, endosonography and intraoperative assessment in TN staging of gastric carcinoma. Gut 1993; 34: 604–10.

53. Dittler HJ, Siewert JR. Role of endoscopic ultrasonography in gastric carcinoma. Endoscopy 1993; 25: 162–6.

54. Maruta S, Tzukamoto Y, Niwa Y, Goto H, Hase S, Yoshikane H. Endoscopic ultrasonography for assessing the horizontal extent of invasive gastric carcinoma. Am J Gastroenterol 1993; 88: 555–9.

55. Dagnini G, Caldironi MW, Marin G, Buzzaccarini O, Tremolda C, Ruol A. Laparoscopy in abdominal staging of esophageal carcinoma. Report of 369 cases. Gastrointest Endosc 1986; 32: 400–2.

56. Gross E, Bancewicz J, Ingram G. Assessment of gastric cancer by laparoscopy. Br Med J 1984; 288: 1577.

57. Stell DA, Carter CR, Stewart I, Anderson JR. A prospective comparison of laparoscopy, ultrasound and computed tomography in the staging of the gastric cancer. Br J Surg 1996; 83: 1260–2.

58. Bruce DM, Anderson DN, Campbell S, Park KGM. Interoperative laparoscopic ultrasonography in the staging of gastro-oesophageal malignancy. Br J Surg (Suppl. 1) 1996: 83: 13.

59. Fok M, Chong SWK, Wong J. Endosonography in patient selection for surgical treatment of esophageal carcinoma. World J Surg 1992; 16: 1098–103.

60. Molloy RG, McCourtney JS, Anderson JR. Laparoscopy in the management of patients with cancer of the gastric cardia and oesophagus. Br J Surg 1995; 82: 352–4.

61. Japanese Research Society for Gastric Cancer. The general rules for the gastric cancer study in surgery and pathology. Jpn J Surg 1981; 11: 127–39.

62. Kennedy BJ. TNM classification for stomach cancer. Cancer 1970; 26: 971–83.

63. Beahrs OH, Henson DE, Hunter RVP, Kennedy BJ (eds) Manual of staging of cancer. Philadelphia: JB Lippincott, 1992.

64. Hermanek P, Sobin LH (eds) UICC:TNM classification of malignant tumours, 5th edn. Berlin: Springer-Verlag, 1996.

65. Japanese Society for Esophageal Diseases. Guide for the clinical and pathological studies on carcinoma of the esophagus. Jpn J Surg 1976; 6: 69–78.

66. Wayman J, O'Hanlon D, Hayes N, Shaw IH, Griffin SM. Fibrinogen levels correlate with stage of disease in patients with oesophageal cancer. Br J Surg 1997; 84: 185–8.

4 Anaesthetic aspects of oesophageal and gastric cancer surgery

Ian H. Shaw

Introduction

The anaesthetist has to consider a variety of factors when presented with a patient for upper gastrointestinal surgery for carcinoma. Careful preoperative evaluation and preparation can have a significant influence on the perioperative well-being of the patient. The key to this is early communication between the surgeon and the anaesthetist particularly when patients fall into ASA groups 2 and above (Table 4.1). The intention should be to have the patient optimally fit for anaesthesia and surgery within the constraints of time imposed by the carcinoma.

Preoperative assessment

The preoperative evaluation of patients presenting for upper gastrointestinal surgery is an important aspect of their anaesthetic care. The preoperative assessment should identify those factors amenable to appropriate management and so improve the preoperative status of the patient. Where no correctable factors can be identified the preoperative assessment still allows the anaesthetist to make an evaluation of

Table 4.1 *American Society of Anesthesiologists assessment of physical status*

Grade	Definition
ASA 1	normal healthy patient
ASA 2	patient with a mild systemic disease
ASA 3	patient with a severe systemic disease that limits activity but is not incapacitating
ASA 4	patient with incapacitating disease that is a constant threat to life
ASA 5	moribund patient not expected to survive 24 h with or without surgery

Table 4.2 *Preoperative anaesthetic assessment in patients presenting for upper gastrointestinal surgery*

Previous anaesthetic history
Family history
Past medical history
Cardiorespiratory symptoms and examination
Medication and allergy
Social habits
Oesophageal reflux
Examination of airway
Examination of neck and jaw movement
Investigations

the risks of anaesthesia and establish a reference point which will be important in managing the patient in the operative and postoperative period. Those aspects of the patient's medical history that are of most interest to the anaesthetist are given in Table 4.2.

Previous anaesthetic history

Details of any previous anaesthetics can be of great value. Patients may be unaware or have misunderstood problems which occurred during a previous anaesthetic. Consequently it is important to have past anaesthetic charts made available for the anaesthetist whenever possible.

Family history

Fortunately inherited conditions of concern to the anaesthetist are rare. The most important, however, are pseudocholinesterase deficiency, porphyria and malignant hyperpyrexia. The latter being a potentially fatal condition if unknown to the anaesthetist. A patient known to be suffering from any of these conditions must be made known to the anaesthetist in good time.

Previous medical history

Although a detailed discussion of the assessment of anaesthetic risk is outwith the scope of this chapter several factors are of particular importance. It is helpful for surgical colleagues to have some appreciation of the concerns of the anaesthetist regarding oesophageal and gastric surgery. If during the preoperative staging and workup a surgical colleague can identify a potential anaesthetic problem the staging period can be used simultaneously to optimise the patient's preoperative status thereby reducing the anaesthetics risks. Again the value of good communication between the anaesthetist and the surgeon is

Table 4.3 *Computation of the Goldman cardiac risk index*

Criteria	Points
History	
Age > 70 years	5
MI within 6 months	10
Physical examination	
S3 gallop or jugular venous distension	11
Significant aortic stenosis	3
Electrocardiogram	
Rhythm other than sinus rhythm or premature atrial contractions on last preoperative ECG	7
> 5 premature ventricular contractions/min documented at any time before operation	7
General status	
$Pao_2 < 8$ kPa or $Paco_2 > 6.6$ kPa, potassium < 3 or $HCO_3 > 20$ mmol/l, blood urea nitrogen > 50 mg/dl, creatine > 3 mg/dl, abnormal aspartate amino transferase, signs of chronic liver failure or bedridden from non-cardiac disease	3
Operation	
Intraperitoneal or thoracic	3
Emergency	4
Total possible	53

Of the patients scoring greater than 26 points 56% died from a cardiac cause and 22% sustained life-threatening complications.

self-evident. Although all past medical history may be of interest to the anaesthetist, in the context of gastric or oesophageal surgery particular emphasis is placed on any past or present cardiorespiratory illness. A careful assessment of the patient's cardiorespiratory function is essential. Goldman *et al.*[1] were the first workers to critically evaluate the significance of pre-existing disease on perioperative outcome. It was apparent that the largest single cause of perioperative death in patients was pre-existing cardiovascular disease. Since Goldman *et al.* reported their findings there have been several attempts to improve the predictability of preoperative risk assessment as regards postoperative outcome. Although none of the published risk indexes are totally predictive several factors have been repeatedly identified (Table 4.3).

Other authors have modified the Goldman risk index to include prolonged operations and extensive elective surgery such as gastrectomy and oesophagectomy. For a critical discussion of preoperative cardiac risk assessment the reader should consult the review by Juste *et al.*[2]

Hypertension

It is generally accepted that preoperative hypertension is associated with increasing perioperative morbidity. Hypertension is still one of the most common reasons for the postponement of anaesthesia and surgery. All patients should have their blood pressure measured when first seen in the clinic. This will allow for the efficient use of the time between presentation and surgery in treating any pre-existing hypertension. Poorly controlled hypertension is characterised by haemodynamic instability which may have some relationship with morbidity. This instability can be exaggerated by surgical stimulation and manipulation of the mediastinum as well as changes in posture and hypovolaemia. It is important, therefore, to ensure the patient's medication is optimal and continued up to the day of surgery. Hypertension is invariably associated with systemic complications and evidence of co-existing peripheral vascular disease, cardiac, cerebral and renal impairment should be sought.

Providing one is circumspect, setting perioperative haemodynamic variables for any given patient can be helpful. To this end 4 hourly blood pressure and pulse measurements during the preoperative period, particularly during sleep, can be of value in setting acceptable limits.

Ischaemic heart disease

All authors agree that ischaemic heart disease is associated with an increased perioperative morbidity and mortality. Limited cardiopulmonary reserve in the presence of myocardial ischaemia is a very ominous preoperative finding and needs very careful evaluation. Of particular concern is a myocardial infarction within 6 months of any proposed surgery, unstable or significant angina, heart failure and advancing age.[3] Reinfarction following surgery after a recent myocardial infarction carries a considerable mortality. A history of chest pain, dyspnoea at rest or on minimal exertion, paroxysmal nocturnal dyspnoea, orthopnoea, palpitations and syncope should be sought. Where a patient is identified as 'at risk' then further non-invasive investigations can be worthwhile. Where patients are identified as 'high risk', for example known ischaemic heart disease with unstable angina or after a recent myocardial infarction, or where potentially correctable factors such as angina, heart failure, hypertension and palpitations have been identified, early referral to a cardiac physician would be prudent.

Since the majority of the patients with oesophageal and gastric cancer are smokers and fall into the older age group a significant proportion can be assumed to have underlying ischaemic heart disease even though they may be asymptomatic. The finding of carotid bruits, left ventricular hypertrophy, cardiomegaly, intermittent claudication and an abnormal electrocardiogram should raise suspicion.

Chronic obstructive airway disease

Chronic obstructive airway disease (COAD), as typified by a history of dyspnoea on exertion, orthopnoea, cough and sputum retention requires careful evaluation if a thoracotomy and one lung anaesthesia is being considered. A substantial amount of work has been published which attempts to identify reliable preoperative predictors of postoperative outcome in patients with COAD, much of it conflicting. Nunn et al.[4] in a study of patients with COAD undergoing non-thoracic surgery, demonstrated that an arterial oxygen tension of 75% or less than that predicted for age and dyspnoea at rest, or on minimal exertion, were ominous preoperative findings. Pulmonary function tests appeared to have a limited predictive value.

Sputum retention, inefficient bronchial clearance and airway irritability are well recognised in patients with COAD. Bronchospasm, precipitated by intubation, in particular carinal or bronchial stimulation during the positioning of an endobronchial tube can be troublesome and may occasionally require therapeutic intervention before surgery can commence.

Every effort should be made to optimise respiratory function during the preoperative period, if necessary seeking the advice of a chest physician. Often a short course of treatment under specialist supervision can bring about an appreciable improvement in pulmonary function and exercise tolerance. Preoperative sputum samples should be cultured and any infection identified and treated appropriately.

Smoking

A significant number of the patients presenting with oesophageal and gastric carcinoma are heavy smokers. Smoking has long been regarded as a major aetiological factor in perioperative morbidity, in particular pulmonary complications. Smoking is commonly associated with ischaemic heart disease, chronic obstructive pulmonary disease, emphysema, mucus hypersecretion, impaired bronchial clearance and poor lung compliance. Following upper abdominal or thoracic surgery the inability to clear bronchial secretions proficiently can lead to significant postoperative complications, in particular atelectasis and subsequent hypoxia. Inhaled carbon monoxide associated with smoking decreases the amount of haemoglobin available to bind oxygen and a left shift of the oxygen dissociation curve results decreasing the availability of oxygen to the tissues.

Table 4.4 *Effects of stopping smoking prior to surgery (from Erskine and Hanning[5])*

Abnormality	Time to return to normal
Nicotine	3–4 h
Carboxyhaemoglobin	2–3 half-lives
Ciliary function	4–6 days with some improvement over months
Sputum production	2–6 weeks
Small airway function	6 weeks minimum
Laryngeal hypersensitivity	5–10 days
Platelet function	3 days
Hb, RBC, Hct, WBC	24 h
Immune function	6 weeks minimum
Microsomal enzyme induction	6–8 weeks
Postoperative pulmonary morbidity	8 weeks

Cigarette smokers often have an elevated haemoglobin concentration, haematocrit and red and white cell counts. An increase in blood viscosity, fibrinogen, platelet numbers and reactivity can all contribute to an increased thromboembolic tendency in the postoperative period. All the evidence to date suggests that it is beneficial for patients to stop smoking preoperatively (Table 4.4). With this in mind the surgeon should impress upon the patient the importance of abstinence at the earliest opportunity. For a detailed appraisal of the effects of smoking and its significance during the perioperative period the reader should consult Erskine and Hanning.[5]

Gastro-oesophageal reflux

Gastro-oesophageal reflux is a major predisposing factor in pulmonary aspiration, a potentially lethal complication of general anaesthesia.[6] Anaesthesia obtunds the protective upper airway and cough reflexes. The greatest risk of aspiration is during induction prior to endotracheal intubation. Difficulties with bag and mask ventilation or intubation and any subsequent hypoxia can all predispose to pulmonary aspiration. Obese patients are at particular risk in this respect. In addition patients undergoing oesophageal and abdominal surgery are known to be at a greater risk from aspiration. Patients in whom dysphagia is a prominent symptom are of particular concern. A relatively small amount of inhaled acidic gastric fluid can give rise to severe pneumonitis and pulmonary oedema.

Many of the drugs used in daily anaesthetic practice can reduce lower oesophageal sphincter tone thereby increasing the potential for silent regurgitation of gastric contents. Of particular note are the volatile anaesthetic agents enflurane and halothane, the anticholinergics atropine and glycopyrrolate, the induction agent thiopentone and the opiate analgesics. Several of these drugs also reduce gastric emptying.

The anaesthetist will wish to establish if the patient has symptomatic reflux and in particular if it is in any way postural. The availability of recent endoscopy reports is helpful in this respect where evidence of oesophagitis or of a hiatus hernia may be found. The presence of gastro-oesophageal reflux in a patient about to undergo upper gastrointestinal surgery has a significant influence on the conduct of the anaesthetic and prophylactic measures to protect the patient from aspiration have to be considered.

Evaluation of the airway

The patency and accessibility of the patient's airway is of obvious importance to the anaesthetist. Any anatomical or pathological factors which may impede endotracheal intubation should be noted. The position of the trachea, temporomandibular joint and neck movement should be carefully assessed. Prominent or irregular dentition can make visualising the glottis during direct laryngoscopy incomplete or impossible. Other factors of concern include a receding jawline, a marked upper incisor overbite, limited mandibular movement, poor neck extension and obesity. Oesophageal surgery often necessitates the passing of a double lumen endobronchial tube and this can be particularly difficult in the presence of any of the above findings.

The nasal airway should be checked for patency as any obstruction may make passing a nasogastric or nasotracheal tube difficult. This is of particular relevance in a patient with a history of asthma where coexisting nasal polyps are extremely common. Nasotracheal intubation is preferred if the patient is to be electively ventilated postoperatively on an intensive care unit.

Preoperative investigations

Following a comprehensive clinical assessment and examination of the patient the preoperative investigations which will be of most interest to the anaesthetist are given in Table 4.5. Working to an established preoperative protocol is sensible as this will facilitate a comprehensive workup and minimise the risk of any omission.

Preoperatively the anaesthetist has to establish if the patient undergoing oesophageal surgery will have sufficient cardiopulmonary reserve to tolerate a period, often up to 2 or 3 hours, of one lung anaesthesia. Much of the published work on the relationship between preoperative cardiopulmonary assessment and postoperative outcome relates to patients undergoing varying degrees of lung resection. It is important to appreciate that deflation of a healthy lung during oesophageal surgery is to facilitate surgical access only. In consequence this has profound implications for the anaesthetist in attempting to maintain adequate oxygenation during surgery where the compen-

Table 4.5 *Suggested preoperative investigations for a patient presenting for upper gastrointestinal surgery*

Haematological
  Haemoglobin
  Full blood count
  Coagulation profile
Biochemical
  Urea and electrolytes
  Blood glucose
  Liver function tests
  Arterial blood gases
Electrocardiogram
Pulmonary function tests
Radiology
  Chest radiography
Exercise test

---

satory mechanisms seen in those patients with primary pulmonary disease are not evident.

Arterial blood gases should be assessed with the patient breathing room air. Hypoxia suggesting the presence of an intrapulmonary shunt may be of even greater significance during any subsequent one lung anaesthesia. Hypercarbia is indicative of ventilatory impairment and as a consequence the patient may be at a greater risk of postoperative morbidity and mortality. In one study[7] it was demonstrated that a low preoperative oxygen saturation correlated with postoperative hypoxaemia following a thoracotomy for hiatus hernia repair.

Where the results of pulmonary function tests are suboptimal any reversibility of airflow obstruction should be identified by repeating the tests after inhaled bronchodilator therapy. If a degree of reversibility has been identified consideration should be given to a preoperative course of vigorous physiotherapy, bronchodilator and steroid therapy. The forced expiratory volume in 1 s (FEV_1) may have some predictive value in patients undergoing lung resection but its significance in a patient undergoing transient one lung anaesthesia is less clear. There is some evidence that the closer the measured preoperative FEV_1 is to the predicted value, the greater the degree of ensuing hypoxia during one-lung anaesthesia. It must be borne in mind that the results of pulmonary function testing are the composite of the function of both lungs rather than the function of an individual lung.

An appreciable increase in mortality has been noted following pneumonectomy in patients with an FEV_1 of less than 2 l whereas an FEV_1 of less than 0.8 l was regarded as a contraindication to pulmonary resection. A peak expiratory flow rate of less than 70% of the predicted value suggests the patient's ability to clear bronchial secretions postoperatively will be impaired. In patients with chronic obstructive lung disease undergoing non-thoracic surgery the FEV_1 was a very poor prognostic indicator of postoperative complications.[4] Indeed several patients with a grossly abnormal FEV_1 had a totally uneventful postoperative course.

In conclusion, pulmonary function tests do have a role in the preoperative investigation of patients presenting with upper gastrointestinal carcinoma but the results have to be considered in association with the clinical findings and the arterial blood gas analysis, especially the PaO_2. It is generally accepted that there is no one test result which absolutely contraindicates surgery.

Exercise testing

The value of preoperative exercise testing remains controversial but has been positively postulated by Smith et al.[8] and others. Exercise tolerance, as an evaluation of cardiopulmonary reserve, can be assessed in its simplest form by asking the patient to walk up two flights of stairs having first established baseline blood pressure, respiratory and pulse rates.

Bronchoscopy

In some circumstances preoperative bronchoscopy can be helpful to the anaesthetist in assessing any anatomical or pathological abnormalities; in particular where radiological evidence exists of carinal or bronchial involvement with any adjacent oesophageal tumour which can result in displacement of the main bronchus so making endobronchial intubation more difficult or impossible. It is for this reason that some anaesthetists advocate bronchoscopy immediately after induction of the anaesthetic and before intubation. The chest radiograph and the CT scan report should also be made available for the anaesthetist.

Anaesthesia for gastric and oesophageal surgery

Preoperative preparation

The choice of the anaesthetic technique for upper gastrointestinal surgery is largely one of individual preference taking into account the medical status of the patient. A technique utilising nitrous oxide and oxygen, a volatile anaesthetic agent supplemented by opiate analgesics, neuromuscular paralysis and intermittent positive pressure ventilation is by far the most common.

Premedication where given, is again a matter of individual preference. Where dysphagia is troublesome soluble and liquid preparations should be used. H2-antagonists should be administered to those patients felt to be at risk from aspiration. With the exception of oral hypoglycaemics, anticoagulants and monoamine oxidase inhibitors, the patient's current medication should be given up until and including the day of surgery. This is especially important for cardiorespiratory therapeutic agents. Thromboembolic prophylaxis in the form of antithromboembolic stockings and subcutaneous unfractionated heparin (5000 units twice daily), or one of the low-molecular-weight heparins should be prescribed. The latter is longer acting and has the advantage of only requiring administration once a day. These measures can be consolidated by the use of automatic calf compressors perioperatively.

Rapid sequence induction

Where there is an appreciable risk of pulmonary aspiration the anaesthetist will elect to perform a rapid sequence induction and intubation in order to protect the airway during the induction of anaesthesia. A rapid sequence induction involves washing the nitrogen out of the lungs by preoxygenation with 100% oxygen for 3 min or more. This reservoir of oxygen allows the induction and intubation, after the administration of a short-acting depolarising muscle relaxant, to be performed in the apnoeic patient. An assistant protects the airway by gently pushing the cricoid ring against the adjacent cervical vertebral body so occluding the oesophageal lumen. Oesophageal occlusion is maintained until the trachea has been isolated by endotracheal intubation.

Endobronchial intubation

Both gastric and oesophageal surgery can be performed in a patient intubated with a standard endotracheal tube. However, since oesophageal surgery usually involves a thoracotomy, unilateral lung deflation to facilitate surgical access is preferred. An appropriate double lumen endobronchial tube is selected (Fig. 4.1). Irrespective of the side of the intended thoracotomy, a left-sided double lumen tube is the most popular. The right upper lobe bronchus is particularly susceptible to occlusion during right-sided endobronchial intubation owing to its close proximity to the carina.

Malposition of the endobronchial tube is excluded by auscultation of the chest and demonstration that both lung fields can be isolated from each other and ventilated adequately. During auscultation it is important to confirm that the left upper lobe bronchus is not compromised by the tube, otherwise one lung anaesthesia will be associated with severe hypoxaemia. There is published evidence that shows malposition is less likely if the position of the double lumen tube is confirmed by fibreoptic bronchoscopy. However, the lumen of many of the smaller double lumen tubes are too small to allow the passage of a fibreoptic bronchoscope and this limits its use in practice.

Double lumen tubes are bulky and can interfere with the passage of a nasogastric tube. Some anaesthetists advocate passing the nasogastric tube before intubation although in a patient with dysphagia this may increase the risk of pulmonary aspiration.

Figure 4.1 *A Robertshaw double lumen endobronchial tube for isolating the left lung during the thoracic stage of an oesophagectomy. Photo by courtesy of Pheonix Medical Ltd.*

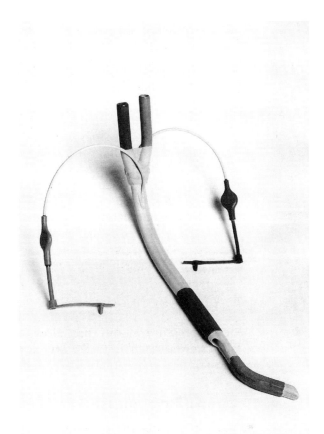

During a two-stage oesophageal operation when lung deflation will not be required for several hours, it is desirable to deflate the endobronchial cuff in order to minimise the risk of mucosal damage as a consequence of prolonged cuff inflation. After repositioning the patient in the lateral position for the second thoracic stage of the procedure it is essential to recheck the function of the double lumen tube. With the patient in the left lateral position the dependent lung is ventilated through the longer endobronchial limb. To aid surgical access the non-dependent right lung is collapsed by occluding the gas flow through the tracheal limb and opening the lumen to the atmosphere. The endobronchial portion of the tube in the dependent bronchus is especially prone to displacement during surgical manipulation of any tumour adjacent to the carina and excessive movement of the tube can have an effect on the ventilation delivered to the dependent lung.

Peroperative monitoring

The peroperative monitoring of patients undergoing oesophageal and gastric surgery should be comprehensive taking into consideration the patient's medical status (Table 4.6). Thoracotomy and one lung anaesthesia will necessitate invasive cardiovascular monitoring. Invasive

Table 4.6 *Suggested operative anaesthetic monitoring of a patient during oesophageal and gastric surgery*

Vital functions
 Electrocardiogram
 Blood pressure: non-invasive or invasive
 Central venous pressure
 Urine output
 Oximetry
 Core temperature
Ventilation
 End tidal carbon dioxide
 Inspired oxygen concentration
 Airway pressure
 Tidal volume

blood pressure monitoring allows the anaesthetist to detect immediately cardiovascular instability associated with one lung anaesthesia and surgical manipulation of mediastinal and hiatal structures.

Peroperative anaesthetic management

From the anaesthetist's viewpoint gastric and oesophageal surgery have many aspects in common. Several large-bore intravenous cannulae provide venous access. Precautions have to be taken to avoid excessive dehydration and hypovolaemia. The maintenance of satisfactory urine output is important in this respect. Hiatal and mediastinal manipulation are poorly tolerated in hypovolaemic patients.

Heat conservation is an important aspect of anaesthetic management during major surgery. Hypothermic patients are more intolerant to pain and discomfort postoperatively and exhibit cardiovascular instability particularly as they vasodilate on rewarming. Shivering causes a substantial increase in oxygen consumption which can lead to hypoxaemia unless adequate supplementary oxygen is given.

Oesophageal surgery

The anaesthetic management of the first stage of a two-stage oesophagectomy is identical to the management of an abdominal gastrectomy. Most of the difficulties for the anaesthetist arise from the need for one lung anaesthesia during the second stage of the procedure.

Cardiovascular instability

Surgical manipulation of the hiatus and mediastinum is often associated with sudden cardiovascular instability. Excessive peritoneal traction can cause an increase in vagal tone manifest as a profound bradycardia. Manipulation of the heart can precipitate unstable dysrhythmias. A misplaced retractor, hand or surgical pack can result in a sudden reduction in venous return and a fall in cardiac output and blood pressure. Delivering the stomach through the hiatus into the chest is especially hazardous in this respect. There is some evidence that the more extensive the hiatal dissection and diaphragmatic resection during the abdominal stage of a two-stage oesophagectomy, then the less disruption there is to the cardiovascular system during the delivery of the stomach into the thorax during the second stage. If this cardiovascular instability is associated with a period of relative hypoxia during one lung anaesthesia the situation can become potentially life threatening if uncorrected. Again good communication between the surgeon and the anaesthetist is of paramount importance.

One-lung anaesthesia during oesophagectomy

During the thoracic stage of an oesophagectomy the patient is placed in the lateral position and the non-dependent lung collapsed by selectively stopping ventilation. As a consequence the area available for respiratory exchange is reduced substantially. In adopting the lateral position gravity allows the less compliant dependent lung to be preferentially perfused. Blood perfusing the collapsed lung is no longer oxygenated and will mix with oxygenated blood from the ventilated dependent lung in the heart causing venous admixture and a fall in arterial oxygen tension.

The aetiology of hypoxia during one-lung anaesthesia is multifactorial (Table 4.7) and may necessitate compensatory manoeuvres on the part of the anaesthetist (Fig. 4.2). Hypoxia during one-lung anaesthesia for oesophageal surgery is generally of a greater magnitude than during surgery for primary lung disease.[9] Diseased lung is often poorly perfused and the ensuing hypoxia activates the hypoxic pulmonary vasoconstrictor response, an important homeostatic mechanism that serves to direct blood flow to better oxygenated parts of the lungs. In a patient undergoing an oesophagectomy a healthy lung is suddenly deflated and a substantial imbalance of ventilation and perfusion occurs (i.e. a shunt). The hypoxic pulmonary vasoconstrictor response has been shown to be rendered less responsive by hypocarbia

Table 4.7 *Circumstances which precipitate peroperative hypoxia during oesophageal surgery (after Gothard[11])*

One-lung anaesthesia in a patient with healthy lungs
Pre-existing disease in the dependent lung
Displaced or partly occluded endobronchial tube
Low cardiac output secondary to hypovolaemia or mediastinal manipulation
Peroperative deterioration in the dependent lung
Massive blood transfusion

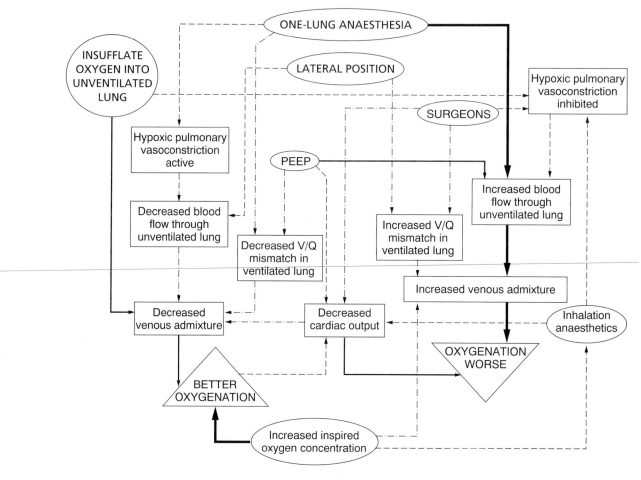

Figure 4.2 *Interactions between various factors which can affect arterial oxygenation during one-lung anaesthesia for an oesophagectomy. Physiological influences are placed in oblong boxes in the centre and the resultant effect on oxygenation indicated by the orientation of the triangles. Relevant extrinsic factors are placed in ovals round the periphery. The thickness of the connecting arrow indicates the relative importance of the effect. Most of these factors can have both beneficial and detrimental effects and the difficulty in predicting the behaviour of an individual patient lies in the varying balances between these effects. During an oesophagectomy in particular, surgical manipulation can be of major significance. After Kerr,[12] with permission.*

($Pa_{CO_2} < 4.0$ kPa) and inhalational anaesthetic agents. This latter observation does not appear to be significant at the inhaled anaesthetic concentrations commonly used during surgery. For a more detailed discussion of the hypoxic pulmonary vasoconstrictor response the reader should consult the review by Eisenkraft.[10]

One-lung anaesthesia does not appear to impair the efficiency of the lungs to remove carbon dioxide from the body. This is reflected by the observation that no major compensatory adjustments of the minute ventilation are necessary when switching from two lung ventilation.

During an oesophagectomy the ventilated lung is subjected to compressive forces which can result in a degree of pulmonary atelectasis. Surgical manipulation, the effects of gravity on mediastinal structures, the weight of the abdominal contents acting through a paralysed diaphragm and the weight of the patient lying on the dependent lung all contribute in this respect. A fall in functional residual capacity and compliance in the dependent ventilated lung ensues. In consequence patchy atelectasis within the dependent lung is a not uncommon finding on a postoperative chest radiograph.

Anaesthetic techniques during one-lung anaesthesia

One of the anaesthetist's primary objectives during the thoracic stage of an oesophagectomy is to match ventilation with perfusion in the dependent lung. With this in mind several manoeuvres have been proposed (Table 4.8). Provided the double lumen tube is correctly positioned and cardiac output maintained, adequate oxygenation can often be achieved simply by increasing the fractional inspired oxygen concentration to 0.5. If hypoxia persists, increasing the oxygen concentration further to 100% is often sufficient. Provided adequate anaesthesia is maintained awareness is not a problem. If hypoxia persists the anaesthetist has several options available, not all of which have been fully substantiated as totally beneficial.

The application of 5–15 cmH$_2$O positive end expiratory pressure (PEEP) to the dependent ventilated lung has been advocated as a means of preventing atelectasis. PEEP increases the area available for gas exchange and improves the functional residual capacity by recruiting collapsed alveoli so reducing any existing shunt. PEEP cannot, however, be regarded as benign. It increases the pulmonary vascular resistance within the ventilated lung and can redirect blood through the non-ventilated lung and the risk of barotrauma is ever present. Combined with any detrimental effects PEEP might have on cardiac output, there can in some circumstances be an exacerbation of the hypoxia. It has been postulated that the beneficial effects of PEEP

Table 4.8 *Anaesthetic techniques to reduce the ventilation/perfusion mismatch during the thoracic stage of an oesophagectomy*

Dependent ventilated lung
  Increasing the inspired oxygen concentration
  Positive end expiratory pressure
Non-dependent collapsed lung
  Oxygen insufflation
  Continuous positive end expiratory pressure
Both lungs
  Intermittent two lung ventilation
Circulation
  Maintenance of an adequate cardiac output

can be enhanced by applying continuous and expiratory pressure (CPAP) to the collapsed lung. In practice, however, this combined manoeuvre is often associated with a reduction in cardiac output.

The insufflation of 2–5 l min^{-1} of 100% oxygen to the collapsed non-dependent lung is a simple and often effective way to maintain adequate oxygenation during one-lung anaesthesia. Too high a flow can result in reinflation of the lung and obscure the surgical field. Insufflation of oxygen into the collapsed lung can also obtund the homeostatic hypoxic pulmonary vasoconstrictor response. The application of less than 10 cmH$_2$O CPAP to the collapsed lung is said to have a similar beneficial effect.

An important aspect of the anaesthetic management of the second stage of an oesophagectomy is the maintenance of an adequate cardiac output, blood pressure and organ perfusion. Changes in cardiac output will effect arterial oxygenation even in the presence of optimal pulmonary ventilation. Where an appreciable shunt already exists (> 30%) a fall in cardiac output will exacerbate any systemic hypoxia.[13] Surgical behaviour is an important factor in the well-being of the patient. During an oesophagectomy inadvertent surgical compression of the inferior vena cava or the right atrium can precipitate a sudden reduction in cardiac output with deleterious effects on oxygenation and organ perfusion.

When the anaesthetist is unable to maintain adequate oxygenation despite the above measures then two lung ventilation, either intermittently or continuously with retraction of the non-dependent lung, will have to be adopted. Unquestionably this will make the surgery considerably more difficult and reidentifying the surgical plane on deflation can be difficult (S. M. Griffin, personal communication).

On completion of the surgery the collapsed lung is aspirated and reinflated by hand ventilation under direct vision. Failure to reinflate the lung fully can be a major cause of postoperative hypoxia. Difficulty in reinflation may be encountered if endobronchial secretions are especially tenacious and suction bronchoscopy is then indicated.

The anaesthetist has to be vigilant when moving the patient from the lateral to the supine position as this can be associated with a sudden fall in blood pressure due to improved perfusion of the non-dependent tissues.

Postoperative care

The postoperative care of patients who have undergone upper gastrointestinal surgery must be of a high standard if the skills of the anaesthetist and surgeon are to be consolidated. The aim of postoperative monitoring is to facilitate prompt intervention so as to prevent complications arising which increase morbidity or mortality. Where a patient is nursed will depend on the nature of the surgery, the medical status of the patient and the facilities available within the hospital. The options are generally on a surgical ward familiar with upper gastrointestinal surgery, in a high dependency unit (HDU) or an ICU.

The latter two have the advantage of a higher nurse to patient ratio and the facilities to use more sophisticated invasive monitoring systems. The first 48 h postoperatively are extremely important.

Patients who have undergone an uncomplicated gastrectomy can usually be extubated in theatre and then nursed in a ward or HDU. Where a period of postoperative ventilation is indicated than transfer to an ICU is mandatory. Following thoracotomy the patient will need nursing in an HDU or an ICU. The major concerns during the immediate postoperative period after upper abdominal or thoracic surgery are hypoxia, cardiovascular stability and analgesia.

Postoperative hypoxia

Postoperative hypoxia is a common sequelae to upper gastrointestinal surgery. At arterial oxygen tensions of less than 8 kPa or 90% oxygen saturation end organ hypoxia can ensue if left uncorrected. All patients must receive humidified oxygen appropriate to their needs postoperatively and have their oxygen saturation monitored as the provision of oxygen by a face mask alone may be insufficient. Obesity, old age, smoking and pre-existing cardiorespiratory disease can further exacerbate hypoxia. The aetiology of postoperative hypoxia is multifactorial and interested readers should consult Sabanathan et al.[14]

In the immediate postoperative period the residual effects of anaesthesia can cause hypoxia. Diffusion hypoxia is a well-recognised transient short-lived phenomena observed at the cessation of anaesthesia. When nitrous oxide is discontinued this highly diffusible gas enters the alveoli and dilutes the alveolar air resulting in a fall in Pao_2 unless supplementary oxygen is administered. Opiate analgesia and inhalational anaesthetics also depress the ventilatory response to carbon dioxide and hypoxia.

Upper abdominal and thoracic operations are detrimental to ventilatory mechanisms and gas exchange. Both the vital capacity and functional residual capacity (FRC) are reduced. As the FRC falls it encroaches on the closing volume such that airway closure occurs during tidal ventilation in the dependent parts of the lungs. The resultant pulmonary shunt gives rise to hypoxia. Among the contributory factors are persistent pain, posture, inadequate expectoration and subsequent atelectasis. This alteration of pulmonary function can persist for many days or weeks. Several measures to minimise postoperative hypoxia and pulmonary complications following upper gastrointestinal surgery have been advocated: adequate analgesia, a semi-erect posture which increases FRC, continuous humidified oxygen for four consecutive days and regular physiotherapy.[15] Alternatively a brief period of postoperative ventilation on ICU for patients who have undergone an oesophagectomy can be of value in allowing for the vital functions to be optimised, to aid lung expansion, for efficient endobronchial suction and physiotherapy to be performed without distress.[17]

Cardiovascular instability

Fluid and blood requirements have to be carefully monitored during the immediate postoperative period. Patients who have undergone a prolonged oesophagectomy often require appreciable volumes of fluid in the immediate postoperative period. Central venous pressure monitoring can be useful in the evaluation of the patient's fluid requirements. A fall in systemic vascular resistance coinciding with rewarming after prolonged surgery can be associated with systemic hypotension and an inadequate urine output. An acceptable haemoglobin concentration must be maintained for adequate oxygen transport. Although common practice, blood transfusion is a potentially hazardous procedure and blood should only be given when absolutely necessary. Stored blood has a high affinity for oxygen as a result of a decrease in erythrocyte 2,3-diphosphoglycerate. The oxygen dissociation curve (ODC) is displaced to the left and impaired tissue oxygen delivery can result. This effect is further exacerbated by hypothermia and alkalosis. Apart from the risk of transfusion reactions and transmission of infection, blood transfusion can also be associated with electrolyte disturbances, coagulopathies and impaired gas exchange secondary to pulmonary microaggregate deposition. Provided the patient is kept normovolaemic and pulmonary gas exchange is unimpeded, a degree of postoperative haemodilution will be tolerated by most patients.[18] Adequate tissue oxygenation can be maintained at a haematocrit of 25–30%. Tissue blood flow will be maintained by a combination of increased stroke volume and cardiac output and a fall in viscous flow resistance. Maintaining normovolaemia is very important as hypovolaemic patients can demonstrate exaggerated hypotensive response to opiate analgesics. New dysrhythmias in the postoperative period must be evaluated carefully. Atrial fibrillation in particular may herald early mediastinitis and an anastomotic leak. Chest drains which have been inserted too far can also precipitate atrial fibrillation. There is no evidence that prophylactic digitalisation is of any value in patients who have undergone an oesophagectomy.

Postoperative pain

Pain can be considerable after upper abdominal and thoracic surgery. Pain inhibits movement and coughing leading to sputum retention, atelectasis and chest infection.[18] Effective pain relief has been consistently shown to improve pulmonary function postoperatively as assessed by measured improvements in FEV_1 and vital capacity. The elected method of pain relief after gastrectomy and oesophagectomy will depend on the expertise and facilities available.

Patient controlled analgesia (PCA)

A small bolus of intravenous morphine delivered on patient demand by a preprogrammed syringe driver is considerably more efficacious than 'as required' intramuscular injections. The technique is flexible, painless and well received by patients who can attain more consistent analgesia largely because any individual variation in opiate pharmacokinetics and pharmacodynamics is compensated for by the patients themselves. The infusion should be administered through a dedicated cannula or a one-way valve to avoid retrograde accumulation of opiate when administered in conjunction with an intravenous infusion. A constant background infusion of opiate is associated with a higher incidence of complications and is best avoided, particularly outwith an area of high dependency nursing. A prerequisite to PCA following upper gastrointestinal surgery is adequate monitoring of respiratory function and the conscious state. PCA is only effective if the patient has the ability to cooperate and comprehend. Although a safe technique, before using any PCA system staff training is mandatory as any technical errors can be fatal.

Extradural analgesia

Extradural analgesia, using either an opiate, local anaesthetic or a combination of both, can provide extremely effective analgesia and improve respiratory function after surgery.[19] The level of the extradural catheter will depend on the dermatomes to be rendered analgesic. Ideally the level at which the epidural catheter is sited should represent a central dermatome of the surgical incision.

Extradural analgesia is a potentially dangerous technique and requires a high degree of skill, particularly in the thoracic region, and the patient must be closely observed by competent staff thereafter. Both medical and nursing staff have to be totally familiar with possible side effects, especially in recognising an excessively high block, hypotension, CNS and respiratory depression. Although ward-based epidurals may become more common with the deployment of dedicated pain teams, it is advisable to nurse these patients in an ITU or HDU with adequate monitoring.

Bilateral sympathetic autonomic blockade and subsequent hypotension is common after extradural bupivacaine, particularly in the thoracic region. An element of motor blockade is not uncommon. Hypotension is exacerbated by hypovolaemia and limited cardiovascular reserve. Consequently patients unable to tolerate fluid loads may not be ideal candidates for extradural analgesia employing local anaesthetics. Extradural opiates are devoid of these cardiovascular effects but can be associated with central respiratory depression of an unpredictable and insidious onset. The risk of respiratory depression by cephalad spread of the extradural opiate appears to be related to the lipid solubility of the drug. Morphine, an opiate of low lipophilicity, can cause respiratory depression of late onset in contrast to highly soluble fentanyl which can precipitate the early onset of respiratory depression. The central depressant effects of extradural opiates are potentiated by systemic opiates and the two should not be administered concurrently. In an attempt to reduce the risks of these side

Table 4.9 *Comparison of opiates and local anaesthetics when given via the extradural route (from Wilson and Smith,[17] with permission)*

	Opiates	Local anaesthetics
Cardiovascular	Usually no effect	Often causes hypotension due to sympathetic block
Respiratory depression Unusual unless block		Early: from systemic
	absorption Late: from rostral spread in CSF augmented by age/dose/posture/aqueous solubility/additional systemic opiate	involves depression of intercostal muscles of diaphragm
Nausea/vomiting	Similar to i.m. administration	Only as sequelae to hypotension
Itching	More common with morphine than fentanyl or diamorphine. Possibly central mechanism, relieved by naloxone or antihistamine	No
Urinary retention	Varies from 20%. Improved by naloxone	Common with lower blocks
Sedation	Associated invariably with severe form of late respiratory depression	Occasionally mild as a result of decreased input to the reticular activating system

effects combinations of opiates and local anaesthetics have been used with some success. However, the sympathetic block does not seem to be readily amenable to changes in drug combination.

Extradural analgesia can be administered by bolus or by continuous infusion. The latter, although effective, has a higher incidence of CNS depression when opiates are given. The choice of therapeutic agent for extradural analgesia after upper gastrointestinal surgery should be made only after consideration of all the potential side effects (Table 4.9).

Local analgesia

Infiltration of the wound with local anaesthetic at the end of surgery is more effective for somatic pain than visceral pain but may help to reduce the patient's opiate requirement. Bupivacaine (0.25% without adrenaline), to a maximum dose of $2 \, \text{mg kg}^{-1}$, is the most popular.

Conclusion Upper gastrointestinal surgery for carcinoma presents the anaesthetist with a challenge. Good communication between the surgeon and the anaesthetist is important for the well-being of the patient. During the preoperative surgical workup the patient's cardiopulmonary status should be optimised, if necessary recruiting specialist advice. Upper abdominal and thoracic surgery have significant effects on respiratory mechanics which have implications for the postoperative care. During one-lung anaesthesia surgical manipulation of an oesophageal tumour and adjacent mediastinal structures can have a major impact on cardiovascular stability and oxygenation. Successful surgery can only be consolidated by a high standard of postoperative care. Effective postoperative analgesia is necessary to improve pulmonary function.

References

1. Goldman L, Caldera RN, Nussbaum SR *et al*. Multifactorial index of cardiac risk in non-cardiac surgical procedures. N Engl J Med 1977; 297: 845–50.

2. Juste RN, Lawson AD, Soni N. Minimising cardiac anaesthetic risk. Anaesthesia 1996; 51: 255–62.

3. Detsky AS, Abrams HB, McLauchlin JR. Predicting cardiac complications in patients undergoing non-cardiac surgery. J Gen Intern Med 1986; 41: 211–19.

4. Nunn JF, Milledge JS, Chen D, Dore C. Respiratory criteria of fitness for surgery and anaesthesia. Anaesthesia 1988; 43: 543–51.

5. Erskine RJ, Hanning CD. Do I advise my patient to stop smoking preoperatively? Curr Anaesth Crit Care 1992; 3: 175–80.

6. Black GW. Aspiration pneumonitis and its prevention. Hosp Update 1994; May: 1–7.

7. Entwistle MD, Roe PG, Sapsford DJ, Berrisford RG, Jones JG. Patterns of oxygenation after thoracotomy. Br J Anaesth 1991; 67: 704–11.

8. Smith TP, Kinasewitz GT, Tucker WY, Spillers WP, George RB. Exercise capacity as a predictor of post thoracotomy morbidity. Am Rev Resp Dis 1984; 129: 730–4.

9. Kerr JH, Crampton-Smith A, Prys-Roberts C *et al*. Observations during endobronchial anaesthesia II: oxygenation. Br J Anaesth 1974; 46: 84–92.

10. Eisenkraft JB. Anaesthesia and hypoxic pulmonary vasoconstriction. In: Atkinson RS, Adams AP (eds) Recent advances in anaes-thesia, Edinburgh: Churchill Livingstone 1994; Vol. 18, pp. 103–22.

11. Gothard JWW. Principles of thoracic anaes-thesia. In: Gothard JWW (ed.) Anaesthesia for thoracic surgery, 2nd edn. Oxford: Blackwell Scientific Publications, 1993, pp. 60–80.

12. Kerr JH. Ventilation and blood flow during thoracic surgery. In: Gothard JWW (ed.) Baillière's clinical anaesthesiology: thoracic anaesthesia. London: WB Saunders, 1987, pp. 61–78.

13. Kerr JH. Physiological aspects of one-lung (endobronchial) anaesthesia. Int Anaesthesiol Clin 1972; 10: 61–78.

14. Sabaratnam S, Eng J, Mearns AJ. Alterations in respiratory mechanics following thoraco-tomy. J R Coll Surg Edin 1990; 35: 144–50.

15. Hayes N, Shaw IH, Griffin SM. Timing of extubation after oesophagectomy. Br J Surg 1994; 81: 921–2.

16. Wilson IG, Smith G. The management of acute pain. Hosp Update 1993; April: 214–22.

17. Messmer K. Hemodilution. Surg Clin North Am 1975; 55: 659–70.

18. Sutton BA. Postoperative management and the provision of pain relief. In: Gothard JWW (ed.) Anaesthesia for thoracic surgery, 2nd edn. Oxford: Blackwell Scientific Publications, 1993, pp. 105–49.

19. Shulman M, Sandler AN, Bradley JW, Young PS, Brebner J. Post thoracotomy pain and pulmonary function following epidural and systemic morphine. Anesthesiology 1984: 61: 569–75.

5 Surgery for cancer of the oesophagus

S. Michael Griffin

Introduction Oesophageal cancer is well recognised as being one of the most challenging pathological conditions confronting the surgeon. This is not only due to the versatility required in surgical reconstruction but also the magnitude of the surgical procedure, dealing with wide areas of the neck, mediastinum and abdomen. No other modality to date has consistently been shown to provide a chance of cure in this increasingly common cancer. Many efforts have been made to increase the cure rate whilst maintaining the safety of the procedure, but despite this, the overall survival for oesophageal cancer remains around 10% in most countries. Although treatment for cancer of the oesophagus is of necessity multidisciplinary, surgery, whenever possible, is the primary mode of therapy. The surgical procedure required may differ in each case, depending on the nature of the tumour, the condition of the patient, the method of approach and the extent of resection and dissection.

The disease often presents at a stage when increasing obstructive symptoms have been present for several months and the tumour has evolved over many months or years. Patients with oesophageal cancer have to be considered either for radical treatment or for palliative therapy in those who are too elderly, unfit or have tumours too far advanced. At this stage the disease has not only spread into the lumen and wall of the oesophagus, but also beyond the muscularis propria and probably to distant lymph nodes and organs. Although surgery at this stage is unlikely to lead to long-term survival, it nevertheless provides symptomatic relief for the patient suffering from progressive dysphagia, loss of weight and increasing retrosternal discomfort. As the disease predominantly affects the elderly, treatment must be associated with a low morbidity and mortality. Although surgical intervention may not be tolerated well in the very elderly, neither indeed are radiotherapy or chemotherapy regimens, both of which can cause debilitating systemic effects for long periods.

Several modalities of therapy are available to the clinician dealing with oesophageal cancer. A combination of these modalities may well have to be used in the future management of these patients. Although randomised multicentred clinical trials are essential in assessing new therapeutic regimens, the experienced surgeon managing a patient with oesophageal malignancy must exercise judgement in the choice of the appropriate combination of therapies. These will depend on patient age, fitness, symptoms, prognosis and the histopathological characteristics of the malignancy itself.

Surgical pathology

The majority of oesophageal neoplasms are epithelial in origin. They arise from the squamous lining of the mucosa, but increasingly also from metaplastic columnar epithelium, resulting in glandular carcinomas affecting specialised epithelium in the lower oesophagus. Tumour site and histology are two crucial factors requiring assessment during the management of oesophageal malignancy. Tumours arising from different sites in the oesophagus vary in their behaviour. Squamous cell carcinoma and adenocarcinoma arising from the cervical oesophagus, thoracic oesophagus and cardia, differ in their mode of spread and response to therapeutic modalities. This has been discussed in detail in Chapter 1. It is essential, therefore, that the anatomical regions of the oesophagus are described such that the different therapeutic surgical procedures adopted for tumours at each site can be understood.

Surgical anatomy

The oesophagus is a mid-line hollow viscus, starting at the cricopharyngeal sphincter at the level of the 6th cervical vertebra, entering the chest at the level of the suprasternal notch and traversing the posterior mediastinum and entering the abdomen through the oesophageal hiatus in the diaphragm to join the stomach at the cardia. It bears a close relationship to the trachea and pericardium in front and the vertebral column posteriorly. The vagus and its branches are in close proximity over its entire length. There is no serosal covering. The thoracic duct enters the posterior mediastinum through the aortic opening in the diaphragm. It lies on the bodies of the thoracic vertebrae posterolateral to the oesophagus and between the aorta and the azygos vein. The left atrium and the inferior pulmonary veins lie in intimate contact with the left wall of the lower third of the oesophagus.

The TNM classification has been proposed and revised in 1992[1] to combine the salient features of the staging process. This classification has divided the oesophagus into discrete anatomical regions (Fig. 5.1).

Hypopharynx and cervical oesophagus

The region between the level of the pharyngo-epiglottic fold and the inferior border of the cricoid cartilage is known as the hypopharynx; that above, as the oropharynx. The cervical oesophagus begins at the lower border of the cricoid cartilage and terminates at the level of the thoracic inlet or jugular notch. Surgical management of carcinomas in these regions differs from that of other parts of the oesophagus, because tumour extension in these two areas commonly overlap. This is considered separately later in the chapter.

Figure 5.1
Anatomical regions of the hypopharynx, oesophagus and gastric cardia.

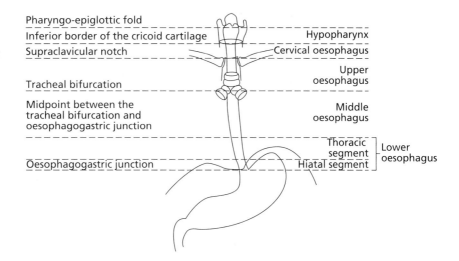

Pharyngo-epiglottic fold	
Inferior border of the cricoid cartilage	Hypopharynx
Supraclavicular notch	Cervical oesophagus
	Upper oesophagus
Tracheal bifurcation	
Midpoint between the tracheal bifurcation and oesophagogastric junction	Middle oesophagus
	Thoracic segment
Oesophagogastric junction	Hiatal segment
	Lower oesophagus

Upper oesophagus

This segment of the oesophagus extends between the level of the jugular notch and the carina.

Middle oesophagus

This section of oesophagus extends from the tracheal bifurcation to the mid-point between the tracheal bifurcation and the oesophago-gastric junction.

Lower oesophagus

This is composed of both the lower thoracic oesophagus and the hiatal segment of the oesophagus. The latter segment is often termed the 'abdominal oesophagus'. The oesophagogastric junction is a somewhat nebulous term and the anatomy depends on the differing viewpoints of surgeons, endoscopists, radiologists, pathologists and anatomists. It is further complicated by the presence of a hiatal hernia and the presence or absence of a columnar lined oesophagus.

Blood supply and lymphatics

Blood supply is derived directly from the aorta in the form of oesophageal vessels together with branches adjacent to or from organs such as the pulmonary hilum, trachea, stomach and thyroid gland. The venous drainage is through tributaries draining into the azygos and hemi-azygos system in the chest, via the thyroid veins in the neck and the left gastric vein in the upper abdomen.

The lymphatics of the oesophagus are distributed predominantly in the form of a submucous plexus and a paraoesophageal plexus. Both plexi receive lymph from all parts of the respective layers of the oesophageal wall. The plexi communicate through penetrating vessels which traverse the longitudinal and circular muscle walls. The paraoesophageal plexus drains into the paraoesophageal lymph nodes

Table 5.1 *Lymph nodes of the oesophagus*

Paraoesophageal nodes (on the wall of the oesophagus)	Cervical (101)[a] Upper thoracic (105) Middle thoracic (108) Lower thoracic (110)
Perioesophageal nodes (in immediate apposition to the oesophagus)	Deep cervical (102) Supraclavicular (104) Paratracheal (106) Subcarinal (107) Para-aortic or posterior mediastinal (112) Diaphragmatic (111) Left gastric (7) Lesser curvature (3) Coeliac (9) Right cardiac (1) Left cardiac (2)
Lateral oesophageal nodes (located lateral to the oesophagus)	Posterior triangle of the neck (100) Hilar (109) Suprapyloric (5) Subpyloric (6) Common hepatic (8) Greater curvature (4)

[a] For location see Chapter 3, Fig. 3.5.

which are situated on the surface of the oesophagus and also into perioesophageal lymph nodes, situated in close proximity to the oesophagus. Lymphatics also drain from the perioesophageal nodes to the lateral oesophageal nodes or directly from the para- to the lateral oesophageal nodes, skipping the perioesophageal group[2] (Table 5.1 and Fig. 3.5).

Preoperative surgical preparation

Meticulous preoperative evaluation and estimation of surgical risk is a prerequisite to successful surgical outcome in this disease. Postoperative complications may be either patient or surgeon related. Patient-related factors include extreme age, malnutrition secondary to malignancy in general or to dysphagia, immunosuppression secondary to bone marrow depression that may result from adjuvant chemotherapy and lastly, associated systemic diseases which are more common with increasing age.

Nutritional support

Significant malnutrition with depletion of protein and fat stores as well as dehydration are frequently seen in patients with oesophageal

narrowing and should be corrected preoperatively. Nutritional deficiency can be corrected either enterally or parenterally. Enteral feeding
is simpler and safer, using high calorie and protein liquid feeds of
known volume and composition, given either by mouth or via fine
bore tube placed endoscopically. The routine use of parenteral nutrition (TPN) is controversial on general and immunological grounds
and should be avoided in order to minimise nosocomial infection and
associated sepsis. There is well-established evidence that increased
nosocomial infections are found when the GI tract is not used for nutrition in the pre- and postoperative periods.[3] In those patients who have
failed to show satisfactory improvement, it may be necessary to
construct a feeding jejunostomy either before or at the time of surgery
in order to continue hyperalimentation via the enteral route.

Respiratory care

Optimisation of respiratory function is vital in preventing the serious
pulmonary complications associated with prolonged surgery and
thoracotomy.[4] Smoking ought to be discouraged as early as possible.
Preoperative physiotherapy with coughing exercises and effective use
of the diaphragm by restoration of muscle strength through ambulation is encouraged. Poor risk patients should also be provided with
vigorous physiotherapy with or without bronchodilators prior to
surgery. Orodental hygiene is also relevant in preventing a source of
chronic sepsis that could disseminate infection to the tracheobronchial
tree during intubation.

To reduce the incidence of thromboembolic complications, prophylactic low dose heparin together with anti-thromboembolism stockings,
must be provided as soon as the patient comes into hospital.

Mental preparation

Every effort must be made to familiarise the patient with the hospital
environment including the intensive care unit, to minimise fear and
apprehension. Patient cooperation is crucial and can be enhanced by
reassurance and good communication. Descriptions of the methods of
pain relief, oxygen and intravenous fluid administration and the
awareness of intercostal tube drainage and the likelihood of prolonged
periods without oral intake, must be adequately explained. All patients
and their relatives should be counselled about the treatment options,
paying particular attention to results and limitations of surgery.

Perioperative preparation and anaesthetic details are highlighted
and explained in depth in Chapter 4.

Surgical objectives Curative surgical resection of oesophageal malignancy is based on the
precept that if all neoplastic tissue can be removed, then resection and
reconstruction could lead to a worthwhile period of survival and

possible cure, but only if operative mortality is low and the life expectancy of the patient is not shortened for other reasons. Provided the tumour is contained within the muscularis propria of the oesophagus and extensive longitudinal submucosal spread has not occurred, then radical removal of the oesophagus by total or subtotal oesophagectomy with clearance of the lymph nodes draining the organ is a justifiable procedure. A more extended radical procedure may be justified if the tumour has invaded the perioesophageal tissues and local lymph nodes in a fit patient. A similar argument would be untenable in an elderly patient in whom a decreased chance of survival would be preferred to the high morbidity and mortality that would ensue from an extended radical operation.

Surgical therapy is the only treatment that has repeatedly been shown to provide prolonged survival, albeit in only 10–20% of cases.[5,6] Resection, therefore, must be the chosen method of therapy in fit patients with favourable tumours of the middle and lower thirds of the oesophagus. Survival is related to the stage of disease and with Stage I disease, five-year survivals of greater than 80% have been achieved[7] emphasising the importance of early detection.

An attitude of pessimism has prevailed over many years owing to poor surgical results achieved in small series by non-specialised units. The overall results of surgical resection for all stages of tumour have steadily improved over the past 20 years with falling morbidity and mortality associated with the procedure. The reasons for this are listed in Table 5.2.

Among these is an increased tendency to concentrate the management of such cases in specialist units with the numbers treated allowing the development of a multidisciplinary approach that involves surgeons, gastroenterologists, anaesthetists, radiologists, intensivists as well as physiotherapists and nursing staff. Studies have confirmed that improved results parallel experience in managing this condition[8] and poor results occur when experience is limited. There is now overwhelming evidence to confirm the influence of surgeon case volume on the outcome of site specific cancer surgery.[9] Other reasons for improved outcome include better patient selection, earlier diagnosis by open access endoscopy, screening of Barrett's oesophagus and improved preoperative, operative and postoperative management.

Table 5.2 *Reasons for improved results for oesophageal resection*

1.	Increase in Specialist Units
2.	Multidisciplinary approach
3.	Earlier diagnosis
4.	Better patient selection
5.	Improved perioperative management

Principles of oesophag-ectomy

Resection of primary tumour

Complete resection of an oesophageal cancer not only involves the removal of the primary, but also the concomitant separate lesions which can develop due to longitudinal spread in the submucosal lymphatics. The incidence of positive resection margins reported in the literature is high.[10–12] Fortunately, with new advances in endoscopic and radiological techniques, such as endoscopic ultrasound, the tumour extent and spread, together with the diagnosis of synchronous lesions are now more accurately assessed. It is crucial to obtain accurate information concerning the tumours by careful examination using barium swallow, video endoscopy and endoscopic ultrasound in the preoperative staging process. This will help to determine more exactly the level of resection. It is, however, often difficult to ascertain the length for clear surgical margins, particularly in high lesions, despite exhaustive preoperative investigations.

Rules on resection margins

Much discussion and argument has centred around how many centimetres of macroscopically normal oesophagus should routinely be removed either side of the palpable primary lesion. Skinner *et al.*[13] advocated that a minimum resection margin of 10 cm from the palpable edge of the tumour was essential to minimise the risk of anastomotic recurrence and positive resection margins. This figure, however, does not take into account the nature, pattern and location of the primary cancer. It also fails to discriminate between *in vivo* margins of resection and resection margins measured by the histopathologist when a considerable degree of shrinkage has occurred after fixation in formalin. This shrinkage has been clearly documented in an elaborate study by Siu *et al.*[14] who demonstrated a significant difference between the length of resection margin obtained *in vivo*, and that achieved after fixation with formalin. They also demonstrated that upper resection margins were found to contract more than the lower resection margins and the tumour itself reduced very little in size, even after fixation.

Many studies have also demonstrated that localised tumours require shorter lengths of clearance for safe surgical margins.[15] Not infrequently, primary tumours with multicentric lesions are encountered which require more extensive lengths for safe surgical margins. In squamous cancers, three representative patterns of presentation are encountered[16] (Fig. 5.2). Failure to take this into account may explain the finding of positive resection margins in nearly 40% of specimens when the oesophageal resection margin is limited to only 4 cm and still of 17% when the margin is 10 cm.[11,12] Therefore, 10 cm is a reasonable resection margin to attain in both directions if at all possible. In practice this rule of perfection can rarely be achieved. A 10 cm margin on both sides of a tumour measuring an average of 5.5 cm would require an overall length of specimen exceeding that of the normal human oesophagus. Under

Figure 5.2   *(a) A single cancer; (b) multifocal cancer; (c) intramural vascular spread. There is a high risk of positive resection margins in (b) and (c). Shaded areas represent sub-mucosal spread.*

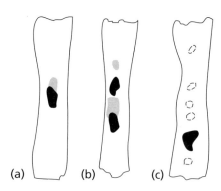

(a)   (b)   (c)

these circumstances it would be necessary in tumours with an upper margin of less than 10 cm from the cricopharyngeus, to require a resection of the distal pharynx and larynx. The choice between a safe margin and the preservation of a patient's voice needs to be carefully considered. In general, preservation of the patient's voice would be the preferred option, especially if resection were deemed palliative and a macroscopically clear margin had been obtained. Much of the published evidence is conflicting and some would suggest that resection margins of 4 cm or more result in anastomotic recurrence in less than 15% of cases.[17] This particular study also showed that if patients were given radiotherapy to the anastomotic site after the operation they did not subsequently develop recurrence. None of those with recurrence had been postoperatively treated with radiotherapy. It is the author's opinion that when only a short resection margin can be obtained through the thoracic exposure, a cervical phase with total oesophagectomy is advisable. If resection margins of less than 4 cm are obtained, consideration should be given to using supplementary adjuvant intraluminal or external beam radiotherapy.[18] Adenocarcinoma of the lower oesophagus commonly infiltrates the gastric cardia, fundus and lesser curve. Extensive sleeve resection of the lesser curve and fundus is necessary to minimise positive distal resection margins. Other studies have demonstrated that patients with microscopically cancer-positive margins undergoing palliative resection died of other manifestations before clinical evidence of locoregional recurrence.[19,20] A tumour-free surgical margin is, therefore, not the only important factor to be considered in radical surgery. Nevertheless, it should be the main goal of every operation. Most authors would agree that in order to make allowance for intramural submucosal spread of squamous and adenocarcinomas a subtotal oesophagectomy should be carried out in patients with tumours at any site.

Resection of lymph nodes

Early experiences of lymphadenectomy for oesophageal cancer[21] have been further reinforced by the results of the Japanese in the treatment of gastric cancer[22] which are now being reproduced in the UK.[23] The evidence for radical lymph node dissection in squamous and adeno-carcinoma of the oesophagus is less extensive, and the extent of lymphadenectomy continues to be an area of considerable controversy.

There is little doubt that some patients with oesophageal cancer who have lymph node involvement could be cured by surgical clearance.[24] The identification of those patients who would benefit is one aspect that provides the preoperative staging process with its greatest challenge. Early experience of endoscopic ultrasonography has suggested that this technique is both highly sensitive and specific in detecting lymph node metastases, in both the para-aortic and paraoesophageal regions. Further experience with this technique may well allow patients to be selected more accurately for radical lymph node dissection.

Many reports describe retrospective series of differing extents of lymphadenectomy in squamous and adenocarcinoma of the oesoph-agus.[13,25-27] These include no formal lymph node dissection as well as one-field, two-field and three-field lymphadenectomies. Unfortunately, very few prospective randomised trials are available for analysis.[28-30] The description of the tiers of lymph nodes in oesophageal cancer has been designed according to the anatomy of the lymphatic draining system of the oesophagus.[2,31-33]

The extent of lymphadenectomy is demonstrated in Fig. 5.3. Many surgeons do not practise a formal lymphadenectomy during either transhiatal or transthoracic approaches to oesophagectomy. A formal one-field lymph node dissection would involve the dissection of the diaphragmatic, right and left paracardiac, lesser curvature, left gastric, coeliac and common hepatic nodes. Two-field dissection includes the para-aortic (mediastinal nodes) together with the thoracic duct, the right and left pulmonary hilar nodes, the paraoesophageal nodes, tracheal bifurcation and the right paratracheal nodes. The extent of extensive three-field dissection includes the first and second fields as well as a dissection in the neck to clear the brachiocephalic, deep lateral and external cervical nodes and including the right and left recurrent nerve lymphatic chains (deep anterior cervical nodes). The fields of nodal dissection should not be confused with the histopathological staging of nodal involvement (see Table 3.13 on TNM staging of oesophageal cancer). Much of the data available on lymph node dissec-tion in oesophageal cancer suffers from poor definition of the terms oesophagectomy and oesophagectomy with lymph node dissection. It is essential, therefore, that all surgical techniques are standardised such that meaningful data can be derived in the future.

There seems little justification for oesophagectomy to be performed with intent to cure without any attempt to clear the first tier of lymph nodes. According to the literature 80% of all squamous oesophageal malignancies have lymph node metastases at the time of surgery.[25] Patients with either squamous or adenocarcinoma of the oesophagus affecting the upper middle and lower regions have lymph node meta-stases in the mediastinal nodes in over 60% of cases.[20,25,27,34] Many

Figure 5.3 *Extent of resection and fields of lymph node dissection routinely carried out for cancer of the oesophagus.*

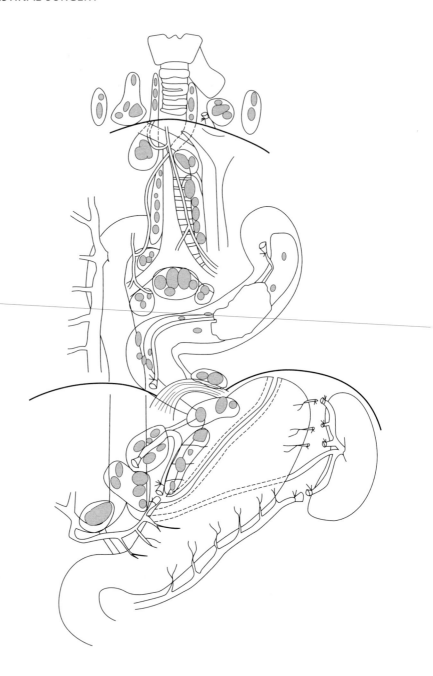

personal series of oesophageal cancer surgery have confirmed that over three-quarters of patients presenting with lower third tumours had positive lymph nodes in the coeliac trunk, left gastric and common hepatic territories. To perform a potentially curative resection for carcinoma in the middle and lower thirds, a dissection of abdominal and mediastinal lymph nodes is essential. Series from Japan as well as Europe, have confirmed that systematic nodal dissection employing meticulous surgical technique, can be performed with acceptable operative morbidity and mortality. Despite these advances in lymph node dissection during the last few decades, there is currently a mood of scepticism as to whether lymph node dissection really contributes to an improvement in survival. It is the author's opinion that two field lymph node dissection is justified on the grounds of the histopathological and surgical data presented by both Japanese and European groups.[24,25,27,35–37].

The role of extensive three-field dissection in oesophageal malignancy is less clear. The difference in tumour spread between squamous cell carcinoma and adenocarcinoma needs to be better reported and understood. Many reports combine these quite separate tumours and, therefore, confuse the results. Akiyama reports nearly a quarter of lower third squamous tumours presenting with metastases in the neck. Five-year survival rates showed no significant difference between two-field and three-field dissection in this group of patients.[25] In adenocarcinoma of the lower oesophagus, dissection of the cervical nodes cannot be justified, as there is no evidence that three-field nodal dissection provides any survival benefit in this group of patients. Although abdominal nodal dissection for cancer of the upper thoracic oesophagus (third tier) has not been shown to be beneficial, dissection in the neck for these upper-third tumours does appear to have some justification.[25]

As for many other solid organ tumours controversy persists as to the value of lymphadenectomy in oesophageal cancer. Two major attitudes exist. First, there is the concept that lymph node metastases are considered simply as markers of systemic disease and the removal of involved nodes will confer no benefit. Some surgeons advocate removal of the primary lesion alone and claim the same survival as with more extensive resections.[38] On the other hand there is the belief that in some patients with positive nodes cure can be obtained by an aggressive surgical approach focusing on wide excision and extended lymphadenectomy using a transthoracic approach. As described earlier the results of different extents of surgery are difficult to compare. Nevertheless the following strong arguments exist for more extensive surgery including lymphadenectomy:

1. Optimal staging
2. Prolonged locoregional tumour control
3. Improved cure rate.

Optimal staging

There can be no doubt that lymph node dissection contributes to the accuracy of the final staging of the disease.[25,36]

Locoregional tumour control

More extensive surgery produces prolonged tumour-free survival. In recent years overwhelming evidence has accumulated that R0 resection (no residual tumour left behind) is a very important prognostic variable after surgical excision.[39] To consistently achieve an R0 resection, organ dissection and lymphadenectomy must be radical. Roder et al.[40] showed in a series of 204 resections, a statistically significant difference between R0 and R1 or R2 (residual disease left behind) resections for squamous cell carcinoma with a five-year survival rate of 35% and below 10%, respectively. Lerut et al.[37] demonstrated a 20% five-year survival for R0 versus zero five-year survival for R1 and R2 resections in advanced Stage III and Stage IV adeno and squamous cell carcinomas.

Locoregional disease-free survival is a difficult, yet important goal to achieve in oesophageal carcinoma as the majority of patients present with advanced disease. Furthermore, recurrent locoregional mediastinal disease can be very difficult to palliate. Clark et al.[41] examined the operative specimens from 43 patients undergoing en bloc oesophagectomy for adenocarcinoma of the lower oesophagus and looked at the pattern of recurrence during follow-up. They found that nodal recurrence occurred within the area of dissection in only 20%. In addition Lerut et al.[37] demonstrated a four-year survival of 22% in patients with Stage IV disease due to distant lymph node metastases. This further endorses the apparent beneficial effect of adequate lymphadenectomy on reducing local recurrence.

Cure
The third argument for extended lymphadenectomy is the contribution to an improved survival. This argument unfortunately suffers from the lack of definite evidence from randomised trials as already discussed. Although many questions relating to surgical technique remain unanswered, several groups accept the value of lymphadenectomy when treating oesophageal carcinoma. It is not yet clear, however, which patients will benefit from such systematic nodal dissection. There is some evidence that patients with early stage oesophageal carcinoma in whom up to 50% have nodal involvement, would also benefit from extensive resection with lymphadenectomy.[42]

Method of reconstruction of the oesophagus

Route of reconstruction
After resection of the cervical, thoracic or abdominal oesophagus, one of three main paths can be used for reconstruction (Fig. 5.4).

Presternal route
Historically the presternal route was the preference of many surgeons. The presternal route is approximately 2 cm longer than the retrosternal route which in turn is approximately 2 cm longer than the posterior mediastinal route. As a result, the popularity of this route of reconstruction has declined over recent years. There seems little indication for using this route unless the thorax is of extremely small

Figure 5.4 *Three routes of oesophageal reconstruction. (1) Presternal route; (2) retrosternal route; (3) posterior mediastinal route.*

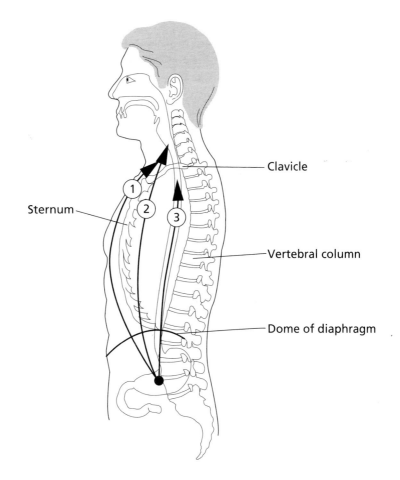

capacity such that a bulky oesophageal substitute could compromise effective respiration.

Retrosternal route (Anterior mediastinal)

The space between the sternum and the anterior mediastinum is easily created with good dissection. There is reported to be a lower incidence of cervical anastomotic dehiscence compared with that of the presternal route.[43] Unfortunately its major disadvantage stems from the somewhat unnatural position of the cervical oesophagus in front of the trachea which results in an unpleasant sensation on swallowing.

A major indication for the use for this extra-anatomical route of reconstruction is in emergency treatment of anastomotic dehiscence or the dehiscence of a gastric substitute which has caused posterior mediastinal sepsis.

The retrosternal route is created by blunt finger dissection through the abdominal and cervical incisions and further developed by insertion of a malleable intestinal retractor. The tip of this instrument is passed up to the neck in direct contact with the back of the sternum.

Care is taken not to deviate from the mid-line. The sternohyoid and sternothyroid muscles are divided in the neck and this allows the passage of the oesophageal substitute easily into the left or right side of the neck.

Posterior mediastinal route

This route provides the shortest distance between the abdomen and the apex of the thorax and also the neck. This is the preferred route of reconstruction in the primary surgical excision of oesophageal cancers. Gastric or colonic substitutes are easily passed through the posterior mediastinum after completion of the oesophageal dissection in the thorax. No attempt is made to close the pleura after this route of reconstruction.

Organ of reconstruction

Reconstruction with stomach

The method of reconstruction should be kept as simple as possible, to minimise complications. Oesophageal replacement is determined by the site of the primary lesion. The stomach is the preferred option as this organ is easy to prepare and involves only one anastomosis.

The patient is positioned supine and exposure obtained using an upper midline incision. There are six broad principles and practices which must be observed in the preparation of the stomach as an oesophageal substitute.

The use of isoperistaltic stomach and vascular integrity The right gastroepiploic and the right gastric artery and veins are vital in the maintenance of viability of the stomach when used as an oesophageal substitute. The greater omentum is opened and the entire course of the right gastroepiploic artery is carefully identified and preserved. The vascular arcade is interrupted at the junction where the right gastroepiploic artery meets the left. The short gastric vessels are ligated and divided (Fig. 5.5).

Excision of the lesser curvature Cancers of the lower two-thirds of the oesophagus require complete clearance of the lesser curve lymph nodes as well as the left gastric, coeliac trunk and common hepatic lymph nodes. The left gastric artery should be ligated at its origin and resection of the proximal half of the lesser curvature of the stomach, including the cardia, is performed. The right gastric artery contributes to the maintenance of the gastric intramural vascular network and should be preserved if possible. In carcinoma of the cervical oesophagus the entire arterial arcade along the lesser curvature of the stomach can be preserved. In this situation, all of the stomach is used for reconstruction.

Figure 5.5 *Main arteries of the stomach and points of division of vessels and stomach for oesophageal substitution.*

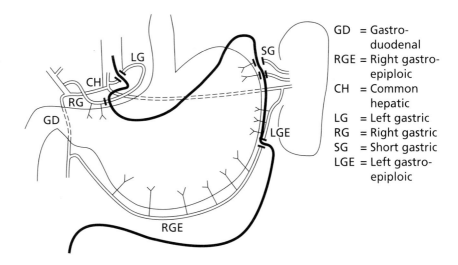

GD = Gastro-
　　　duodenal
RGE = Right gastro-
　　　epiploic
CH = Common
　　　hepatic
LG = Left gastric
RG = Right gastric
SG = Short gastric
LGE = Left gastro-
　　　epiploic

Preservation of the intramural vascular arcade Extensive intramural arterial anastomoses between the vascular arcade of the lesser and greater curvatures exist. This has been well demonstrated by El-Eishi *et al.*[44] and Thomas *et al.*[45] This extensive vascular network must be preserved during resection of the left gastric area of the lesser curvature and the cardia of the stomach. The extent of the resection of the lesser curvature is determined by a line connecting the highest point of the fundus (Fig. 5.6) and the lesser curvature at the junction of the right and left gastric arteries. This allows the removal of all potentially involved lymph nodes, yet preserves the arterial network to the fundus. There is no evidence to suggest that the trunk and descending branches of the left gastric artery running along the lesser curve needs to be preserved and from an oncological view point it is essential that these

Figure 5.6 *The high point of the stomach.*

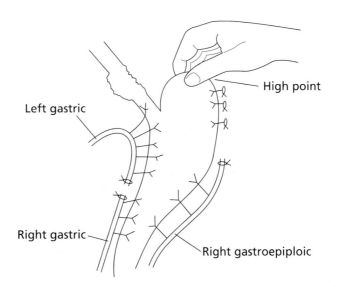

are excised with the specimen. Care should be taken to ligate the short gastric vessels away from the greater curvature of the stomach so as not to damage the intramural network. The right gastroepiploic artery provides an adequate blood flow to maintain vascularity in the region of the fundus which is the area used for anastomosis.[46]

The high point of the stomach   The stomach is a flexible and capacious organ. The high point of the stomach is the logical and sensible point at which to fashion an anastomosis with the remaining oesophagus. It is easily identified by applying traction with the surgeon's fingers in an upward direction after all preparations have been completed. The stomach is transected as described previously (Fig. 5.6).

Gastric drainage   The role of pyloroplasty after gastric reconstruction is contentious. As truncal vagotomy is inevitable, pyloroplasty should be required because of the resulting gastric stasis. Many surgeons believe that a pyloroplasty is essential following an oesophagogastric resection but the situation is not identical to truncal vagotomy for duodenal ulcer disease, because the pyloroduodenal area is almost always normal and the pylorus comes to lie vertically after the operation, aiding gastric emptying. Nevertheless, delay in gastric emptying has been reported in patients not undergoing pyloroplasty. As complications of pyloroplasty are minimal, it is the author's view that this should be performed routinely to prevent life-threatening complications of early gastric stasis and aspiration and the less serious ones of late vomiting and bloatedness.[47,48]

On occasions the upper anastomosis may need to be as high as the back of the tongue, so methods of stomach lengthening must be considered.

Methods of lengthening the stomach

1. Kocher manoeuvre: This is essential and allows the distance between the first part of the duodenum and the hiatus to be reduced.
2. Excision of lesser curve of stomach. When the lesser curve of the stomach is unusually short, an increase in length of the gastric substitute can be obtained, by dividing the lesser curve between curved clamps, before its resection. If absolutely necessary, a tense right gastric artery may be sacrificed by division at the level of the pylorus. The right gastro–epiploic artery can maintain an adequate blood flow along the greater curvature.
3. Incision of the serosa on the gastric wall. Multiple incisions placed in the gastric serosa may lengthen the stomach. A longitudinal incision placed along the resection line allows this to occur.[48] The indications for this procedure are extremely rare.
4. Reversed gastric tube: this method was originally described by Gavriliu, but is very rarely necessary.[49]

Table 5.3 *Indications for colonic reconstruction*

1.	Previous gastric resection
2.	Tumours with extensive gastric involvement
3.	Failed gastric transposition

Reconstruction with colon

The principal indication for the use of colonic interposition is for tumours close to the gastro-oesophageal junction which need an extensive oesophageal as well as gastric resection. A small proportion of patients will present with oesophageal malignancy who have had a previous gastric resection for peptic ulcer disease, precluding the use of stomach as the oesophageal substitute. The choice of an oesophageal replacement under these circumstances lies between colon and jejunum. The colon is often recommended because of its advantage of having a greater capacity as a reservoir than the jejunum. Rarely it may be used in an emergency after failed gastric interposition.

Indications for colonic reconstruction   These are shown in Table 5.3. It is preferable to use the colon in an isoperistaltic fashion. Unfortunately, the vascular pattern of the colon varies and careful selection of the correct vascular pedicle to ensure viability of the transverse colon is essential. Each case requires evaluation on its own merit because of variations in anatomy. Not infrequently, the marginal artery is found to be of insufficient calibre to maintain viability of the transposed colon. Although the vascular appearance determines the appropriate colonic segment for use in each individual, the two possibilities for effective use of isoperistaltic colon are: (a) transverse colon based on the left colic vessels and (b) right colon based on the middle colic vessels.

The disadvantage of transverse colon is that an abnormally narrow marginal artery may exist at the splenic flexure, thus compromising the blood supply of the proximal colonic segment. Preoperative assessment by angiography of the colonic vascular pathway has been suggested,[50] but careful intraoperative observation of the vascular anatomy with temporary occlusion of vessels before division is a simple manoeuvre which is effective in most cases.

Surgical technique Preoperative mechanical bowel preparation is necessary and oral antibiotic cover to sterilise the bowel for 48 h prior to surgery. The omentum is freed from the transverse colon and the hepatic and splenic flexures and the entire colon is mobilised so that it can be placed outside the abdominal cavity for inspection of its vascular blood supply. Mobilising the sigmoid colon provides additional length so that the transverse colon can be tunnelled into the chest, to reach the neck. The proximal colon should be divided and after anastomosis to the oesophagus, placed on sufficient stretch to prevent redundancy within the chest or in the substernal area. The colon should then be anchored in the straightened position by sutures to the crural margin of the hiatus, although not circumferentially. Continuity of the large bowel is re-established by end-to-end anastomosis, which is conveniently performed before the colojejunostomy or cologastrostomy for anatomical reasons. Excellent technical descriptions for the use of various segments of colon have been described by Demeester[51] and Belsay et al.[52]

Jejunal reconstruction

Replacement of the lower oesophagus is accomplished using either a Roux-en-Y technique or by segmental interposition. Replacement of the upper oesophagus is accomplished by free jejunal transfer with microvascular anastomosis of the jejunal pedicle to neck vessels. It is sometimes possible to create a long loop for replacement of the entire thoracic oesophagus. The jejunum should be considered the third choice, after colon and stomach, and chosen only when the other two organs were unsuitable or absent.

No specific measures are required to prepare the small bowel preoperatively other than to ensure that patients are not known to have small bowel pathology. A loop of jejunum is identified in the upper segments within the first 25 cm after the duodenojejunal flexure. Typical jejunal vascular pattern of arterial arcades are encountered in this area and the veins and arteries are close together but bifurcate at separate levels making individual division of the veins and arteries essential. Transillumination of the mesentery helps to identify the jejunal vascular tree precisely. It is important to appreciate that during the creation of a jejunal loop, it is the length of the free edge of the mesentery which will determine the length of the loop created rather than the length of the jejunum itself. The jejunum is usually longer than the mesentery and will, therefore, have a tendency to become redundant.

The technique of microvascular free jejunal transfer for reconstruction of the upper oesophagus is well described elsewhere.[53] The specific indications for such a reconstruction are usually after pharyngolaryngectomy performed for carcinoma of the hypopharynx, postcricoid region, and cervical oesophagus. The operation is usually performed with a radical neck dissection as part of the primary treatment programme, or as palliative surgery following recurrence after radiotherapy.

Method of surgical approach

The preceding discussion has described the method and rationale behind the surgical objectives of treating oesophageal cancer. The aims of resecting the primary tumour together with the lymph nodes and producing the oesophageal reconstruction must be achieved safely and effectively and with ease of access. The method of surgical approach to obtain these objectives must be considered in each individual case. The choice of the surgical approach is dependent on the tumour location, the extent of spread, the fitness, age and build of the individual patient and whether surgical intervention is to be curative or palliative.

Carcinoma of the hypopharynx and cervical oesophagus – pharyngolaryngo-oesophagectomy

Resection of squamous lesions in this area is achieved by removal of the larynx, the lower pharynx, cervical trachea, one or both lobes of the thyroid gland and cervical oesophagus. If the tumour is located in the hypopharynx only (postcricoid region), the thoracic oesophagus may be conserved and a free graft of jejunum transferred by micro-vascular anastomosis, as previously described. If tumour has extended onto the lower part of the cervical oesophagus, a total pharyngo-laryngo-oesophagectomy and gastric transposition, with immediate pharyngogastric reconstruction is the treatment of choice.

The patient is placed in the supine position with the neck hyper-extended. A 'U' shaped incision in the neck provides excellent access. It allows the construction of a permanent tracheostomy with ease and can be extended into a Y-shaped incision ready for a median steno-tomy if required. The resection includes a radical lymph node dissection in the neck. The thyroid and parathyroid glands are also removed en bloc with the internal jugular vein and the deep internal cervical nodes. The common carotid artery, vagus nerve and the sympathetic trunk are carefully protected.

Two-stage subtotal oesophagectomy via a right thoracotomy for carcinomas of the middle and lower thirds of the oesophagus

There has been much disagreement concerning the ideal approach to the thoracic oesophagus. The left thoracotomy was used for the first oesophagectomy and was a standard approach until the 1960s.[54] The advantage of the left thoracotomy is that it provides better access to the lower few centimetres of oesophagus, but satisfactory exposure of the upper and middle thoracic oesophagus, trachea and surrounding tissue is restricted by the intervening aortic arch and descending aorta. It has been argued that access to the left paratracheal nodes and hilum of the left lung is restricted in the right thoracotomy approach. Experienced oesophageal surgeons have encountered no difficulty in dissecting the left mediastinum from the right side. Two-stage right thoracotomy (initially described by Ivor Lewis and Tanner) is now becoming accepted as the approach of choice to the thoracic oesoph-agus.[25,46] A right thoracotomy and laparotomy through an upper midline incision is performed for carcinomas situated in the thoracic oesophagus. Both resection and reconstruction of the oesophagus are carried out in one stage. After completion of the mediastinal dissec-tion through the right thoracotomy, the stomach is delivered into the chest and an anastomosis fashioned at the thoracic inlet.

The procedure is started with exploration of the abdomen to exclude the presence of gross distant metastases and to determine whether resection is indicated. After performing routine gastric mobilisation, which has been described earlier, the coeliac trunk together with its branches, namely the common hepatic and the roots of the splenic and left gastric arteries are then skeletonised by complete removal of the surrounding lymph nodes. The left gastric artery is divided and ligated at its origin and each nodal group marked with a silk suture to help identification when the stomach is delivered into the chest. The patient is then placed in the left lateral decubitus position and is held firmly in place by a moulding mattress. Two sandbags are placed under the axilla and thorax to facilitate elevation of the rib cage. The pelvis is strapped to the operating table. The right arm is fixed on an arm rest whilst the left is stretched out on an arm support. All pressure points must be protected by padding.

The incision is made in line with the 5th intercostal space, beginning at the lower angle of the scapula and extending to the border of the sternum. The 4th intercostal space may be preferred for tumours of the middle third. The superior mediastinal pleura is incised along the course of the right vagus nerve and is extended upwards towards the brachiocephalic and subclavian arteries. The right recurrent larygeal nerve is preserved and meticulous dissection is then applied to the lymph node chain alongside it. The pleura is incised along the border of the superior vena cava and the right paratracheal lymph nodes located between the trachea and the vein are then dissected free. Care is taken not to dissect circumferentially around the trachea, as this may prejudice its blood supply. Routine resection of the arch of the azygos vein is crucial for adequate exposure. The right and left bronchial and carinal nodes are dissected. This continues towards the right pulmonary hilum and may result in some troublesome bleeding from bronchial arteries. It is advisable to avoid diathermy in this region due to the vulnerability of the membranous part of both the trachea and bronchi. The thoracic duct through which the lymph flows is rarely the site of metastases, except in extensive disease. There are, however, numerous lymph nodes scattered along the length of the duct in the para-aortic region. To remove these, en bloc resection together with the duct is necessary. The duct is easily identified after minimal sharp and blunt dissection in the inferior mediastinum on the right aspect of the descending thoracic aorta. The duct is ligated at this point along with the proximal end after resection in the superior mediastinum, along the posterior border of the oesophagus. Chylothorax secondary to inadvertent and undetected damage to the thoracic duct is therefore prevented. The oesophagus is then transected at the thoracic inlet. The stomach is delivered into the chest and the specimen removed after careful sleeve resection of the lesser curvature en bloc with the coeliac, left gastric, lesser curve, splenic artery and hepatic artery nodes. Oesophagogastric anastomosis is fashioned in the apex of the thorax.

Combined synchronous two team oesophagectomy

Modification of the standard access for oesophagectomy has been described wherein mobilisation of the stomach and abdominal oesophagus proceeds synchronously with mobilisation of the thoracic oesophagus via a right thoracotomy using a second operating team.[55,56] A reduction in operating and anaesthetic time was suggested as a possible reason for decreased operative morbidity and mortality rates in Hong Kong Chinese patients. Patients in the study had a lower incidence of pulmonary and cardiovascular disease than those with oesophageal cancer in the West. A comparison of the synchronous two team approach with conventional two-stage subtotal oesophagectomy was performed in Western patients. Not only was there a higher incidence of complications and a higher mortality rate but nodal dissection in larger more obese patients was technically very difficult.[57]

Three-stage subtotal oesophagectomy for tumours of the upper middle third of the oesophagus

Some surgeons prefer to expose and divide the oesophagus in the neck. This certainly provides excellent access for a relatively easy anastomosis, although it often does not allow resection of much more oesophagus than can be removed by the two-stage approach. This is because the cervical oesophagus is relatively short and it is difficult to perform an anastomosis unless a stump of oesophagus is left, hence the term, subtotal oesophagectomy. McKeown[58] recommended cervical anastomosis on the grounds that a cervical anastomotic leak was less catastrophic than a thoracic leak. This is probably an overstatement and is now of limited significance as overall oesophageal anastomotic leakage is uncommon – approximately 1–2% in practised hands. The three-phase operation takes longer to complete and is also associated with early postoperative difficulty in swallowing. This is probably because of the extensive proximal mobilisation of the cervical oesophagus. Proponents of the three-phase operation claim that a more complete oesophagectomy is achieved. The need for a subtotal oesophagectomy regardless of the site of the primary tumour was justified by pathological studies, which apparently indicated extensive proximal submucosal spread of tumour. Only if the tumour cannot be resected with adequate longitudinal margins should the three-stage technique be employed.

The first stage of this operation is routine gastric mobilisation with dissection of the nodal groups as described before. The second stage should mirror the dissection described in the preceding section but adding the mobilisation of the oesophagus in the apex of the thorax. The right thorax is closed and the patient turned supine once again. Through either a left or right sided cervical incision, the whole of the thoracic oesophagus can be removed and the stomach delivered into the neck and an oesophagogastrostomy fashioned.

Left-sided subtotal oesophagectomy for middle and lower third oesophageal cancers

For many years the left thoracotomy has been adopted, not only for carcinoma of the lower oesophagus and cardia, but also for carcinoma of the upper and mid-thoracic oesophagus. The left thoracoabdominal approach continues to maintain an established position as an appropriate surgical approach to resection of tumours at the cardia. Although many thoracic surgeons continue to use the left approach to lesions of the lower and mid-oesophagus, the access to the abdominal nodal dissection through a diaphragmatic incision is thought to be inadequate. Advocates of the left thoracotomy approach have failed to quote data about nodal status, or incidence of mucosal resection margins.[59,60] Randomised studies comparing the left approach to the right, have never been performed and so no clear survival advantage has emerged for either operative technique. Nevertheless Molina et al.[61] compared a 10-year experience of both the left and right approaches and clearly showed a higher incidence of residual tumour at the line of resection in patients undergoing a left thoracotomy. Others have reported a high incidence of residual tumour at the line of resection when performing a standard left thoracotomy when compared with a more extensive subtotal oesophagectomy.[62,63]

The left-sided approach was modified by Matthews and Steel[34] who described a two-stage procedure with a left thoracolaparotomy followed by a left neck approach. Much more extensive access was achieved by dividing the costal margin of the diaphragm peripherally for 15 cm close to its origin on the ribs. Although this more extensive resection should decrease positive resection margins, no data on the incidence of positive margins was quoted. This left-sided approach is nevertheless absolutely contraindicated if the tumour is situated at or above the aortic arch, for which a standard three-stage right-sided approach is necessary. Although data are limited on the incidence of respiratory complications in the left-sided approach, Molina et al.[61] and Earlam et al.'s[64] comprehensive review suggested an increased incidence of serious chest infections following the left-sided approach.

Transhiatal oesophagectomy for upper and lower third tumours of the oesophagus

There is still controversy about the role of oesophagectomy without thoracotomy in oesophageal cancer surgery. Proponents of the technique argue that most cancers are already locally advanced at the time of surgery and that 'cures' are fortuitous and dependent on the stage at presentation rather than the operative technique employed. Opponents claim improvements in survival for a small proportion of patients undergoing radical en bloc resection for more favourable tumour stage.[36,65] Its safety and benefits may be questioned if applied inappropriately. The original technique was described as a blind procedure, which therefore defied one of the most fundamental principles of surgery; that surgical procedures should always be carried out under direct vision.[66–68] Nevertheless refinements to the technique have been made and the operation has developed and gained many advocates.[69]

A modified technique of transhiatal oesophagectomy under direct vision has been described[70] using a modification of the transhiatal technique described by Pinotti.[71] In this technique almost the entire procedure is undertaken under direct vision and the anastomosis performed in the neck as a combined synchronous operation. The operation attempted to ensure adequate local clearance by avoiding direct contact with the tumour as well as carrying the majority of the procedure out, under direct vision. The authors demonstrated no evidence of proximal or distal resection margin involvement with tumour and an acceptable morbidity and mortality. Details of the surgical procedure are clearly described elsewhere.[71]

At present there are only selected indications for transhiatal oesophagectomy.

Carcinoma of the hypopharynx and cervical oesophagus, if the tumour is well localised, the incidence of mediastinal metastases is low and the thoracic oesophagus remains morphologically normal. Oesophagectomy without thoracotomy can, therefore, be safely performed by blunt dissection. Radical neck dissection with phayngolaryngo-oesophagectomy is carried out at the same time and reconstruction fashioned using the stomach through the posterior mediastinal route. A further advantage to this technique is that it ensures that no synchronous early lesions within the oesophagus are left behind, as would happen if a free jejunal graft were used in the neck. Some authors describe transhiatal oesophagectomy as the procedure of choice in *intraepithelial carcinoma of the oesophagus.* These tumours rarely disseminate via the lymphatics.[16] With substantial progress being made in endoscopic techniques using epithelial dye staining and endoscopic ultrasonography, early tumours can be more accurately staged. When tumour penetration is confined to the epithelial layer, resection by transhiatal oesophagectomy is entirely feasible. A few enthusiasts have even advocated transhiatal oesophagectomy for middle third tumours, although most would consider these tumours to represent a contraindication. Nevertheless, *advanced adenocarcinoma of the lower oesophagus* has been successfully treated for many years by blunt transhiatal oesophagectomy.[26]

The debate over which operative procedure is most appropriate for the treatment of lower third oesophageal carcinoma will continue. Randomised studies have never been performed and no clear survival advantage has emerged for any particular operative technique.[5] Alderson *et al.*[70] confirm that radical transhiatal oesophagectomy is not as radical a procedure as that proposed by Skinner.[13] The dissection does not include the thoracic duct and para-aortic nodes. Randomised controlled trials of radical transhiatal oesophagectomy against two-field lymph node dissection for lower third tumours should be performed to establish the role of each in the surgical treatment of cancer of the oesophagus.

Endoscopically assisted oesophagectomy for cancer

A number of techniques have been described to reduce the severity of the surgical insult and complications produced by formal thoractomy. These include thoracoscopic dissection within the chest,[72] laparoscopic mobilisation of the stomach for oesophageal replacement[73] and a mediastinoscopic technique.[74] Although endoscopic mobilisation is entirely possible, the length of time for the procedure appears prohibitive. Experience with thoracoscopically assisted oesophagectomy has not been uniformly encouraging. Although this technique avoids thoracotomy and dissection and haemostasis are performed under direct vision, prolonged deflation of the right lung contributes to the frequency of postoperative respiratory problems. The hospital stay has not been shown to be shortened and respiratory complications overall were increased when compared with experience using the open technique.[72] Widespread adoption of this technique cannot be recommended at present.

The mediastinoscopic technique allows the entire operation to be performed without changing the position of the patient, but dissection of the lower third of the oesophagus is extremely difficult. Lymph node dissection cannot accurately be performed and the technique has not achieved widespread acceptance.

Overall preliminary results from minimally invasive techniques do not show a clear benefit over open surgery in terms of mortality and morbidity although as yet it is too early to evaluate overall survival.

Technique of anastomosis

There have been no major changes in suturing techniques of the intestinal tract for many years. Meticulous technique is essential in achieving good results after oesophageal anastomosis. Morbidity and mortality for many years were related to anastomotic leakage.[75] The surgical principles relating to oesophageal anastomoses are the same as those in other parts of the alimentary tract. Emphasis is placed on (a) adequate blood supply, (b) absence of tension in the anastomosis, (c) accurate approximation of epithelial edges and (d) precise layer to layer suturing with primary healing. One layer and two layer anastomoses have been described, but no conclusive randomised controlled studies have been reported. Skinner[76] advocates a single layer anastomosis with a monofilament suture. A two layer oesophagogastric anastomosis is advocated by Akiyama[43] who emphasises the importance of the absence of a serosal layer, which he believes would reinforce strength at the anastomotic site. He therefore advocates a carefully preserved adventitia, which provides sufficient strength to support sutures. Others have even suggested a three-layer anastomosis[77] using adventitia to 'ink well' the stomach around the oesophagus.

Stapling devices were introduced into gastrointestinal surgery by Ravitch and Steichen.[78] These instruments have been further developed for ease of introduction and application. The latest instrument adopts a low profile head which permits a larger diameter anvil to be introduced into the oesophageal stump. A larger diameter anastomosis is thereby fashioned, reducing the main drawback to stapled oesophageal anastomoses – that of benign anastomotic stricture. These anastomotic fibrotic strictures are frequent after both manual and mechanical anastomosis but a higher rate of benign stricture is seen using the mechanical stapler.[79] These strictures are particularly associated with anastomoses constructed with a staple gun of 25 mm or less.[80] The author routinely uses stapling instruments for intrathoracic oesophageal anastomoses but continues to use a hand suture in the anastomosis of the cervical oesophagus and in circumstances where mechanical instruments are impractical.

Anastomotic leakage is more frequent in the neck than in the chest although the related mortality rate has not been shown to be different. The incidence of leakage does not depend on any suture material, or on technical modalities used to perform the anastomosis. Indeed the anastomosis is a technical procedure and suture healing is independent of the patient's biological condition. There has been no significant difference demonstrated between leakage rates using hand sewn and mechanical anastomoses. Higher overall incidence of leak rates is found in collective reviews rather than in reports from specialist units.

Postoperative management

A detailed account of immediate postoperative care after oesophageal cancer surgery is described in Chapter 4 and a summary is given in Tables 5.4 and 5.5. Meticulous attention to the maintenance of fluid balance and respiratory care are essential in the immediate postoperative

Table 5.4 *Routine postoperative measures*

1.	Fluid balance
2.	Intensive physiotherapy
3.	Analgesia
4.	Anti-thromboembolic measures
5.	Nutrition

Table 5.5 *Routine sequence of events after extubation*

1.	25 ml water/h from day 1
2.	4 × daily intensive physiotherapy for days 1–4
3.	Antibiotics days 0–2
4.	Mobilisation at day 2
5.	Nasogastric suction for days 1–5
6.	Non-ionic contrast swallow on day 5
7.	Chest drains removed days 5 and 6

period. Pain control and physiotherapy are crucial. Although some authors advocate the routine use of a feeding jejunostomy, most patients will be feeding normally on the fifth postoperative day once the anastomosis has been checked radiologically using a non-ionic fat-soluble contrast medium. Only if respiratory or surgical complications develop should early provision of enteral nutrition become essential. A feeding jejunostomy by either an open or percutaneous route is the preferred mode of administration under these circumstances. Early mobilisation is important in preventing venous thrombosis and pulmonary embolus. It also enhances ventilation, clearance of sputum and early bowel movement. It is the author's practice to remove the chest drains on the fifth and sixth postoperative days once oral feeding has recommenced. Some surgeons remove drains 48 h after surgery.

Routine nasogastric decompression is continued for five days until contrast radiology confirms oesophagogastric integrity. Patients are allowed 25 ml of water every hour soon after extubation. Subcutaneous low-dose heparin is administered routinely, until the patient is discharged. Chest physiotherapy is commenced in Intensive Care and continued 4 hourly for the first three days. Systemic antibiotics are commenced on the morning of surgery and continued for 48 h as a prophylactic measure. All patients are counselled by the surgeon, an oesophageal nurse practitioner and a dietician prior to discharge.

Postoperative complications

Postoperative complications can be subdivided into those that are common to any major surgical procedure in an elderly population and those specific to oesophageal resection. The complication rate of oesophageal surgery is relatively high. Early recognition of such complications and the rapid proactive management is essential to achieve good results.

General complications (see also Chapter 4)

These complications can be minimised by improved patient evaluation preoperatively and adopting prophylactic measures to counteract the predisposing factors. Respiratory complications constitute the largest proportion of this group.[4,81] Pain from the extensive incisions is the major contributor to decreased ventilation and atelectasis which leads to bronchopneumonia and respiratory failure. Mucous plugs may result in lobar collapse. Impaired diaphragmatic movement is caused by incisions placed on the diaphragm and extensive lymphadenectomy can cause poor lymphatic drainage of the pulmonary alveoli, leading to parenchymal fluid retention resulting in a form of acute pulmonary oedema. Significant respiratory complications occur in 25–50% of cases following subtotal oesophagectomy.[82]

Thromboembolic complications are not uncommon in malignant disease in the elderly age groups. These complications are comparatively rare in Oriental patients but not infrequent in Western series.

Serious thromboembolic complications in oesophageal cancer surgery occur in less than 10% of all procedures.[82]

Myocardial ischaemia and cerebral vascular episodes are specific to the age group undergoing surgery and are precipitated by hypoxia and hypotension and underlying vascular occlusive disease.

Haemorrhage is relatively uncommon and blood loss during surgery should range from 250 to 1500 ml. Acute primary bleeding from major vessels is uncommon. Secondary haemorrhage is also rare and is almost always associated with a mediastinal infection from a specific complication such as an anastomotic leakage. Wound infections are uncommon because of perioperative antibiotic prophylaxis and in particular when meticulous aseptic technique is used during surgery.

Specific complications

The second group of complications following oesophageal surgery for cancer are specific to the procedure.

Anastomotic leakage and leakage from the gastric resection line

Early disruption (within 48–72 h) is due to a technical error. If disruption occurs within the first 48–72 h and the general condition of the patient is good and the diagnosis confirmed, then the patient should be re-explored for correction of the technical fault. Later disruptions manifest themselves between days 5 and 9 postoperatively and are due to ischaemia of the tissues or tension on the anastomotic line. Further operative intervention is likely to be hazardous and detrimental. Conservative treatment with nasogastric suction, persistent chest drainage, therapeutic antibiotic regimens and early enteral nutrition via a jejunostomy are all essential. Late anastomotic leakage should not result in a high mortality if aggressively managed. Dehiscence of the gastric resection line is more unusual and usually dramatic. Re-exploration is essential as the extent of leakage is frequently large.[83] The incidence of anastomotic leakage is influenced by a variety of conditions including cancer hypermetabolism, malnutrition, anastomotic vascular deficit, anastomotic tension and surgical technique. The incidence of anastomotic leakage has decreased significantly over the last ten years and rates of well under 5% should be expected.[5,83] Total gastric necrosis can occur with catastrophic consequences. The condition must be diagnosed early, resuscitation immediate and the patient returned to theatre for the formation of a cervical oesophagostomy and closing off the gastric remnant. The establishment of a feeding jejunostomy is essential. At a later date, when the patient has stabilised a colonic interposition is used to restore intestinal continuity.

Chylothorax

The thoracic duct can often be damaged during mobilisation of advanced oesophageal cancers, whether via a right thoracotomy or through the transhiatal route. A comprehensive review[84] reports chylothorax occurring in up to 10% of patients after blunt transhiatal oesophagectomy. An incidence of 2–3% during open resection is commonly reported.[82,84] Accidental damage to the thoracic duct can be prevented by identification during dissection as previously described and ligating the duct low in the inferior mediastinum on the right lateral aspect of the descending thoracic aorta. Chylothorax usually presents in the first seven days after surgery when the patient has commenced oral intake, especially of fat containing nutrients. A massive increase in chest drainage occurs which results in malnutrition and significant immune suppression from the subsequent white cell loss. Immediate re-exploration is recommended as the damaged thoracic duct is easily identified at the time of re-exploration. Pre-exploratory intake of enteral fat helps to locate the leaking duct. Prolonged total parenteral nutrition has been used but patients rapidly become malnourished and frequently require a long hospital stay.

Recurrent laryngeal palsy

The incidence of recurrent laryngeal palsy has increased over recent years due to the increase of cervical oesophagogastric anastomoses. It is often unilateral and can be transient. Recurrent layrngeal nerve palsy is extremely rare when the anastomosis is constructed in the apex of the chest via the right thoracotomy route for subtotal oesophagectomy. If the palsy is transient but unilateral, the opposite cord may well compensate. The use of a percutaneous tracheostomy or a temporary formal tracheostomy may be required to safeguard the airway. If the palsy is permanent, teflon injection of the cord or a formal thyroplasty can restore adequate voice volume and a satisfactory cough.[85]

Gastric outlet obstruction

Gastric outlet obstruction is prevented by the routine use of a pyloroplasty. In the author's experience there have been no cases of gastric outlet obstruction following subtotal oesophagectomy and pyloroplasty in over 150 consecutive resections. Acid or akaline reflux is common but not troublesome provided the anastomosis is in the apex of the thorax. Procedures which leave part of the stomach as an abdominal organ and part of the stomach as a thoracic organ, predisposes to gastro-oesophageal reflux. Prokinetic agents such as cisapride, metoclopramide and erythromycin can improve gastric emptying and minimise these complications. Dumping after oesophagogastric reconstruction is relatively common but usually resolves by twelve months after surgery. It is adequately treated by the avoidance of high carbohydrate loads (see Chapter 12, p. 348).

Benign anastomotic stricture

Benign anastomotic stricture is a late complication following any form of anastomosis – either mechanical or hand sewn. These strictures are extremely easy to treat and respond to a single dilatation performed with the flexible endoscope under sedation.[80] Stenoses after stapled anastomosis are becoming increasingly rare now that larger diameter staple guns are being routinely used.

Overall results of single modality resectional therapy

Overall results of surgical therapy in oesophageal cancer can be analysed in terms of hospital mortality and patient survival. Assessment of quality of life during this period is essential, but data at present available, although interesting, are preliminary.[86,87]

Hospital mortality

Two comprehensive reviews during the last two decades shed some light in trends in both hospital mortality and overall survival.[5,64] Although individual units have achieved considerably better results, the analysis of the literature on oesophageal carcinoma during the 25-year period from 1953 to 1978 can be compared with an analysis of 1201 papers of surgical treatment for oesophageal carcinoma from 1980 to 1988. Muller's[5] review confirmed that the average hospital mortality rate following resection had halved during the past decade when compared with the figures reported by Earlam and Cunha Melo[64] in 1980. The overall mortality rate was quoted as 13% and this decrease from the earlier report of 28% was attributed to the introduction of prophylactic antibiotics, perioperative parenteral and enteral nutrition and by improvements in anaesthesia, surgical technique and intensive care medicine. Some authors have differentiated their results for oesophageal resection relating to changes in operative technique and peroperative management over a certain time span. Hospital mortality rates in these units dropped from a median of 22% to a median of 5% from their first descriptions to their latest series. No evidence has been provided to relate tumour biology to mortality rate following oesophageal resection. There was also no difference in mortality rates between resections for squamous cell carcinoma and adenocarcinoma. Overall mortality rates in many series can be confusing because of variations in definitions. 'In hospital' and not 30 day mortality rates should be quoted in all papers but unfortunately, this is not the case. Mortality rates of 10% and above in the present decade are no longer acceptable for the continued practice of this complicated and demanding surgical procedure. There is certainly no place for the occasional oesophagectomist in the management of this serious disease.[8,88]

Comparison of hospital mortality rates for different resection techniques reveals only minor differences. In the review by Muller the lowest mortality rate was found with transhiatal oesophagectomy with a median figure of 8%. These data, however, are not strictly comparable because transhiatal resection was the most recent surgical development and, therefore, benefited from the experience of recent advances in perioperative care.

Survival figures

In the review of the last decade, Muller *et al.* found that 56% of all resected patients survived the first postoperative year, 34% the second, 25% the third, 21% the fourth and 20% the fifth year after resection. These figures were very similar to those collected by Earlam and Cunha Melo, revealing that despite improved hospital mortality overall, long-term prognosis had remained unchanged. No differences in 5-year survival rates has been noted between different techniques of resection but en bloc resections have showed a significantly better long-term prognosis.[35,36] The primary determinants of overall outcome appear to be the stage of the tumour and the cell type. Prognosis is excellent with tumours invading the lamina propria or submucosa only and 32% of the patients with these tumours described in Muller's review survive 5 years if the tumour was confined to the muscularis propria at the time of presentation. If lymph node involvement was confirmed the five-year survival rate reduced to 13%. Better results with resection and two-field lymphadenectomy for node positive tumours have been achieved in specialist units.[6,13,28–30,35,36] There is considerable evidence to suggest that adenocarcinomas within Barrett's epithelium tend to fare worse than squamous lesions, although this may simply reflect the more advanced stage at which these lesions tend to present.[34,89]

Summary and future research

Cancer of the oesophagus is a depressing condition which is rapidly increasing in incidence, and has a poor overall survival rate. At present there is no ideal treatment for this carcinoma and each patient requires treatment strategies designed to suit their specific problems. At present surgical resection provides the only prospect of long-term survival. It is nevertheless still associated with significant risk although this has dramatically decreased over the last two decades. During the same time period, however, the cure rate of both squamous and adenocarcinoma of the oesophagus have failed to improve significantly. There is considerable evidence to suggest that early cancer of the oesophagus (primary tumour confined to the oesophageal wall without lymph node metastases) is associated with a much better prognosis than more advanced tumours. These patients have a good chance of cure with radical surgery. Any operation for carcinoma in the gastrointestinal tract must be designed to minimise the risk of anastomotic and locoregional recurrence. Subtotal oesophagectomy with two-field lymph node dissection seems to satisfy there criteria. Nevertheless, other surgical approaches including radical transhiatal oesophagectomy may well achieve the same goal.

The majority of patients will still die of their disease and genuine efforts must be made to determine if patients with a short survival time can be identified and spared unnecessarily aggressive attempts at cure and palliation. Referral of all patients with oesophageal malignancy to centres with a specialist interest should be encouraged, such that these centres can take part in large prospective trials, focusing on both attempted curative and palliative treatments. Clinical research must concentrate on randomised trials incorporating:

1. The separate assessment of squamous and adenocarcinoma. The rapid increase in incidence of adenocarcinoma in the West requires urgent assessment of other therapeutic modalities prior to surgery;

2. The assessment of T and N staging by endoscopic ultrasonography;

3. The standardisation of surgical procedures, pathological examination and treatment protocols.

Scientific research should focus on molecular biological techniques and the development of effective and less toxic preoperative neo-adjuvant regimen. Future clinical research must focus on prospective studies assessing the role, extent and timing of different therapeutic modalities. Until these studies are concluded, however, the data suggest that the best option for a patient with an oesophageal cancer is to have a surgical resection performed safely and effectively.

References

1. Hermanec KP, Sobin LH. UICC TNM classification of malignant tumours, 4th edn (2nd Rev). Berlin: Springer, 1992, pp. 45–8.
2. Japanese Society for Oesophageal Diseases. Guidelines for the clinical and pathological studies on carcinoma of the oesophagus. Part 1. Clinical Classification. Jpn J Surg 1976; 6: 64–78.
3. Moore FA, Feliciano DV, Adrassy RJ *et al.* Early enteral feeding compared with parenteral, reduces post operative septic complications. The results of a meta-analysis. Ann Surg 1992; 216: 172–83.
4. Nagawa H, Kobori O, Muto T. Prediction of pulmonary complications after transthoracic oesophagectomy. Br J Surg 1994; 81: 860–2.
5. Muller JM, Erasmit T, Stelsner M, Zieren U, Pichlmaier H. Surgical therapy of oesophageal cancer. Br J Surg 1990; 77: 845–57.
6. Lerut T. Oesophageal cancer – past and present studies. Eur J Surg Oncol 1996; 22: 317–25.
7. Bonavina L. Early oesophageal cancer: results of a European multicentre study. Br J Surg 1995; 82: 98–101.
8. Matthews HR, Powell DJ, McConkey CC. Effect of surgical experience of the results of resection for oesophageal cancer. Br J Surg 1986; 72: 621–8.
9. Steele RJC. The influence of surgeon case volume on outcome in site-specific cancer surgery. Eur J Surg Oncol 1996; 22: 211–13.
10. McKeown KC. Trends in oesophageal resection for carcinoma. Ann R Coll Surg Engl 1972; 51: 213–39.
11. Hill S, Cahill J, Wastell C. The right approach to carcinoma of the cardia, preliminary results. Eur J Surg Oncol 1992; 18: 282–6.
12. Giuli R. Surgery for squamous carcinoma of the oesophagus – an overview. In: Jamieson GG (ed) Surgery of the oesophagus. Edinburgh: Churchill Livingstone, 1988, pp. 585–95.
13. Skinner DB. En bloc resection for neoplasms of the esophagus and cardia. J Thorac Cardiovasc Surg 1983; 85: 59–71.
14. Siu KF, Cheung HC, Wong J. Shrinkage of the oesophagus after resection of carcinoma. Ann Surg 1986; 203: 173–6.
15. Akiyama H, Tsurumaru M, Watonabe G, Ono Y, Ukagawa H, Suzuki M. Development of surgery for carcinoma of the oesophagus. Am J Surg 1984; 147: 9–16.
16. Akiyama H. Surgery for cancer of the oesophagus. Baltimore: Williams and Wilkins, 1990, pp. 43–4 and 223–4.
17. Tam PC, Siu KF, Cheung HC, Ma L, Wong J. Local recurrences after subtotal oesophagectomy for squamous cell carcinoma. Ann Surg 1987; 205: 189–94.

18. Wong J. Esophageal resection for cancer: the rationale of current practice. Am J Surg 1987; 153: 18–24.

19. Mandard AM, Chasle J, Marney J et al. Autopsy findings in 111 cases of esophageal cancer. Cancer 1981; 48; 329–35.

20. Sons HU, Borchard F. Cancer of the distal oesophagus and cardia. Incidence, tumourous infiltration and metastatic spread. Ann Surg 1986; 203: 188–95.

21. Moynihan B. Abdominal operations, Vol. 1. Philadelphia, London: WB Saunders, 1916, pp. 285–317.

22. Maruyama K. Results of surgery correlated with staging in cancer of the stomach. In: Preece PE, Cuschieri A, Wellwood JM (eds) Cancer of the stomach. London: Grune and Stratton, 1986, pp. 145–63.

23. Sue Ling H, Johnstone D, Martin IG et al. Gastric cancer – a curable disease in Britain. Br Med J 1993; 307: 591–6.

24. Skinner DB. Selection of operations for esophageal cancer based on staging. Ann Surg 1986; 204: 391–400.

25. Akiyama H, Tsurumaru M, Udagawa H, Kajiyama Y. Radical lymph node dissection for cancer of the thoracic oesophagus. Ann Surg 1994; 22: 364–73.

26. Orringer M. Transthoracic versus transhiatal esophagectomy. What difference does it make? Ann Thorac Surg 1987; 44: 116–18.

27. Siewert JR, Roder JD. Lymphadenectomy in oesophageal cancer surgery. Dis Oesophagus 1992; 2: 91–97.

28. Goldminc M, Maddern G, Le Prise E, Meunier B, Campion JP, Launois B. Oesophagectomy by a transhiatal approach or thoracotomy: a prospective randomised study. Br J Surg 1993; 80: 367–70.

29. Kato H, Watanabe H, Tachimore Y, Izuka T. Evaluation of neck lymph node dissection for thoracic carcinoma. Ann Thorac Surg 1991; 51: 931–935.

30. Hagen JA, Peter JH, Demeester TR. Superiority of extended en bloc esophago-gastrectomy for carcinoma of the lower esophagus and cardia. J Thorac Cardiovasc Surg 1993; 106: 850–9.

31. Haagensen DC. The lymphatics in cancer. Philadelphia: WB Saunders, 1972, pp. 245–9.

32. Sato T, Sacamoto K. Illustrations and pho-tographs of surgical oesophageal anatomy, specially prepared for lymph node dissection. In: Color atlas of surgical anatomy for oesophageal cancer. Tokyo and Berlin: Springer-Verlag, 1992, pp. 25–90.

33. Tanabe G. Clinical evaluation of oesophageal lymph flow system based on the R1 uptake of removed regional lymph nodes following lymphoscintigraphy (written in Japanese). J Surg Soc 1986; 87: 315–23.

34. Matthews HR, Steel A. Left sided sub total oesophagectomy for carcinoma. Br J Surg 1987; 74: 1115–17.

35. Siewert JR, Hoelscher AH, Adolf J, Bartels H. Oesophageal carcinoma en bloc oesophagec-tomy with mediastinal lymphadenectomy in oesophageal reconstruction with delayed urgency. In: Siewert JR, Hoelscher AH (eds) Disease of the oesophagus. Berlin: Springer-Verlag, 1987, pp. 427–32.

36. Lerut TE, De Leyn P, Coosemans W, Van Raemdonck D. Cuypers PH. Van Cleyenbreughel B. Advanced esophageal carcinoma. World J Surg 1994; 18: 379–87.

37. Lerut T, De Leuyn P, Coosemans W, van Raemdonck D, Scheys I, Le Saffre E. Surgical strategies in esophageal carcinoma with emphasis on radical lymphadenectomy. Ann Surg 1994; 216: 583–90.

38. Orringer MB, Marshall B, Stirling MC. Transhiatal oesophagectomy for benign and malignant disease. J Thorac Cardiovasc Surg 1993; 105: 265–77.

39. International Union against Cancer (UICC). Hermanek P, Henson T, Hutter RVP, Sobin LH (eds) Supplement 1993, Berlin/Heidelberg, New York.

40. Roder JD, Bucsh R, Stein JH, Fink U, Siewert JR. Ratio of invaded to removed lymph nodes as a predictor of survival in squamous cell carcinoma of the oesophagus. Br J Surg, 1994; 81: 410–13.

41. Clark GWB, Peters JH, Ireland AP et al. Nodal metastasis and sites of recurrence after en bloc oesophagectomy for adenocarcinoma. Ann Thorac Surg 1994; 58: 646–54.

42. Kato H, Tachimori Y, Mizobuchi S, Igaki H, Ochiai A. Cervical, mediastinal and abdomi-nal lymph node dissection (three field dissection) for superficial carcinoma of the thoracic oesophagus. Cancer 1993; 72: 2879–82.

43. Akiyama H. Surgery for cancer of the oesophagus. Baltimore: Williams & Wilkins, 1990, pp. 74–5.

44. El Eishi HI, Ayoob SF, Abet el Khalek M. The arterial supply of the human stomach. Acta Anat 1973; 86: 565–80.

45. Thomas DM, Langford RM, Russel RCG, Le Quesne LP. Anatomical basis for gastric mobilization in total oesophagectomy. Br J Surg 1979; 166: 230–233.

46. Belsay R, Hiebert CA. An exclusive right thoracic approach for cancer of the middle third of the oesophagus. Ann Thorac Surg 1974; 18: 1–15.

47. Cheung HC, Siu KF, Wong J. Is pyloroplasty necessary in oesophageal replacement by stomach? A prospective randomised controlled trial. Surgery 1987; 102: 19–24.

48. Suibi Matchi Gay, Yaita A, Ueno H, Natsuda Y, Innochutchi K. A safer more reliable operative technique for oesophageal reconstruction using a gastric tube. Am J Surg 1980; 114: 471–4.

49. Gavriliu D. Aspects of oesophageal surgery, current problems in surgery. Chicago Year Book Med Publ, 1974, pp. 36–44.

50. Ventemigala R, Caleal KG, Frazier OH, Mountain CF. The role of preoperative mesenteric arteriography in colon interposition. J Thorac Cardiovasc Surg 1977; 74: 98–104.

51. Demeester TR. Indications of surgical technique in long term functional results of colon interposition or bypass. Ann Surg 1988; 208: 460.

52. Belsay RHR. Reconstruction of the oesophagus with left colon. J Thorac Cardiovcasc Surg 1965; 49: 33.

53. Sasaki TM. Free jejunal graft reconstruction after extensive head and neck surgery. Am J Surg 1980; 139: 650.

54. Logan A. The surgical treatment of carcinoma of the oesophagus and cardia. J Thorac Cardiovasc Surg 1963; 46: 150–61.

55. Nansen EN. Synchronous combined abdomino-thoracocervical oesophagectomy. Aust N Z J Surg 1975; 45: 340–8.

56. Chung SCS, Griffin SM, Woods SDS, Crofts TJ, Li AKC. Two team synchronous esophagectomy. Surg Gynaecol Obstet 1990; 170: 68–69.

57. Hayes N, Shaw I, Raimes SA, Griffin SM. Comparison of conventional Lewis Tanner two stage oesophagectomy with the synchronous two team approach. Br J Surg 1995; 82: 95–7.

58. McKeown KC. The surgical treatment of carcinoma of the oesophagus. A review of the results in 478 cases. J R Coll Surg Edin 1985; 30: 1–14.

59. Graham JN, Eng JB, Sabanathans S. Left thoracotomy approach for resection of cancer of the oesophagus. Surg Gynaecol Obstet 1989; 168: 49–53.

60. Lu YK, Li YM, Gu YZ. Cancer of the oesophagus at the oesophago-gastric junction. Analysis of results of 1025 resections after 5–20 years. Ann Thorac Surg 1987; 43: 176–81.

61. Molina JE, Lawton BR, Myers WO, Humphrey EW. Oesophago-gastrectomy for adenocarcinoma of the cardia. Ann Surg 1982; 195: 146–51.

62. Papachristou DN, Fortner JG. Anastomotic failure complicating total gastrectomy and esophagogastrectomy for carcinoma of the stomach. Am J Surg 1979; 138: 399–402.

63. Hankins JR, Cole FN, Atar S et al. Adenocarcinoma involving the oesophagus. J Thorac Cardiovasc Surg 1974; 68: 148.

64. Earlam R, Cunha Melo JR. Oesophageal squamous cell carcinoma. 1) A critical review of surgery. Br J Surg 1980; 67: 381–90.

65. Skinner DB, Little AG, Ferguson MK, Soriano A, Staszak DM. Selection of operation for oesophageal cancer based on staging. Ann Surg 1986; 204: 391–401.

66. Turner GG. Excision of thoracic oesophagus for carcinoma with construction of an extra thoracic gullet. Lancet 1933; i: 1315–16.

67. Lequesne LP, Ranger D. Pharyngo-laryngectomy with immediate pharyngo-gastric anastomosis. Br J Surg 1966; 53: 105–9.

68. Ong GB. Carcinoma of the hypo-pharynx and cervical oesophageal. In: Samith R (ed) Progress in clinical surgery, London: J & A Churchill, 1969, series 3, pp. 155–78.

69. Orringer M, Sloan H. Esophagectomy with thoracotomy. J Thorac Cardiovasc Surg 1978; 5: 643–54.

70. Alderson D, Courtney SP, Kennedy RH. Radical transhiatal oesophagectomy under direct vision. Br J Surg 1994; 81: 404–7.

71. Pinotti HW. A new approach to the thoracic oesophagus by the abdominal transdiaphragmatic route. Langenbeck Arch Chir 1983; 359: 229–35.

72. McAnena OJ, Roger J, Williams NS. Right thoracoscopic assisted oesophagectomy for carcinoma. Br J Surg 1994; 81: 236–8.

73. Jagot P, Sauvanet A, Berthoux I, Belghiti J. Laparoscopic mobilization of the stomach for oesophageal replacement. Br J Surg 1996; 83: 540–2.

74. Buess G, Kipfmuller K, Nahrun M, Melzer A. Endoskopis chemikro chirurgische dissektion des oeophagus. In: Buess G (ed) Endoskopie. Koln: Arzte, 1990, pp. 358–75.

75. Hernreck S, Crawford DG. The oesophageal anastomotic leak. Am J Surg 1976; 132: 794–8.

76. Skinner DB. Oesophageal reconstruction. Am J Surg 1980; 139: 810–14.

77. Sweep RH. Thoracic surgery. Philadelphia, London: WB Saunders, 1950, pp. 256–94.

78. Ravitch MM, Steichen RM. A stapling instrument for end to end inverting anastomoses in the gastro-intestinal tract. Ann Surg 1979; 189: 791–7.

79. Bardini B, Asolati M, Ruol A, Bonavina L, Baseggio D, Peracchia A. Anastomosis. World J Surg 1994; 18: 373–8.

80. Griffin SM, Woods SDS, Chan A, Chung SCS, Li AKC. Early and late surgical complications of sub-total oesophagectomy for squamous carcinoma of the oesophagus. J R Coll Surg Edin 1991; 36: 170–3.

81. Fan ST, Lau WY, Yip WC, Poon JP. Prediction of post operative pulmonary complications in oesophagogastric cancer surgery. Br J Surg 1987; 74: 408–10.

82. Watson A. Operable oesophageal cancer. Current results from the West. World J Surg 1994; 18: 361–7.

83. Paterson IM, Wong J. Anastomotic leakage: an avoidable complication of Lewis Tanner oesophagectomy. Br J Surg 1989; 76: 127–9.

84. Bolger C, Walsh TN, Tanner WA, Keeling P, Hennessey TPJ. Chylothorax after oesophagectomy. Br J Surg 1991; 78: 578–87.

85. Griffin SM, Chung SCS, Van Hasselt CA, Li AKC. Late swallowing problems after oesophagectomy for cancer. Malignant infiltration of the recurrent laryngeal nerves and its management. Surgery 1992; 112: 533–5.

86. Blazeby JM, Williams MH, Brooks ST, Alderson D, Farndon JR. Quality of life measurement in patients with oesophageal cancer. Gut 1995; 37: 505–8.

87. O'Hanlon D, Harkin M, Hayes N, Sargeant T, Raimes SA, Griffin SM. Quality of life assessment of patients undergoing treatment for oesophageal cancer. Br J Surg 1995; 82: 1682–5.

88. Bancewicz J. Cancer of the oesophagus. Br Med J 1990; 303: 3–4.

89. Watson A. Cancer of the oesophagus. In: Misiewicz JJ, Pounder RE, Venables CW (eds) Diseases of gut and pancreas. Oxford: Blackwell Scientific, 1994, pp. 159–172.

6 Surgery for cancer of the stomach

Simon A. Raimes

Introduction

The overall cure rate for gastric cancer remains around 10% in most countries. In marked contrast the results from Japan are very much better and overall 5-year survival rates of over 50% are being consistently reported. Surgeons in the West have been unable to produce similar results, though some specialist centres have recently reported significant improvements, apparently as a result of trying to emulate Japanese surgical practice.

Any discussion of gastric cancer surgery has to include an analysis of Japanese practice which is regarded as the 'gold standard' at present. Comparison of 5-year survival figures for similar stages of the disease reveals results that are up to 20% better in Japan than in the West.[1] If surgeons in the West are to strive to produce similar results it is important to understand exactly how the Japanese surgeons have achieved this level of excellence. It is necessary to examine critically the evolution of Japanese practice to determine whether similar results can realistically be achieved by Western surgeons who adopt this practice.

Development of gastric cancer treatment in Japan

Stomach cancer is the most common cause of cancer death in Japan. Thirty years ago the survival rates were little different from those now reported in the West. There are three important changes that have occurred subsequently.

National screening programme for gastric cancer

Mass survey of the population by mobile X-ray units was started in 1960. Barium meal screening of the population over 40 years of age has been a massive undertaking – in 1988 5.2 million people were screened of whom 13% required further investigation. The programme has proved to be cost-effective in those over 65 years of age. Success can be measured by the fact that in 1988 62.4% of cancers detected by screening were early mucosal or submucosal lesions.

Japanese Research Society for Gastric Cancer (JRSGC)

This was established in 1961 to promote basic research and management of gastric cancer. The initial objective was to collect standardised data on clinical (macroscopic) staging at the time of surgery and subsequent pathological (microscopic) staging to allow accurate comparison of results. Recommended surgical techniques and rules for documentation of surgery were published and are regularly updated. Pathological assessment was rigidly standardised and is similarly updated. The JRSGC and the National Cancer Centre in Tokyo started a nationwide collection of data in 1963. Around 10 000 cases are registered annually, though it should be emphasised that this is less than 20% of gastric cancers treated each year in Japan – it is highly selected and certainly represents the very best practice in that country.

Radical gastric cancer surgery

Radical excision of the stomach and its lymphatic drainage had previously been practised in specialist centres in both Japan and the West. Publication by the JRSGC of precise definitions of radicality and standardisation of operations in the 'General Rules' reinforced this concept and led to the widespread adoption of radical gastric surgery in Japan. It has been proposed that this surgical attitude has been a major factor in the improvement in results. Remarkably, this has never been tested in a randomised trial and Japanese surgeons claim that to try to do so now would be unethical.

The real question is to what extent has each of the above factors contributed to the overall improvement in survival. These measures were introduced concurrently and the Japanese have not been able to separate the respective contributions of earlier diagnosis, improved pathological staging and radical surgery. This analysis is very important in understanding how practice should evolve in the West.

Development of gastric cancer treatment in the West

Screening for gastric cancer

A UICC Workshop held in the UK in 1990 concluded that asymptomatic screening of the population for gastric cancer was only cost-effective in countries with a high incidence of the disease. It could not be recommended as a public health policy in the West.

Screening of symptomatic 'dyspeptic' patients does increase the proportion of early gastric cancers diagnosed.[2] Increased availability of endoscopic services, including open and direct access endoscopy, also improves the stage at which cancers are diagnosed.[3] However, it must be emphasised that there is a significant difference in outcome between symptomatic cancers diagnosed at an earlier stage and that of screen-detected asymptomatic cancers included in Japanese series. In Japan there is a significantly improved long-term survival after surgery in asymptomatic cancer cases when compared with those presenting with symptoms.[4]

Shift to the left phenomenon   The presentation of gastric cancer can be considered to produce a spectrum of disease with the worst stages to the right. Asymptomatic screening and to a lesser extent symptomatic screening not only increase the proportion of early cancers at the far left end of the spectrum, but also shift the whole spectrum to the left. Staging simply divides the spectrum of the disease into four sections. The shift to the left phenomenon may mean that all stages contain a higher proportion of patients in the more favourable left side of the stage. This may partly explain why the survival of all stages of gastric cancer is better in screened populations and particularly in the Japanese asymptomatic screened population. It is also postulated that increased population awareness of the risk of gastric cancer, such as has occurred in Japan, also contributes to a shift to the left phenomenon even in the non-screened population as more patients recognise the potential significance of their symptoms and report them earlier.

It may be more meaningful to compare Western results with those of symptomatic Japanese patients only – this would allow a more accurate prediction of the likely effects of the widespread adoption of radical surgery in the West.

Effects of radical surgery and improved pathology on staging

The staging systems used in the West have not been as clearly defined or standardised as those in Japan. Accurate comparison of results was not possible until 1985 when the UICC and AJCC agreed a unified staging system (Chapter 3).

It should be realised that there are also other more subtle effects on the process of staging that affect comparisons of Western and Japanese practice.

Stage migration phenomenon   The extent of lymph node involvement (N factor) is an important aspect of staging. The Japanese Rules for Pathology require very detailed sampling of each defined node group and multiple sections of each node. The detection of nodal micrometastases by this type of obsessive sampling is much more likely than in standard Western pathological assessment. If the same principles were applied in the West a proportion of cancers would be allocated to a worse stage on the basis of the true N factor (Chapter 3). Present Western pathological analysis produces overoptimistic staging of cancers and this is one reason why long-term survival is not as good as the comparable Japanese figures of the same stage. Many specialist centres have already addressed this shortcoming and nodal staging is now much more accurate.

Another very important factor in the accurate staging of cancers on the basis of lymph node involvement is the extent of the lymphadenectomy. If only the first tier of nodes is excised then the N factor could not be more than N_1. In the best Japanese centres all second tier and possibly some third tier nodes are also excised en bloc and so if there are metastases in these nodes the cancer will be correctly staged N_2 or N_3. Examination of 5-year survival figures (5YSR) in Japan reveals the importance of correctly determining the N factor by more radical lymphadenectomy:[5]

e.g. $T_2N_1M_0$ – 71% 5YSR $T_2N_2M_0$ – 52% 5YSR

$T_3N_1M_0$ – 46% 5YSR $T_3N_2M_0$ – 23% 5YSR

It is noteworthy that correct staging of a node-positive cancer may decrease the 5-year survival expectancy by about 20%. It is still not clear what proportion of the 'benefit' of radical lymphadenectomy is due to removal of nodal tissue as opposed to that attributable to the correct pathological staging of the cancer. This not only affects comparison of Japanese and Western results, but is also an important factor that should be allowed for in randomised studies comparing D1 and D2 lymphadenectomy.

Different disease in the West?

It has been observed that gastric cancer in the West may be a different disease from that in Japan.[6] There is not much evidence to support this hypothesis. The natural course of the disease, the modes of spread and areas of recurrence are similar. If early gastric cancers are excluded then most prognostic factors are similar.[7] However, there are two factors that may be of some significance.

Lauren histological type   Many studies show a higher proportion of intestinal-type cancers in Japan. This type has a better prognosis than the diffuse-type that is more commonly seen in the West.

Proximal cancers   Cancers of the proximal third of the stomach have a worse prognosis than those in the distal two-thirds.[8] The factors responsible include a higher incidence of diffuse-type cancers in the proximal stomach and more frequent nodal spread. Recent Western series report a 40–50% incidence of proximal cancers compared to 20–30% in Japan. The incidence of proximal cancers is increasing more rapidly in the West and it is possible that this will negate the beneficial effects of other factors that are being improved.

Perioperative mortality of radical surgery in the West

Although the Japanese specialist centres report mortality rates of 1–3% for radical gastric surgery, this is considerably higher in the West and particularly for total gastrectomy.[9] Even centres of excellence in the West report a mortality rate of 5–10% for curative surgery and this is even higher for palliative procedures.[10] The results are improving, but are unlikely ever to equal the Japanese figures because Western patients are, on average, 10 years older and have a higher incidence of cardiovascular disease than those with gastric cancer in Japan. Japanese patients are thinner and have a very low incidence of postoperative thromboembolic complications. The higher incidence of proximal cancers in the West means that the proportion of total gastrectomies is higher and it should be remembered that this operation is associated with a mortality of about twice that of a subtotal resection.

Role of radical surgery in Western practice

It is apparent from the previous analysis that the results obtained in gastric cancer treatment in Japan are superior to those in the West for multiple and complex reasons. It has to be accepted that comparison of overall survival rates is of little meaning. Even now that there is a uniform staging system there are subtle reasons why Japanese patients may do better, related to the 'stage migration' and 'shift to the left' phenomena and the higher incidence of proximal cancers in the West.

Past experience with radical gastric resection in the West produced variable and usually disappointing results with any therapeutic gain being negated by the high mortality of the surgery. Only a few specialist centres have pursued the concept of radical excision as practised by the Japanese. Most surgeons have restricted their surgical effort to limited resections that can be achieved with a lower operative mortality. The basic philosophy should be that the additional risks of radical and extended gastric resections must be shown to be less than the survival advantage. The Leeds General Infirmary experience is presently closest to Japanese practice in the UK (Table 6.1). They are reporting stage-specific survival rates nearer to those of best Japanese practice, at least for earlier stages, and with an acceptable mortality.[10] Unfortunately the actual contribution of radical surgery remains uncertain because, in addition to adopting this surgical policy, they have concurrently introduced pathology reporting along Japanese lines and an enhanced endoscopy service for the rapid investigation of symptomatic patients. Despite this reservation the Leeds practice is now the 'gold standard' in the UK and will remain so while the results of randomised studies comparing different surgical strategies are awaited. It is certainly more meaningful to compare UK results with Leeds rather than Japan.

Table 6.1 *Five-year survival after potentially curative gastric cancer surgery. Comparison of results from Leeds[11] and Tokyo[37]*

	Cumulative 5-year survival (%)	
	Tokyo	Leeds
All potentially curative resections	75	54
Early gastric cancer	91	91
Stage I	91	87
Stage II	72	65
Stage III	44	18

The remaining unanswered question is what advantage does radical surgery actually produce? It seems reasonable to assume that there is some survival benefit but that this may be variable depending on the stage of the disease. It is possible that the advantage in Western patients could be offset by the increased mortality of radical surgery. In addition more extensive resections are associated with increased postoperative morbidity, long-term sequelae and nutritional conse-quences.

Modern practice in gastric cancer surgery should evolve on the basis of the following philosophy at least until there is more information.

1. A nihilistic approach to gastric cancer is no longer acceptable even if radical surgery only has a limited role and is only part of a 'package' of measures to improve survival. It is an oversimplifica-tion to attribute improvement of results to the extent of the lymphadenectomy alone.
2. There has to be continued effort to reduce the postoperative mortality and morbidity of radical gastric resections.
3. Randomised studies must continue to explore the role of radical surgery – these should be undertaken by surgeons already experi-enced in the techniques to be studied.
4. Present surgical practice should be based on an understanding of the disease and in particular how treatment failure occurs.

Areas of failure after gastric cancer surgery

A rational approach to surgery for gastric cancer requires an under-standing of the modes of spread of this cancer and how it recurs after surgery. This knowledge is essential to define the aims and limitations of radical surgery.

Metastatic pathways

Direct extension
There may be direct extension into adjacent organs or structures that may be excised en bloc with the stomach as part of a potentially curative resection.

Lymphatic spread
Lateral spread occurs in the submucosal and subserosal lymphatic plexuses depending on the depth of penetration of the cancer. Drainage is then to the perigastric nodes and subsequently along the lymphatics that accompany the arteries to the stomach back to the coeliac trunk. This is discussed in detail in the section on lympha-denectomy. Lymphatic spread can occur at any stage, but becomes more common the deeper the invasion through the stomach wall. Between 60 and 80% of patients with evidence of intra-abdominal metastatic spread will have lymph node involvement.[12] Lymphatic spread is the most common mode of dissemination in both the

intestinal and diffuse types of gastric cancer, emphasising the potential importance of adequate nodal excision.

Peritoneal spread

This should only occur once the cancer has breached the serosal surface when cells can be shed into the peritoneal cavity. There is evidence that the likelihood of retrieving viable shed cells is proportional to the area of serosa that is invaded.[13] There is experimental evidence that shed cells can adhere to and infiltrate intact peritoneum.[14] Since more than 75% of cancers in the West are serosa-positive a large number of patients have the potential for intraperitoneal recurrence by cell implantation in the gastric bed or elsewhere in the peritoneal cavity. Peritoneal seeding is much more common in diffuse-type cancers (45–75% versus 10–30% for the intestinal-type).[12] Surgery that includes removal of the intact lesser sac peritoneum may possibly be of value for a localised cancer with only posterior wall serosal invasion, but in general surgery has no curative role in treating this mode of spread. It is very important to appreciate this limitation in treating the majority of patients with gastric cancer in the West.

Haematogenous spread

Despite the rich vascular supply of the stomach, liver metastases at the time of diagnosis are relatively uncommon, even in advanced cancers. It has been postulated that gastric cancer is inefficient in metastasising via the haematogenous route and this may apply to the diffuse-type particularly. The alternative explanation is that diffuse-type cancers spread rapidly by other routes and that although haematogenous spread may occur, the patient dies of other forms of metastasis before liver and distant metastases become clinically apparent.

Concept of gastric cancer as a locoregional disease

It has been observed that even in cancers that are locally advanced at the time of diagnosis the disease is still confined to the area of the stomach, the retroperitoneum and peritoneal cavity – liver and distant metastases are frequently not detected. This concept is supported in a study by Wangensteen and his co-workers of reoperation data in patients who had previously undergone 'curative' gastric resection. This is reported in a paper by Gunderson and Sosin that should be regarded as essential reading.[15] The reoperations were mainly elective procedures in patients thought to be at high risk of recurrence. At second look, over 80% had evidence of recurrence. Looking at those with recurrence, the most important finding was that although 29.3% had haematogenous spread, in only 6.1% was this the only mode of recurrence – all the patients had additional gastric bed or peritoneal disease. In total, 87.8% had disease in the gastric bed and anastomosis and a third of these patients had distant peritoneal seedlings.

Importantly, virtually all those who had serosa-positive (T_3 and T_4) cancers at the time of their first resection had intra-abdominal recurrence. It was apparent that the extent of resection had little effect on the incidence or type of recurrence. Wangensteen concluded that radical surgery had produced little benefit in this group of patients. These findings have subsequently been confirmed in other studies.[16,17]

The pattern of recurrence is quite different in serosa-negative (T_1 and T_2) cancers and especially early gastric cancers. Unlike serosa-positive cancers which tend to recur early (within 2 years), if recurrence does occur it does so later and much more frequently as haematogenous metastases without local recurrence.

The high incidence of serosa-positive cancers in the West explains why the overall outlook after gastric resection is still poor. Recurrence occurs early and within the abdomen – most of these patients probably do not live long enough to show evidence of blood-borne metastases. It is possible that improved locoregional control of serosa-positive cancers will not prevent patients dying later of distant metastases. However, control of locoregional recurrence would improve the prognosis in a large number of patients even if cure was not achieved. The value of the symptom-free interval in those patients who cannot be cured by surgery should not be underestimated.

It has been postulated that there is a biphasic pattern of recurrence in gastric cancer. There is a first early phase of local failure in the gastric bed, anastomosis and peritoneal surfaces most commonly seen in serosa-positive cancers and diffuse-type cancers in particular. The second later phase of failure is due to haematogenous metastases to the liver or distant organs. This is more commonly seen in earlier cancers and intestinal-type cancers that have not recurred locally in the first phase. The role of surgery is limited to complete removal of curable lesions that have not disseminated at the time of diagnosis and to minimising the early phase of locoregional recurrence.

Strategies to minimise locoregional failure

Local or gastric bed recurrence
There are three factors to consider:

1. Complete resection of the primary lesion to ensure that all resection margins are free of malignant cells. This includes extending the resection line in continuity to adjacent structures and organs if feasible and safe.
2. En bloc resection of all potentially involved lymph nodes within the normal lymphatic pathways from the stomach.
3. Prevention of implantation of free cancer cells in the gastric bed. A 'Tumour Cell Entrapment Hypothesis' has been proposed which suggests that cells shed before or during surgery can implant on and remain viable in the deperitonealised resection site. These cells may already be present in the peritoneal cavity at the time of

surgery in serosa-positive cancers or may be shed during resection from the tumour surface and cut lymphatics and blood vessels.[18]

It is apparent that appropriate radical surgery has a definite role in the control of the first two factors. However, it will have only a minimal effect in preventing cell implantation on the gastric bed, especially in serosa-positive and more advanced cancers with lymphatic spread into the second tier of nodes or beyond. Analysis of survival benefit from radical lymphadenectomy shows a statistically insignificant advantage for T_3 and T_4 cancers.[19] A significant benefit is most apparent in stages II and IIA cancers, producing both a decrease in the rate of local recurrence and increased rate of cure.[20–22]

Peritoneal dissemination

Viable cancer cells may be shed preoperatively and during or soon after surgery. Meticulous surgical technique with en bloc resection of the stomach, affected adjacent organs and intact gastric lymphatic chains is important to prevent 'iatrogenic' cell spillage into the peritoneal cavity. Measures to destroy free cells in the perioperative period will be required in addition to surgery in patients who have serosal involvement and/or metastases in the second lymph node tier. There is increased interest in intraperitoneal chemotherapy in the West. This is already commonly utilised in Japan as part of the multimodality treatment of advanced cancers.[23,24] This treatment is of most value if started during or immediately after surgery. Delayed postoperative treatment does not improve survival. This is thought to be because cells have already implanted in the gastric bed and are protected by a fibrinous coagulum.[25]

Summary

The most important objective for the surgeon is to define the point of diminishing returns in gastric cancer surgery.[12] Appropriate radical surgery with complete resection of the primary lesion is the first priority and in potentially curable cases radical excision of lymph nodes and adjacent organs.

It is important to realise that in the future surgery will probably be one part of the multimodality treatment of gastric cancer. The potential roles of chemotherapy and radiotherapy are discussed in more detail in Chapter 7. A recent review of multimodality treatment of resectable gastric cancer by Averbach and Jacquet is recommended.[12]

Principles of gastric cancer resection   There are certain basic principles that should be adhered to when resecting gastric cancer. There is now considerable evidence on which to base standardised procedures. However, each case is different and there are multiple factors that affect the operative tactics. The stage of the cancer, evidence of spread, mode of spread, the patient's health, age and build all have to be taken into account in 'designing' the appropriate procedure for each patient. These are considered under the following headings:

1. Extent of the gastric resection
2. Lymphadenectomy
3. Splenectomy
4. Distal pancreatectomy
5. Extended resections
6. Lesser resections

Extent of gastric resection

The most fundamental aim of gastric cancer surgery is to adequately excise the primary lesion. The type of gastrectomy required to achieve this depends on the position of the cancer and the margin necessary to be certain not to leave malignant cells at the anastomotic line.

Lateral spread in the gastric wall occurs by direct invasion and by spread within the submucosal and subserosal lymphatics. Once the submucosa has been penetrated there may be extensive lateral spread within the abundant lymphatic plexus. Diffuse-type cancers are particularly prone to spread in this way, in the most aggressive forms most or all of the submucosa may be infiltrated so producing a linitis plastica. It is important to realise that both the oesophagus and duodenum can be infiltrated by spread in the mural lymphatics – in the former via the submucosal channels and the latter via the subserosal channels. This must be taken into account when planning the extent of resection if there is palpable tumour at either end of the stomach.

It is often stated that diffuse-type cancers require a larger resection margin than the intestinal-type.[26] Some European surgeons recommend a total gastrectomy for any diffuse-type lesion.[1] This concept is debatable as examination of resection margins has shown that a 5 cm margin from the palpable edge of the tumour is sufficient for both intestinal and diffuse-types.[27] Cancers that have penetrated the serosa require a wider margin and 6 cm from the palpable edge of the tumours or infiltrated wall has been recommended.[28]

Serosa-negative cancers, particularly of the intestinal-type, may be resected with a smaller margin in elderly or high risk patients. The place of limited resections is discussed later.

Type of gastrectomy (Fig. 6.1)

Distal third cancer (A and AM)
A subtotal (80%) gastrectomy with resection of the first part of the duodenum is recommended.[29] A total gastrectomy is only indicated for large tumours or when there is submucosal infiltration to within 7–8 cm of the oesophagogastric junction.

Figure 6.1 *Extent of gastric resection.*

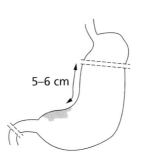

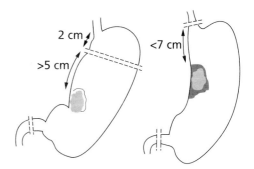

Antral carcinoma
Subtotal gastrectomy and resection of first part of duodenum

Carcinoma of middle third
Subtotal or total gastrectomy depending on proximal margin of resection

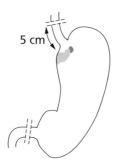

Carcinoma of cardia
Total gastrectomy and resection of lower oesophagus

Middle third cancer (M and MA)

In most cases a total gastrectomy will be necessary, but this depends on the amount of stomach remaining below the oesophagogastric junction after excising an adequate margin of stomach proximal to the palpable edge of the tumour. A minimum of 2 cm is needed and so for a serosa-negative cancer there must be a 7 cm margin from the oesophagogastric junction and at least 8 cm for a serosa-positive cancer.

Proximal third cancer (C, CM and MC)

The choice of resection is between a proximal subtotal or a total gastrectomy. Anastomosis of the distal stomach to the oesophagus produces a poor functional result; alkaline reflux in particular can be very troublesome and difficult to control.[30] Total gastrectomy is recommended as a better cancer operation and results in fewer significant side-effects.

Extensive cancers (CMA)

Total gastrectomy is indicated provided there is a chance of worthwhile palliation in this type of advanced cancer. Adequate proximal and distal margins are important in linitis plastica.

Total gastrectomy de principe for distal cancers

The absolute indications for removal of the whole stomach have been listed above – in these circumstances this is a 'total gastrectomy de necessite'. There are surgeons who argue that all cancers of the stomach, even those in the distal third, should be treated in the same way – 'total gastrectomy de principe'. It is important to understand the arguments for and against such a policy.

1. *Less risk of positive proximal resection margin.* Provided the rules on safe margins of resection are adhered to this is rare. If the margins are still positive despite an adequate margin then this usually indicates an aggressive malignancy and anastomotic recurrence as the only site of recurrence is unusual.
2. *Multicentric cancer and gastric mucosal 'field change'.* The incidence of stump cancer, even in long-term survivors, is low. However, an important part of the preoperative work-up before a subtotal gastrectomy is careful endoscopic examination and biopsy of the proximal stomach. If this shows evidence of a premalignant field change, there are multiple gastric polyps or the patient has pernicious anaemia then total gastrectomy is advised.[31]
3. *Adequacy of lymphadenectomy.* It has been argued that total gastrectomy allows a more certain D2 lymphadenectomy. The only difficult nodes to remove en bloc in a subtotal gastrectomy are the left paracardial group. It is still possible to resect these nodes, though, since they are positive in less than 5% of distal cancers, there is not really a significant therapeutic advantage in doing so. Survival of these patients with positive left paracardial nodes is very poor and there is no demonstrable therapeutic advantage in doing so in distal cancers.

There are no studies that prove a significant survival benefit for total gastrectomy de principe. Against this is a higher mortality for total gastrectomy which in most Western reports is about twice that of subtotal gastrectomy. Even in the best hands the mortality of total gastrectomy is 5% and is on average nearer 10%. There is an increased risk of long-term nutritional problems after total gastrectomy, particularly in older patients. Quality of life assessments also show that subtotal gastrectomy is significantly better in the long term.

On the basis of the available data there is no support for the concept of total gastrectomy de principe for cancers in the lower half of the stomach.

Lymphadenectomy

Lymph node metastasis is the most common mode of spread in gastric cancer. The pattern of spread should in theory divide into four zones based on the arterial blood supply of the stomach. Detailed pathological studies show that lymphatic involvement is not this predictable, mainly due to the abundant blood and lymphatic plexuses in the submucosal layer of the stomach.[32]

Table 6.2 *Lymph node stations: names and locations of the regional lymph nodes of the stomach*

1.	Right cardiac nodes
2.	Left cardiac nodes
3.	Nodes along the lesser curvature
4.	Nodes along the greater curvature
	4sa – nodes along short gastric arteries
	4sb – nodes along left gastroepiploic artery
	4d – nodes along the right gastroepiploic artery
5.	Suprapyloric nodes
6.	Infrapyloric nodes
7.	Nodes along left gastric artery
8.	Nodes along the common hepatic artery
9.	Coeliac artery nodes
10.	Splenic hilum nodes
11.	Nodes along the splenic artery
12.	Nodes in the hepatoduodenal ligament
13.	Nodes on the posterior of pancreas
14.	Nodes at the root of the mesentery
15.	Nodes on the middle colic artery
16.	Para-aortic nodes
110.	Lower thoracic paraoesophageal nodes
111.	Diaphragmatic nodes

The patterns of lymph node involvement have been extensively investigated by the Japanese. As described in Chapter 3 the nodes have been grouped into 16 stations (Fig. 3.4a and b in Chapter 3) and these are listed in Table 6.2. Studies of large numbers of patients treated at the National Cancer Centre in Tokyo have shown the likelihood of involvement of each node station for cancers in different parts of the stomach[33] (Table 6.3).

In planning the extent of lymphadenectomy two factors have to be considered:

1. The likelihood of metastasis at each node station.
2. The possible survival benefit of removing all nodes at that station.

The Japanese introduced the concept of tiers of lymph nodes with lymphatic spread occurring progressively through the tiers. The tiers are allocated an N number:

N_1 – Perigastric nodes closest to the primary lesion
N_2 – Distant perigastric nodes and the nodes along the main arteries supplying the stomach.
N_3 – Nodes outside the normal lymphatic pathways from the stomach. Involved in advanced stages or by retrograde lymphatic flow due to blockage of normal pathways.

Table 6.3 *Incidence of metastasis at each node station for cancers in the proximal, middle and distal thirds of the stomach. Data from the National Cancer Centre Hospital in Tokyo*[33]

Node station	Risk of nodal metastases for advanced gastric cancers (%)		
	Distal (A)	Middle (M)	Proximal (C)
1	7	16	31
2	0	1	13
3	38	40	39
4	35	31	11
5	12	3	2
6	49	15	3
7	23	22	19
8	25	11	7
9	13	8	13
10	0	2	10
11	4	4	12
12	8	2	1
13–16	(0–5 for all)		

The tiers are different for each third of the stomach (Table 6.4).

The JRSGC database has shown that resection of stations 1 to 12 only produces any worthwhile benefit in terms of 5-year survival. The improvement in survival after removal of stations 13 to 16 is so small that any benefit is almost certainly negated by the increased mortality and morbidity associated with the extended radical resection. The station 12 hepatoduodenal ligament nodes are in the third tier for all thirds of the stomach. These nodes are involved in 9% of lower third and 4% of middle third cancers. Five-year survival rates of up to 25% have been reported in Japan for patients who have had positive station 12 nodes resected. This manoeuvre is probably worthwhile in distal cancers where N_2 nodes appear involved. Some surgeons resect these nodes routinely as part of a D2 resection.

Definition of extent of lymphadenectomy
It is important to understand the nomenclature as all too often the extent of nodal dissection is wrongly described in the literature.

D1 – *Limited lymphadenectomy*: all N_1 nodes removed en bloc with the stomach.

D2 – *Systematic lymphadenectomy*: all N_1 and N_2 nodes removed en bloc with the stomach. If any of the second tier stations are not resected then this is technically a D1 resection, but is sometimes represented as a D1/D2 resection.

D3 – *Extended lymphadenectomy*: a more radical en bloc resection

Table 6.4 *Lymph node tiers according to the rules of the JRSGC*

Location	AMC, MAC MCA, CMA	A AM	MA, M MC	C CM
1st tier (N1)	1	3	3	1
	2	4	4	2
	3	5	5	3
	4	6	6	4s
	5		1	
	6			
2nd tier (N2)	7	7	2*	4d
	8	8	7	7
	9	9	8	8
	10	1	9	9
	11		10*	10
			11	11
				5*
				6*
3rd tier (N3)	12	2	12	12
	13	10	13	13
	14	11	14	14
	110	12		110
	111	13		111
		14		

*Notes: 1. Stations 2 and 10 should be excised in a D2 resection for an MC cancer but are optional for M and MA. 2. Stations 5 and 6 resection is optional for C and CM and if not resected the operation is still classified as a D2 resection.

including the third tier nodes. This more commonly includes only some stations, such as the station 12 nodes, and should be represented as a D2/D3 resection.

In the Japanese Rules for Gastric Cancer Surgery the minimum requirement for an effective resection of gastric cancer is a Systematic D2 Lymphadenectomy.

Lymphadenectomy and cure of gastric cancer
This concept is strictly defined in the Japanese Rules:

Absolute curative resection – The surgical D number is greater than the pathological N number.
Relative curative resection – The D number equals the N number.

Effect of the International Unified TNM Staging System on definition of lymphadenectomy
As explained in Chapter 3 the introduction of the agreed staging system has been important in allowing direct comparison of results of

treatment. It has to be recognised that this introduces certain problems with describing the extent of lymphadenectomy in the precise way practised by the Japanese. It is recommended that the JRSGC Rules are still used for describing the extent of the lymphadenectomy and the TNM system for pathological staging of the cancer.

The case for D2 systematic lymphadenectomy

No aspect of gastric cancer surgery has proved more controversial in recent years. Although the Japanese continue to advocate this as a basic requirement of surgery, surgeons in most other countries have been reluctant to adopt this radical approach. There are two factors to consider:

1. The potential improvement in survival and local control of the disease.
2. The additional mortality and morbidity of more radical surgery.

The evidence can be divided into Japanese and that from other countries.

Japanese evidence

The widespread adoption of systematic lymphadenectomy in Japan was based on comparison of the results of this type of resection with that of historical control data. There are published results of uncontrolled studies comparing different levels of node resection, but no randomised controlled studies. The Japanese are so convinced of the value of radical lymphadenectomy that no trials are presently in progress and indeed there are no plans to do any in the future.

The value of D2 lymphadenectomy is stated to be reduction in gastric bed recurrence leading to a longer disease-free interval and increased survival rate.

The extent of lymphadenectomy correlates well with survival in Japanese studies. Multivariate analysis has shown that this is an independent positive variable for survival.[34] On the basis of historical data it has been claimed that the inclusion of a D2/D3 lymphadenectomy in the surgical treatment of 'curable' gastric cancer has doubled the survival rate.[35] There are many other Japanese reports of improved survival after D2 compared with lesser resections.[36,37] As shown in Table 6.5 this applies for all stages of the disease, although as previously explained this simple type of analysis does not take into account the more accurate pathological staging that is inevitable in more extensive nodal resections.

One of the only ways to extract information about the benefit of systematic lymphadenectomy from the Japanese studies is to compare the survival difference for patients with N_1 node involvement only. An incomplete D1 (D0) resection produces a 4% 5YSR, rising to 46% for a D1 resection and with a further 10% benefit for a D2 resection.[38] Importantly this emphasises the value of complete resection of the first

Table 6.5 *Five-year survival related to stage of gastric cancer. New unified TNM categories, % survivors*

Stage	TNM	5YSR (%)
IA	$pT_1\ pN_0\ M_0$	99
IB	$pT_1\ pN_1\ M_0$	90
	$pT_2\ pN_0\ M_0$	88
II	$pT_1\ pN_2\ M_0$	79
	$pT_2\ pN_1\ M_0$	71
	$pT_3\ pN_0\ M_0$	69
IIIA	$pT_2\ pN_2\ M_0$	52
	$pT_3\ pN_1\ M_0$	46
	$pT_4\ pN_0\ M_0$	52
IIIB	$pT_3\ pN_2\ M_0$	23
	$pT_4\ pN_1\ M_0$	26
	$pT_4\ pN_2\ M_0$	16
IV	M_1	10

node tier. It also reveals a modest, but definite, advantage in removing the second tier if only first tier nodes are involved. There is also increasing evidence of an improvement in survival of node-negative (N_0) patients after D2 lymphadenectomy.[39] This seems to be explained by the failure of standard histological stains to identify micrometastases in nodes.[40] It is likely that a proportion of node-negative cases should be classified as having node-positive disease.

It must also be realised that specialist Japanese units report a mortality of 2–3% for gastrectomy with D2 lymphadenectomy. Morbidity is also low, though increased significantly when removal of node stations 10 and 11 is involved if this requires splenectomy and distal pancreatectomy.

Non-Japanese evidence

Many Western surgeons have been unable to reproduce the beneficial effects of radical lymphadenectomy. In attempting to emulate Japanese practice they have encountered higher mortality and morbidity rates than for less radical operations. However, there are now reports from specialist centres in the USA, UK and Europe of D2 lymphadenectomy results that are much closer to those reported from Japan.[11,20,41] More importantly there are a number of prospective controlled studies comparing the different operative strategies. These provide valuable evidence for the role of radical node dissection in gastric cancer surgery.

Table 6.6 *Results of the German gastric cancer study*[42]

	D1 Group Standard node dissection (*n* = 558)	D2 Group Extended node dissection (*n* = 1096)
Morbidity and mortality		
30 day mortality	5.2%	5.0%
Anastomotic leak	8.2%	8.0%
Serious sepsis	3.2%	4.7%
Cardiopulmonary complications	9.5%	9.3%
5 year survival		
Stage IA	86%	86%
Stage IB	72%	69%
Stage II	27%	55%*
Stage IIIA	25%	38%**
Stage IIIB	25%	17%

All results statistically insignificant except: * $P < 0.001$; ** $P < 0.03$.

German gastric cancer study[42]

A prospective but non-randomised study/audit of the practice of D1 and D2 lymphadenectomy was carried out in specialist German surgical units between 1986 and 1989. The definition of a radical nodal resection was based on the number of nodes retrieved from the specimen rather than the surgeon's description or analysis of node stations. This definition is obviously open to question. The overall survival results are shown in Table 6.6. Multivariate analysis revealed that D2 lymphadenectomy was an independent positive factor for survival. More detailed analysis showed that this only applied for those patients who were N_0 or N_1 and not N_2 – this also explains why a significant survival benefit was only detected for stages II and IIIA. Interestingly the Japanese have produced very similar results from the same type of analysis.[33]

There was no significant difference in mortality and morbidity between the two types of resection, though the results were not as good as those from Japan. As previously discussed this is at least partly due to the greater age and higher incidence of concomitant disease in European patients.

Cape Town D1 versus D2 study[43]

This was a small prospective randomised study comparing the results of 21 patients undergoing a D1 resection with 22 having a D2 resection for potentially curable gastric cancer. There was no survival difference between the groups at 3.1 years. There was a significantly higher incidence of complications, greater transfusion requirement and longer hospital stay in the D2 group.

Chinese University of Hong Kong D1 versus D3 study[44]

This was a small prospective randomised trial of 55 patients undergoing either D1 subtotal or D3 total gastrectomy with distal pancreatectomy and splenectomy for resectable cancer in the distal half of the stomach. There was no survival advantage for those undergoing the more radical operation. As with the Cape Town study there was a significantly higher complication rate (particularly related to the splenic and pancreatic resection), greater transfusion requirement and longer hospital stay in the D3 group. It should be noted that the Japanese do not recommend routine resection of the spleen and pancreas for node stations 10 and 11 in distal cancers.

Both this and the Cape Town study involved too few patients to demonstrate a statistically significant difference in survival for more radical surgery. However, both confirmed the increased dangers of radical surgery.

Dutch gastric cancer trial[45]

This multicentre prospective randomised trial comparing D1 and D2 lymphadenectomy involved 33 surgical departments coordinated by Leiden University Hospital and recruited 593 patients in each limb. Because most Dutch surgeons were not familiar with the D2 operation a Japanese surgeon from the National Cancer Centre in Tokyo taught and supervised 8 coordinating surgeons who then continued the supervision of the other participating surgeons.

The five-year survival figures will not be available until 1998. At the time of publication in 1995 there was no survival difference. The other important comparisons showed:

	D1	D2
Perioperative mortality (%)	4	10
Significant complications (%)	25	43
Median hospital stay (days)	18	25

Pathological assessment of resected lymph nodes demonstrated the difficulty in adhering rigidly to the JRSGC Rules. A considerable number of patients who had undergone D2 resections had absence of node groups that should have been resected and in the D1 patients there were nodes present that should not have been resected. It is possible that this 'contamination' of the randomised groups may have affected the survival results. Importantly many of the participating surgeons only contributed relatively small numbers of patients at a time when they were still in their 'learning curve' for the D2 operation. This factor may have affected the completeness of the nodal resection and is also likely to have contributed to the increased mortality and morbidity of the more radical operation. This has been refuted by the coordinating surgeons, but nevertheless must be taken into account and is still being debated.

MRC Gastric Cancer Surgical Trial (STO1)[46]

This was a prospective randomised multicentre study comparing D1 and D2 lymphadenectomy with 200 patients in each limb. Uniformity of surgical technique was ensured by the use of standardised descriptions and videos and by monitoring surgeons' reports. This quality control was not nearly as rigorous as that employed in the Dutch Trial. The pathological analysis is also still incomplete. Five-year survival figures are not yet available, but on the basis of survival figures so far it is stated that the detection of a survival benefit for D2 resection is unlikely. The mortality and incidence of adverse events are remarkably similar to the Dutch Trial and also appear related to resection of the spleen and pancreas. It was also accepted that many of the surgeons were in their 'learning curve' for the D2 operation.

	D1	D2
Perioperative mortality (%)	6.5	13
Overall morbidity (%)	28	46
Median (range) hospital stay (days)	14 (6–101)	14 (10–147)

Summary

1. At present there is no evidence from randomised trials that D2 resection confers a survival benefit over D1 resection. None of these trials are from Japan and a major criticism is the lack of experience of the participating surgeons in the D2 technique.

2. Results of non-randomised studies from Japan and other countries, including Germany, strongly support a survival benefit for D2 resection. Analysis of results suggest that the benefit is largely confined to those with N_0 and N_1 disease. The increase in 5-year survival is most obvious for stages II and IIIA.

3. Comparison of results for the TNM stages does not allow for the 'stage migration phenomenon' related to more extensive nodal resection. The relative contributions of the surgical effort and correct pathological staging have not been determined.

4. It is believed that resection of second tier nodes should decrease the incidence of local recurrence in the gastric bed in node-positive patients.

5. The mortality and morbidity of D2 resection is higher than D1 resection. In all countries this is particularly related to removal of the spleen and distal pancreas. In the West there are the additional factors of the age and general health of gastric cancer patients. Another important factor may be the relative inexperience of many surgeons in radical gastric cancer surgery.

Conclusion

Gastrectomy with D2 resection should presently only be performed by surgeons with proven experience of this type of radical surgery.

The balance of evidence supports the use of a D2 or modified D2 lymphadenectomy in stages II and IIIA. Those who are serosa-positive or have N_2 nodal involvement will require adjuvant (or preferably neoadjuvant) chemotherapy.[12] The role of radical surgery in stages IIIB and IV disease has yet to be defined. It may achieve a decrease in local recurrence in the gastric bed and thus a prolonged symptom-free interval, but almost certainly does not significantly improve the chance of cure. The place of D2 resection in patients with stage I disease is not proven, but given the higher incidence of node-positive early cases in the West, rational use in younger and fitter patients is strongly recommended at present.[3,47] The continued use of radical surgery in apparently node-negative cases is also supported by recent research.[40]

The future trend will be towards radical operations tailored to the preoperative and operative staging of each case.[48] Improvements in staging techniques should allow a more rational approach to specific node station resections based on the likelihood of involvement and the potential benefit of en bloc removal of each station. The place of splenic and pancreatic removal as part of a radical lymphadenectomy is now debatable and discussed at length in the next two sections.

Splenectomy

The addition of a splenectomy increases the rate of septic and thrombo-embolic complications after a gastrectomy. It also affects the immunological response to certain bacteria and possibly to gastric cancer.[49] However, this is controversial and a recent study has found that splenectomy is not an independent variable for postoperative septic problems.[50] The evidence for a long lasting adverse immuno-logical effect in cancer patients is theoretical rather than proven. There are both univariate and multivariate analyses that suggest a negative prognostic effect in all stages of gastric cancer except possibly stage IV.[51] However, there are also studies that have not confirmed an independent effect on survival.[52] In view of these concerns there is an increasing trend to avoid splenectomy unless specifically indicated.

Indications for splenectomy

Direct invasion of spleen or tail of pancreas
If all macroscopic disease can be resected and the operation is potentially curative then en bloc splenectomy or pancreatosplenectomy is worthwhile. If the operation is obviously palliative then the likely benefit of splenectomy has to be weighed against the increased morbidity and mortality associated with splenectomy.

Removal of splenic hilum (station 10) lymph nodes
There are two factors to consider.

1. The likelihood of station 10 nodal metastases. There are several excellent Japanese papers documenting the incidence of splenic nodal metastases in advanced gastric cancer.[33,51,53] The summarised mean incidence for the different parts of the stomach are: distal

third (A), < 1%; middle third (M), 10%; upper third (C) 15–20%; and whole stomach, 25%. This analysis can be further refined for proximal cancers by taking into account whether the cancer involves the greater curve, in which case positive nodes are more likely.[33] The incidence of nodal involvement is also related to the depth of invasion and is significantly lower in T_1 and T_2 cancers.

2. The likely survival benefit of removing all station 10 nodes. Even if the splenic nodes are removed the survival of patients with distal cancers and positive station 10 nodes is minimal. In proximal cancers with positive nodes the 5-year survival is up to 25% in the National Cancer Centre in Tokyo.[33]

The indications for splenectomy as part of a radical lymphadenectomy have been tightened in recent years. This should only be considered for cancers in the upper stomach and probably even then restricted to cancers involving the greater curve and fundus of the stomach. In view of the suspected adverse immunological effects of splenectomy in the earlier stages of gastric cancer there is now a good case for not removing the splenic hilar nodes in T_1 or T_2 cancers. Evidence from randomised trials is awaited.

Clearance of station 10 nodes with splenic preservation

This was previously thought not to be feasible. The Japanese have reported a technique of dissecting out the splenic hilar nodes and have confirmed removal of all lymphatic tissue.[54] This technique is still controversial in Japan and there are doubts that the technique can be consistently performed in Western patients. In view of the limited indications for removal of station 10 nodes the real question is not whether the procedure can be done, but whether it is necessary. At present splenic hilar dissection should only be attempted by specialists with training in this technique, until of proven value in Western patients.

Distal pancreatectomy

En bloc pancreatic resection is associated with a significant increase in morbidity and mortality when compared with gastrectomy with or without splenectomy. This has been consistently demonstrated in studies of radical gastric surgery in the West. Complications include pancreatic leakage, abscess formation, fistula and acute pancreatitis. A few patients will become diabetic after distal pancreatectomy. The complications of the associated splenectomy have to be added to those of the pancreatic resection.

Indications for distal pancreatectomy

In view of the high complication rate the indications for resection of the left side of the pancreas have to be carefully analysed.

Direct invasion of tail of pancreas
As previously discussed this should only be contemplated if all macroscopic disease will be removed.

Removal of splenic artery (station 11) lymph nodes
There are two factors to consider.

1. The likelihood of station 11 nodal metastases. About 10% of patients with proximal cancers have positive splenic artery nodes. As with station 10 nodes the highest incidence is seen with greater curve and advanced cancers. In some patients only the nodes closest to the coeliac trunk are involved, this being due to retrograde lymphatic spread rather than antegrade spread along the normal lymphatic pathway. This type of involvement is seen in advanced cancers affecting any part of the stomach and should correctly be staged as N2+. In such cases resection of the nodes around the origin of the artery may reduce local gastric bed recurrence and increase the disease-free interval, but there is no evidence that it will improve the chance of curing the patient.
2. The likely survival benefit of removing all station 11 nodes. The 5-year survival of patients undergoing resection of positive splenic artery nodes is reported to be 15–20% in Japan.[33]

The decision to resect station 10 and 11 nodes, necessitating distal pancreatectomy and splenectomy, has to be made with the realisation that in Western gastric cancer practice the cost–benefit ratio is at best only marginal. This procedure is not indicated for cancers in the distal half of the stomach, though nodes around the origin of the splenic artery may be excised as part of a radical excision of the coeliac trunk nodes. En bloc pancreatic excision should now only be considered in the younger and fitter patient with an advanced proximal cancer where a lesser procedure is anticipated to leave residual cancer. It should also be considered in patients with proximal cancers in whom operative staging has shown the probable involvement of splenic hilar nodes.

Pancreas-preserving gastrectomy

This has been described in Japan for excision of station 11 nodes in patients with proximal cancers.[55] It requires splenectomy as the splenic artery and accompanying nodes are dissected off the pancreas and the artery ligated at its origin. Lymphangiographic studies show that the splenic artery lymphatics lie within the subserosal space on the upper and posterior aspect of the pancreas and never within the parenchyma. The arterial supply to the distal pancreas is adequate from the transverse pancreatic artery after ligation of the splenic artery. Preservation of the pancreas significantly reduces the incidence of postoperative complications. There is increasing experience with this technique in Japan. It is contraindicated if there is direct invasion of the pancreas. There is concern that this type of dissection would be difficult to perform consistently in Western patients. At present this procedure should only be attempted by those with specialist training and in a research setting.

Extended resections

The concept of gastric cancer remaining a locoregional disease with relatively late distant spread has already been discussed. It is theoretically possible that in some patients with locally advanced disease it is still possible to produce prolonged survival and perhaps cure by radical surgery, though such cases have to be carefully selected.[56] Extended resection is defined as any dissection beyond a D2 subtotal or total gastrectomy. It is advocated by the Japanese for resectable advanced cancers with no evidence of distant spread.[37]

There are two categories of extended resection to be considered.

En bloc resection of involved adjacent organs

This can occur in two different ways:

1. *Intramural spread* either by direct growth or via lymphatics into the oesophagus or duodenum. Extending the resection margin either proximally or distally is certainly worthwhile as cure is still possible.
2. *Transmural spread* into adjacent organs, e.g. pancreas, spleen, left lobe of liver and transverse mesocolon. Pathological assessment in cases of apparent invasion shows that in about one-third the adherence to another organ is inflammatory rather than neoplastic. Trial dissection and intraoperative biopsy must not be attempted as there is risk of disseminating malignant cells. Resection of the adjacent organ is thus recommended provided the patient is fit enough to undergo the extended procedure. If the patient is unfit or too elderly for a radical excision than gastrectomy is still worthwhile as about a third will still have a clear lateral resection margin.

The results of surgical series of extended resections must be interpreted with care. Transmural spread has a much worse prognosis than intramural spread and series may include different proportions of each.[57] It is also important to determine whether the report includes only patients with pathological confirmation of transmural invasion or all patients with adherence to adjacent organs. It is not entirely surprising that late analysis of the results of extended resection has produced conflicting results. Overall it appears that there is a small survival advantage, but this is only realised if operative mortality is minimised in what are usually very major operations.[58,59] The risks in older patients and those with concomitant diseases must be carefully weighed against the potential survival benefit.[60] Extended resection should only be considered when there will be no evidence of macroscopic residual disease (R0, no residual disease; R1, microscopic residual disease; R2, macroscopic residual disease) after the resection. It must be remembered that these more advanced gastric cancers are almost inevitably node-positive and the minimum level of node dissection in an extended resection should be a D2 lymphadenectomy.[42]

Extended lymphadenectomy
Removal of node stations 13–16 has only been reported to be of benefit in Japan.[37] Resection of third and fourth tier nodes does potentially decrease the risk of gastric bed recurrence and prolong the symptom-free interval. It is uncertain whether this potential benefit is worthwhile in Western patients because of the increased risks of radical resection. It is unlikely that D3 or D4 resections are of any benefit except perhaps in younger patients with T_4 disease. Such patients are more likely to benefit from adjuvant therapy and so at present the place of extended lymphadenectomy remains uncertain.

Super-extended radical gastrectomy
This most radical gastric resection is otherwise known as a left upper quadrant evisceration. It has been advocated for advanced cancers in the proximal stomach and in cancers with invasion of adjacent organs in an attempt to minimise the risk of local recurrence and improve survival.[61]

Limited gastric resections

In the elderly or unfit patient it is reasonable to consider a less radical gastric resection, accepting that although the chance of cure may be reduced there is a lower mortality and serious morbidity rate and a lower incidence of nutritional sequelae. As has already been discussed the value of radical surgery revolves around the cost–benefit issue. Surgeons producing the best results are those who are able to appreciate this and select the appropriate operation for each patient.

In Western practice most limited operations are palliative as cancers tend to be advanced and node-positive. However, in Japan the concept of a reduced or limited resection with curative intent is much more important because of the high incidence of screened early gastric cancers. Early cancers have a much lower rate of nodal metastasis and resection without lymphadenectomy may be a 'relative curative' procedure. In Japan the incidence of positive nodes is 3–5% in cancers confined to the mucosa, but rises to 16–25% for cancers invading the submucosa.[61] The accurate identification of mucosal lesions is said to be possible with endoscopic ultrasound and so a subgroup of patients can be selected for limited resection who may be cured. It must be emphasised that the node-positive rate, especially in early cancers penetrating the submucosa, may be much higher in the West and so limited surgery may not be a logical option in patients being treated with curative intent.[47]

A detailed description of the many different operations described for limited resection of early cancers is not necessary, but they can be simply classified under the following headings.

Endoscopic resection

This is only used for mucosal cancers which can either be destroyed by laser or resected via the endoscope. The latter technique has the advantage that resection margins can be assessed. Laser treatment is easier and quicker and is recommended for the elderly and particularly those with multifocal disease who may need repeated treatments. Careful endoscopic monitoring is mandatory after this type of treatment and it remains controversial. It is stated that all mucosal lesions of < 10 mm diameter and all type I protruding early cancers of < 20 mm diameter may be safely resected endoscopically.[62] Although the mortality of such procedures is extremely low, even in the elderly and unfit, it has been emphasised that the long-term results are not yet known and have yet to be compared with radical surgery in younger patients.

Gastric resection

This includes wedge excision and partial gastrectomy with or without nodal dissection. Various pylorus-preserving procedures have been described for middle third and proximal cancers.[63] Recently there have been a considerable number of reports of laparascopic-assisted limited resections.[64,65] These operations still require an abdominal incision and advocates of minimal incision surgery argue that open limited surgery can be achieved more rapidly and safely and at a lower cost.

There is no doubt that quality of life is better after limited gastric resections and particularly in terms of postprandial symptoms and nutritional sequelae. Comparative studies with radical surgery are in progress in some centres in Japan. A recent survey showed that the majority of cancer centres in Japan now use some form of limited resection for older and less fit patients. This finding alone suggests this is a viable treatment option. Use of these procedures in the West will be limited by the low incidence of early gastric cancer and the higher incidence of nodal spread in such cases. The increasing use of endoscopic ultrasound may open up this treatment option for older Western patients with both early and advanced cancers.

Technique of gastric resection with D2 lymphadenectomy

The aim of this section is not to provide a detailed operative manual, but to summarise the basic steps of the main procedures. More detailed descriptions that can be recommended are those by McCulloch[66] and Craven.[67] Both are strongly influenced by the work of Keiichi Maruyama from the National Cancer Centre in Tokyo.

Incision

Gastric cancers below the cardia can be resected via an upper midline incision. In obese or heavily built patients it is usually necessary to extend the incision below the umbilicus to gain adequate exposure and room to operate. Some surgeons use a left thoracoabdominal approach for radical excision of the upper stomach, but there is an increased morbidity and mortality associated with disrupting the left costal margin and diaphragm and entering the left chest. This type of approach should be reserved for cancers in the cardia where it is necessary to resect more than 5 cm of the lower oesophagus to obtain adequate proximal clearance. Increasingly those with specialist experience are using the abdominal transhiatal approach described for transhiatal oesophagectomy.[68] This involved excision of the crura and oesophagophrenic ligament en bloc with the cardia. In addition, the diaphragm is divided anterior to the hiatal opening thus allowing a wide exposure of the lower mediastinum. With appropriate retraction it is possible to resect 6–8 cm of lower oesophagus together with associated lymphatic tissue.

Intraoperative staging

This has been discussed in detail in Chapter 3. Meticulous staging is essential in deciding the appropriate type of resection and lymphadenectomy. Evidence of serosal invasion, invasion of an adjacent organ, peritoneal seedlings, apparent nodal involvement beyond the second tier and liver metastases must be sought. If any of these is found the radical surgery alone may not cure the patient and a decision has to be made about whether to proceed with the planned dissection, modify the operation with a view to adjuvant therapy or to opt for a lesser palliative procedure. Some additional intraoperative investigations may be helpful in making this decision.

Peritoneal cytology

This is widely used in Japan. The finding of free malignant cells in the absence of macroscopic peritoneal seedlings is now an indication for the additional use of intra- and postoperative intraperitoneal chemotherapy in Japan. This treatment modality is now being investigated in the West where, in view of the higher incidence of T_3 and T_4 cancers, it is likely to become more widely used. Washings are taken from the pelvis before any dissection is started (or preferably at staging laparoscopy). Cells are not detected pre- or intraoperatively when the serosa is intact. More than a third of patients with macroscopic evidence of serosal penetration will have malignant cells detectable in their peritoneal washings.[69] Survival is significantly shorter in the positive cases and this finding is a strong indication for the use of adjuvant early postoperative intraperitoneal chemotherapy.

Frozen-section histology of lymph nodes

It must be stressed that if a D2 resection is being contemplated then no node in the first or second tier should be sampled as all lymphatic tissue must be taken en bloc. If there are nodes in the third or fourth tiers that appear involved these should be sampled as this level of spread is now regarded as distant metastasis and may be a contraindication to D2 resection. The trend towards splenic and pancreatic preservation has led to the dilemma of deciding whether to sample enlarged nodes at stations 10 and 11. In the younger fitter patient it is probably best to proceed with an en bloc radical resection rather than disrupt the lymphatic pathways. In the older or less fit patient the additional risks of splenectomy and distal pancreatectomy make node sampling worthwhile if these organs do not need to be resected as part of the lymphadenectomy.

Frozen-section histology of other tissue

As previously stated apparent direct invasion from the stomach into another organ should not be sampled for fear of disseminating cancer cells. In some diffuse cancers there may be concern about the proximal or distal resection margin and histological assessment may be helpful. In elderly or unfit patients undergoing potentially curative limited resections of the stomach, sampling of the resection margin may be necessary. Any lesions or seedlings found at distant sites in the peritoneal cavity should be sent for histology.

Liver biopsy

Any lesions palpated in the liver or detected with intraoperative ultrasound should be sampled before progressing to a radical operation.

Operative strategy after staging

Three types of resection are considered:

1. Subtotal D2 gastrectomy
2. Total D1/D2 gastrectomy without splenectomy and distal pancreatectomy
3. Total D2 gastrectomy with splenectomy and distal pancreatectomy

Variations on these procedures and extended or limited versions may all be indicated in certain circumstances. These three operations fulfil the requirements for radical treatment of gastric cancer in the majority of patients and are the basic armaments of the specialist gastric cancer surgeon. The initial part of the dissection is common to all three procedures.

Initial dissection

1. Mobilise hepatic flexure of colon and fully Kocherise the duodenum and head of pancreas. This allows examination of retropancreatic and para-aortic nodes.
2. Mobilise splenic flexure of colon and carefully divide any adhesions between omentum and spleen so that the capsule is not torn during the dissection.
3. Separate the greater omentum from the transverse colon along a bloodless line about 1 cm from the bowel. This plane of dissection

is continued onto the anterior leaf of the transverse mesocolon. This leaf can be completely separated from the posterior leaf so that the lesser sac remains intact. This is not always an easy dissection in Western patients and requires some patience. It is especially important for cancers that breach the serosa of the posterior wall of the stomach. The line of dissection continues between the peritoneum over the pancreas and the gland itself and care must be taken not to damage the parenchyma.

4. At the right side this line of dissection leads onto the right gastroepiploic vessels and subpyloric nodes. These nodes are swept up on the vessels which are bared and ligated at their origins.

5. The lesser omentum is divided along the line of the reflection on the liver capsule. There is usually an accessory left hepatic artery in the omentum and this should be ligated close to the liver. The line of dissection is continued upwards proximally over the oesophagogastric junction to include the oesophagophrenic ligament and, in cancers of the cardia, part of the diaphragm. Distally the line of dissection passes down the peritoneum over the hepatoduodenal ligament to the upper border of the duodenum.

6. At this stage the surgeon should perform the optional dissection of the lymphatic tissue in the hepatoduodenal ligament (station 12) nodes. This is only done for cancers in the lower half of the stomach and particularly if there is evidence of involvement of the suprapyloric or common hepatic nodes. The dissection starts at the reflection of the peritoneum in the porta hepatis and includes the peritoneum and all lymphatic tissue from both front and back of the bile ducts, common and right and left hepatic arteries and the portal vein down to the neck of the pancreas. The gall bladder may be removed as part of this dissection.

7. Whether or not the hepatoduodenal ligament has been dissected out, the line of dissection brings the surgeon down onto the common hepatic artery and the origin of the often insubstantial right gastric artery. This is ligated at its origin taking care not to damage or occlude the hepatic artery.

8. The first part of the duodenum is now freed from the head of the pancreas. There are several small vessels running between the gastroduodenal and superior pancreatoduodenal arteries and the duodenal wall. It is important to ligate these individually and not use diathermy in this area as both the pancreas and duodenum can suffer damage leading to leakage. The duodenum should be divided at least 2 cm distal to the pylorus – a wider margin is needed for cancers in the distal stomach. The duodenal stump should be as short as possible and whether closed by suture or staples it is a wise step to invert the closure line with interrupted seromuscular sutures.

9. Lifting the distal stomach up and to the left, the dissection of the lymphatics and peritoneum on the posterior wall of the lesser sac is continued to the left. This includes the tissue on the upper border

of the body of the pancreas, along the common hepatic artery and to the left of the portal vein. Troublesome bleeding is often encountered near the pancreas and the left gastric vein sometimes passes down behind the upper border of the pancreas to the splenic vein. Great care is needed in this area and again vessels should be ligated or transfixed rather then diathermised close to pancreatic parenchyma. The retroperitoneal nodes to the left of the portal vein tend to bleed quite profusely and dissection of these nodes should only be contemplated for upper third cancers – in other cases the peritoneal dissection is continued up onto the posterior aspect of the proximal lesser curve thus exposing the right crus of the diaphragm. Inferiorly the dissection reaches the junction of common hepatic and splenic arteries on the upper border of the pancreas.

10. The lymphatic tissue around the origin of the splenic artery is divided and swept up towards the left gastric artery if the operation is for a distal cancer or if the spleen and pancreas are not to be removed. The nodal tissue around the coeliac trunk is carefully dissected off the artery trying to avoid entering the tough neural and fibrous tissue around the origin of the trunk on the anterior aorta. All this tissue is swept upwards with the lymphatic tissue on the left gastric artery. The left gastric artery is then ligated at its origin leaving the distal coeliac trunk and the origins of the common hepatic and splenic arteries bared completely. The left gastric vein is variable and there may be more than one – it is ligated as found.

At this point the operation strategy depends on the extent of the planned reaction.

Subtotal gastrectomy

All the tissue on the proximal lesser curve from the oesophagogastric junction downwards should be removed with the left gastric pedicle. This starts with ligation of the ascending branch of the artery and vein at the hiatus. Small vessels passing to the stomach wall are individually ligated. If involved nodes are detected in this tissue it is preferable to do a total gastrectomy. There is great debate about the left cardial nodes, but the author's view is that when the patient with a distal cancer has involvement of this node group the resection has no chance of being curative. The effort needed and the small chance of damaging the proximal short gastric vessels during the dissection make it not worthwhile.

The final part of the dissection involves separating the left side of the greater omentum from the splenic flexure of the colon and following the line of resection up to the lower pole of the spleen. The dissection of the anterior leaf of the mesocolon is completed between the middle colic vessels and the splenic flexure. This continues over the distal pancreas up towards the hilum of the spleen. At this point the left gastroepiploic vessels are identified with the artery being the first branch of the splenic artery visible at the hilum. The inferior two or three short

Figure 6.2 *(a) D2 subtotal gastrectomy; (b) D2 total gastrectomy with preservation of spleen and pancreas.*

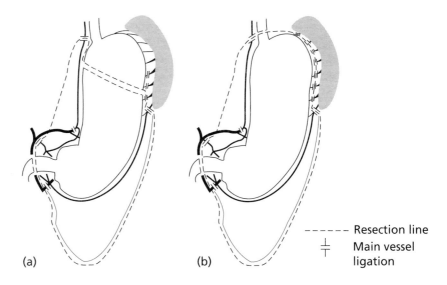

- - - - - - Resection line
+ Main vessel
ligation

(a)   (b)

gastric arteries are also ligated nearer to the stomach to allow full mobilisation of the greater curve. The blood supply of the stomach remnant is entirely from the proximal short gastric arteries (Fig. 6.2).

Total gastrectomy without splenectomy and distal pancreatectomy

The resection is the same thus far. The ligation of the short gastric arteries should be as close to the hilum as is safe. In order to achieve this it is best to divide the peritoneum (lienorenal ligament) lateral to the spleen and mobilise the spleen and tail of pancreas. If there appear to be involved nodes in the hilum, the splenic artery and vein should be dissected off the tail of the pancreas, transfixed and divided so removing the spleen with the stomach.

The nodal dissection is continued up the front of the aorta from the coeliac trunk up into the hiatus, the assistant lifting the stomach up to allow a good view of this area. Two significant vessels are encountered in removing this tissue en bloc with the stomach. The first is the posterior gastric or short gastric artery which passes to the posterior proximal stomach from the splenic artery. The other is the left phrenic artery which should be divided near the upper border of the left adrenal gland to allow the left cardial nodal tissue to be dissected completely off the left crus. The left subphrenic branch of this vessel is divided as it reaches the diaphragm so freeing the lymphatic tissue on the left aspect of the oesophagogastric junction. It is often not realised that the cardia is retroperitoneal in this area and the resection must include all the tissue in the triangle between the upper border of the tail of the pancreas, the left crus and the upper pole of the spleen. Both vagi and the other small vessels around the lower oesophagus are divided so that the stomach is attached only by the oesophagus itself. The length of oesophagus mobilised depends on the resection margin required. The transhiatal approach for cardia cancers has already been described (Fig. 6.2).

Total gastrectomy with splenectomy and distal pancreatectomy

Resection of the spleen and pancreas via an abdominal incision is not technically easy because of limited space. One commonly used manoeuvre is to divide the peritoneum laterally and mobilise the spleen and distal pancreas to the right. The alternative is to mobilise the pancreas where the splenic artery joins it and to divide the pancreas, artery and vein at this point. The dissection is then continued to the left posterior to the pancreas until the lienorenal ligament is divided so freeing the spleen. The dissection is then continued up in the retroperitoneum above the tail of the pancreas as described. When the decision has been made to do a complete D2 resection for a proximal cancer the author finds this latter manoeuvre easier and less bloody than mobilisation of the spleen and pancreas to the right with the limited exposure provided by an abdominal approach. An essential step in the distal pancreatectomy is ligation of the pancreatic duct.

This completes the description of a D2 resection. The next section describes the principles and techniques of reconstruction.

Reconstruction after gastric resection

The stomach is a complex organ that functions as a reservoir for ingested food and is involved in digestion and absorption. One of the most important functions is the ability to dilate to accommodate a meal without a marked rise in intraluminal pressure. However, the most important function is the release of food to the small intestine at a controlled rate that allows adequate mixing with bile and pancreatic juices and does not overwhelm the digestive and absorptive capacity of the small intestine. Control of the rate of delivery of the stomach contents to the small intestine requires an intact and innervated pylorus. Gastric emptying is regulated by a complex neurohumoral feedback from the small intestine. Any gastric resection interferes with all these functions – the aim of the reconstruction is to minimise the disturbance to the upper gastrointestinal physiology.

The two main dangers for a patient undergoing a major gastric resection for cancer are recurrence of the cancer and significant malnutrition. There is a tendency to concentrate mainly on the former and to forget that weight loss and inadequate absorption of essential nutrients can severely affect quality of life after gastrectomy. In recognising that many patients will not be cured by radical surgery it is most important to maximise quality of life while the patient is free of symptomatic recurrence. This is achieved by appropriate reconstruction of the upper gastrointestinal tract and then close follow-up of nutritional status.

The aims of reconstruction are as follows.

1. The construction of the least complex anastomosis to allow adequate nutritional intake.
2. The procedure should be safe and not add to the mortality and morbidity of the gastric resection.
3. The alteration in upper gastrointestinal physiology should be minimised.
4. The reconstruction should not be prone to long-term complications such as bacterial overgrowth.
5. Reflux of bile and alkaline duodenal juices into the oesophagus should be prevented.
6. It should not obstruct at an early stage if there is a gastric bed recurrence.

Reconstructions can be broadly divided into two groups: duodenal bypass and duodenal continuity.

Duodenal bypass

The duodenal stump is closed and the proximal jejunum used to provide continuity. This results in a less physiological mixing of food with bile and pancreatic enzymes and a significant alteration in neuro-humoral feedback from the duodenum. This latter abnormality is not so important after excision of the antrum and pylorus and in any case is probably more important in theory than in reality. The best clinical results are obtained using the Roux-en-Y technique with a 40–60 cm limb of proximal jejunum. There are many variations on this technique, but the important thing is that all prevent the reflux of duodenal contents into the gastric remnant and oesophagus. The disadvantage of a Roux reconstruction is that this segment of proximal jejunum is important for optimum digestion and absorption, but food passing through it has not mixed with bile and pancreatic enzymes. Use of a long jejunal loop instead of a Roux limb 'wastes' even more proximal jejunum and, unless a very long loop is used, is associated with a higher incidence of bile reflux problems.

Duodenal continuity

This is maintained by either joining the gastric remnant to the duodenal stump or interposing a segment of proximal jejunum between the oesophagus or gastric remnant and the duodenal stump. This allows a more physiological mixing of food with bile and enzymes, though this is by no means normal because of the rapid passage of unprepared food through the duodenum. The main disadvantages are an increased risk of symptomatic bile and alkaline reflux and a higher rate of postoperative complications, particularly with the more complex interposition procedures. This type of procedure is not advisable for locally advanced cancers which tend to recur in the gastric bed and may lead to early obstruction of the anastomoses or

Figure 6.3
Reconstruction after gastrectomy.

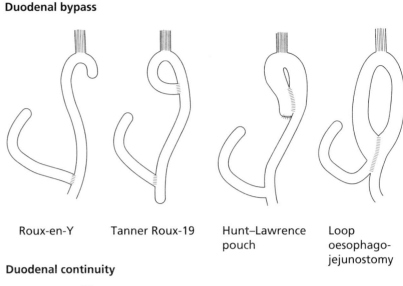

Duodenal bypass

Roux-en-Y   Tanner Roux-19   Hunt–Lawrence pouch   Loop oesophago-jejunostomy

Duodenal continuity

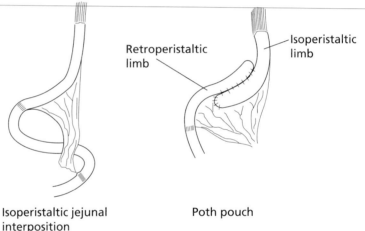

Isoperistaltic jejunal interposition   Poth pouch

interposed jejunum. Cuschieri[69] gives a very good account of these procedures which is recommended.

Examples of the various reconstruction procedures for subtotal and total gastrectomy are shown in Fig. 6.3.

Jejunal pouch reconstruction

The most common symptom after total gastrectomy is early satiety. This restricts food intake and makes it difficult for patients to maintain an adequate calorie intake. Various operations have been devised to increase the reservoir capacity of the proximal jejunum. Initially such operations were used as remedial procedures in patients with severe restriction of intake or with disabling postprandial symptoms. They are now used routinely by some gastric cancer surgeons, either as modifications of the Roux limb or as formal jejunum pouches.[70]

Despite the theoretical advantages of these operations there is no good evidence that they significantly improve nutrition.[71] Rigorous dietetic surveillance is probably of more value than the actual type of reconstruction in ensuring optimal nutrition after a gastrectomy.[72,73]

Early post-operative complications

As with any abdominal surgical procedure these can be divided into general complications and those specifically associated with gastric resection and reconstruction. The general complications of major gastric surgery are covered in Chapter 4. The complication rate is higher after total gastrectomy and particularly if the spleen and distal pancreas have been resected. A basic principle in radical gastric surgery is to recognise complications early and deal with them in a proactive way. This is especially important for intra-abdominal complications within the first few days of surgery. One of the important lessons learnt from the Japanese is to 'look and see' rather than 'wait and see'. A second-look laparotomy when the patient is still stable is considerably safer than waiting until the condition of the patient has deteriorated. An early operation may allow correction of the problem whereas a delay may make this impossible.

The following are the more common intra-abdominal complications specific to gastrectomy for cancer.

Haemorrhage

This may be reactive, within the first few hours of surgery, or secondary, caused by partially or inadequately treated intraabdominal sepsis. Early relaparotomy is advocated for definite or even suspected reactive haemorrhage. It must be remembered that drains can occlude with blood clot and the clinical suspicion of bleeding in a haemodynamically unstable patient is sufficient indication to operate. Even if the bleeding stops spontaneously the presence of blood clot in the gastric bed acts as a potential site for secondary infection and it is preferable to remove this. Secondary haemorrhage is truly life-threatening and the old adage that prevention is better than treatment could not be more true for this complication. Any intra-abdominal sepsis must be treated aggressively and, in particular, collections around the coeliac trunk as erosion of the main arteries in this area is extremely dangerous. If the radiological facilities are adequate then embolisation may be attempted. The author's experience is that in full-blown secondary haemorrhage there is little time to take definitive action and immediate laparotomy is a safer option. This is not to say that surgical control of secondary haemorrhage is easy, but temporary control may save the patient's life while preparation is made for definitive control. Haemorrhage from the coeliac trunk vessels usually requires cross-clamping of the aorta. Since the hiatus is filled by the reconstruction it is often safer to clamp the aorta above the diaphragm using a left thoracic or thoracoabdominal approach and so avoid damage, or further damage, to the anastomoses. This complication most commonly occurs about two or more weeks after the gastrectomy when postoperative adhesions are dense and maturing – in the heat of the moment significant damage can occur. Suture of the eroded vessels is often difficult in the presence of infection and a non absorbable monofilament material is recommended. It is most important that the infected area is adequately debrided and drained prior to closure.

Duodenal stump leak

This may be due to technical error, afferent limb obstruction or ischaemia of the duodenal margin. The role of drains in abdominal surgery is always debatable, but a silastic tube drain to the duodenal stump is strongly recommended. In early leaks the appearance of bile-stained fluid in the drain is an indication for re-exploration and it is frequently possible to correct the problem completely. Conservative management of early leaks produces a less predictable outcome and so intervention is far safer.

Delayed leaks can often be treated conservatively if the duodenal contents come out through the drain and the patient is not obviously septic. In this situation it may be safer to apply gentle suction to the drain for the first few days to ensure the leak remains localised and a fistulous tract is established. Parenteral nutrition is not necessary if the leak is controlled as it is preferable to give an enteral elemental-type diet and to suppress pancreatic secretion with a subcutaneous somatostatin-analogue infusion. Drainage should be continued for at least 14 days and the drain then gradually pulled back from the duodenum. Provided the tract has matured, the resistance in the tract will be greater than that in the duodenum and the fistula should close rapidly. If the fistula output is greater than 200 ml/24 h without suction then drainage should be continued for longer and contrast studies obtained to determine whether there is a technical problem with the reconstruction. In delayed leakage that does not appear in the drain the patient usually presents with a subhepatic abscess. In this situation percutaneous radiological drainage may be sufficient provided the patient's clinical condition responds to drainage. Drainage is continued until the fistula dries up and although this may take weeks it is worthwhile persevering. The patient can continue on enteral nutrition, with or without a subcutaneous somatostatin-analogue, and need not stay in hospital if otherwise well. Any patient who remains septic and unwell despite drainage requires surgical exploration, debridement of the cavity and placement of a drain close to the point of leakage. If there is a major defect than a Foley-type catheter can be placed in the duodenum with a plan to form a controlled fistula. It is unwise to try and suture the duodenum if the presentation is delayed because of the poor tissue condition due to associated sepsis.

Anastomotic leak

This may occur because of technical error, ischaemia of the tissues or tension on the anastomotic line. In fact all these causes are 'technical errors'. If identified within the first 72 h then re-operation is advised. At worst this will allow placement of a drain right up against the point of leakage and also the construction of a more distal feeding jejunostomy. At best the anastomosis can be repaired or patched before sepsis is established in the surrounding tissues. Early leakage in more complex reconstructions may be from any of several suture lines and, even more importantly, may be due to jejunal ischaemia. This must be dealt with before complete disruption occurs when the chance of survival diminishes rapidly.

The management of a delayed presentation anastomotic leak is more controversial. If the leak is contained and only identified on a contrast study prior to beginning enteral feeding then it is wise to keep the patient on a liquid diet and repeat the contrast study every 7 days to confirm resolution of the cavity. However, if the patient is septic then a drain must be placed in the cavity. The dilemma is whether to do this radiologically and risk incomplete drainage or to explore the cavity surgically and risk a very difficult operation. Surgical exploration has the advantage that a feeding jejunostomy can be constructed and the septic area debrided, but the whole upper abdomen is often 'glued up' with new adhesions at this time – it is not an operation for the inexperienced surgeon.

There is no doubt that with appropriate surgical action, modern antibiotics, expert radiological assistance and enteral feeding techniques anastomotic leakage is no longer a surgical disaster. However, it is still the most common surgical cause of death and can be avoided by adhering to basic surgical principles.

Intra-abdominal sepsis

This may present at any time in the first 2 weeks after a gastrectomy. It may be due to anastomotic or duodenal leakage, pancreatic necrosis due to pancreatic parenchymal damage during the resection or leakage from the pancreatic stump. Sepsis is statistically more common after splenectomy, although whether this is an immunological effect or simply reflects damage to or resection of the pancreas as part of the operation is unclear.

Computed tomography with both intravenous and intraluminal contrast is important in defining the site and cause of the sepsis. The choice between radiological and surgical drainage has already been discussed. The dangers of incompletely drained sepsis with deterioration of the patient's condition and the risk of secondary haemorrhage makes adequate drainage essential.

It is not unreasonable to start with radiological drainage unless there is significant tissue necrosis identified on the scans. Percutaneous drainage may be only a temporising measure while the patient's condition is improved and the surgeon must always be prepared to abandon this method of drainage and opt for surgical debridement. It should also be remembered that sepsis after gastrectomy is usually in the gastric bed or high up under the left diaphragm and in both situations there are bowel loops between the abdominal wall and the cavity. Safe drainage of this type of abscess is often difficult and there is a serious risk of damage to the intervening structures. Surgical exploration and drainage through a left subcostal incision is often safer and avoids interfering with the reconstruction or having to dissect through adherent loops of jejunum and transverse colon. It also allows reasonable access to the pancreatic tail or stump.

Pancreatic fistula

This usually presents as a left upper quadrant abscess. It may occur after damage to the tail of the pancreas during splenectomy or following distal pancreatectomy. There is often associated necrosis of the pancreatic and peripancreatic tissue. The principle of treatment is outlined above – surgical drainage with debridement of necrotic tissue and placement of a silastic tube drain to the point of leakage is recommended. Since the proximal pancreatic duct is not obstructed this type of leak will close spontaneously. Subcutaneous infusion of a somotostatin analogue is usually helpful in reducing the volume of the leaked juice more quickly.

Postsplenectomy infections

Left subphrenic abscess after splenectomy has already been discussed. There is increasing evidence that splenectomy predisposes the patient to an increased risk of bacterial infections in both the early postoperative period and for at least 2 years after surgery. Immediate prophylaxis with twice daily oral penicillin is now recommended for patients of all ages. The patient should also be immunised with vaccines against pneumococci, meningoccus and *Haemophilus influenzae*. If the splenectomy has been planned as part of a radical procedure these vaccines are most effective if administered preoperatively. The patient should have an annual influenza vaccine and an updated pneumococcal vaccine every 2 or 3 years.

Late sequelae and complications

The place of follow-up clinics after cancer surgery is a subject that generates considerable discussion and debate. In this section it should become apparent that methodical follow-up of patients who have had a gastrectomy for cancer is mandatory if they are to realise their maximum quality of life, even if survival is likely to be limited. Quality of life is a difficult concept to define. Although there are several 'tools' for the measurement of quality of life after surgery, these are mainly useful in the research setting. Regular follow-up by the surgeon and other trained personnel is the best way of identifying and solving problems that affect the patient's physical and psychological well-being after major cancer surgery.

The main long-term problems and complications can be divided into three groups:

1. Side effects and postprandial sequelae
2. Nutritional problems
3. Recurrence of cancer

Side effects and postprandial sequelae

Early fullness

Loss of the reservoir function of the stomach results in a feeling of early satiety and in some patients, upper abdominal pain. Although the proximal jejunum dilates after a gastrectomy it can never completely replace the gastric reservoir and all patients have to limit their meal size to some extent. Good dietary advice is important to ensure an adequate calorie intake in more frequent smaller meals. The role of gastric pouches has already been discussed and they do apparently decrease the incidence of early satiety. Early dumping is a common cause of postprandial fullness and requires appropriate dietary manipulation. A rarer cause of fullness in some patients who have had a Roux-en-Y reconstruction is a defect of normal peristalsis in the long limb. This produces hold-up in the propulsion of the meal and results in an unpleasant pain during eating and involuntary, or often voluntary, regurgitation of the meal.[74]

Early dumping syndrome

The rapid filling of the proximal small intestine with hypertonic food leads to rapid movement of fluid into the gut from the extracellular fluid compartment. It also triggers a complex neurohumoral response that in some patients produces a variety of unpleasant gastrointestinal and cardiovascular symptoms. The aetiology and treatment of this complication is discussed more fully in Chapter 12. The main importance of the dumping syndrome is that it leads to food avoidance whether because of fullness or other unpleasant symptoms. In severe cases the patient is incapacitated after eating or suffers profuse diarrhoea that prevents normal activities after meals. Quality of life may be very severely restricted and malnutrition can occur rapidly in these patients.

It is perhaps fortunate that patients who have had a total or subtotal gastrectomy have a small reservoir and are usually unable to eat a large hypertonic load. The syndrome is much more common and troublesome in those who have an intact stomach, with the pylorus destroyed or bypassed, or after a partial gastrectomy. Many gastrectomy patients have some dumping symptoms in the first few weeks after surgery, but in most these are relatively mild and improve considerably with simple dietary adjustments which the patients often discover for themselves. During early follow-up it is important to identify significant dumping symptoms. A careful history should be taken and in less clear cases the patient asked to keep a diary recording foods eaten and symptoms experienced. Any patient with postprandial pain in the first few months after gastrectomy should be suspected of suffering from early dumping as this is much more likely than recurrent disease. It is not that unusual for postprandial symptoms to be interpreted wrongly as being due to early recurrence and the author has seen patients started on morphine to help control their 'pain'.

Most patients can be treated quite simply by appropriate dietary adaptation. It is important to involve a qualified dietician in the management of patients with dumping.

Reactive hypoglycaemic attacks

This is often incorrectly termed 'late dumping'. In many patients this occurs without early dumping symptoms. Symptoms of hypoglycaemia, including in the most profound cases blackouts and grand mal fits, occur about two hours after the last meal. The patient often experiences a craving for sweet food early in the attack.

Dietary assessment is the first step and the patient then advised to decrease the carbohydrate load in their main meals and to take small amounts of carbohydrate between main meals. Careful explanation of the problem is usually sufficient to reassure the patient they do not have a serious disorder. Those with frequent attacks should carry dextrose tablets to eat at the first sign of symptoms.

Diarrhoea

There are several causes for diarrhoea after a gastrectomy for cancer:

Truncal vagotomy

This is discussed in Chapter 12.

Early dumping

Diarrhoea not infrequently occurs towards the end or even after a dumping attack and is part of the symptom-complex. Unlike postvagotomy diarrhoea the attack follows a large hypertonic load and has other associated symptoms.

Bacterial overgrowth

This is relatively common after gastrectomy when there are complex reconstructions or pouches producing a blind limb.[75] Overgrowth in the proximal small intestine may also occur after a Roux-en-Y reconstruction. It is the combination of the loss of gastric acid, which destroys pathogenic ingested bacteria, and the formation of 'blind loops' that allows overgrowth of both aerobic and anaerobic organisms that are usually only present in the large intestine. These faecal bacteria produce toxins that damage the brush border enzymes vital for digestion. They may also utilise important nutrients such as the B vitamins. Pathogenic anaerobes deconjugate and dehydroxylate bile acids that are essential for normal fat absorption in the proximal small intestine.

Faecal fat levels are markedly elevated and in the worst cases the patient has steatorrhea and loses weight rapidly. The diagnosis can be confirmed by intubation of the proximal jejunum and aspiration of intestinal juice for culture. The best non-invasive test for the detection of overgrowth is the [^{14}C]glycocholate breath test. Proven bacterial overgrowth that causes diarrhoea and malnutrition should be treated with oral antibiotics such as neomycin or metronidazole. Fresh unpasteurised yoghurt or lactobacillus preparations should be given with and after a course of antibiotics to inhibit recolonisation by pathogenic bacteria. Only in very resistant cases should further surgery be contemplated.

Steatorrhoea

This may be due to bacterial overgrowth or relative pancreatic insufficiency caused by poor mixing of duodenal contents with food in reconstructions where the duodenum is excluded. Patients with fat malabsorption complain of unpleasant flatus and large bowel colic and pass bulky greasy stools that float and are difficult to flush away. A carefully taken history will identify the problem. If bacterial overgrowth has been excluded or treated then persistent fat malabsorption may respond to pancreatic enzyme supplements taken before or preferably mixed with food.

Bile reflux

Reflux of bile and alkaline juices into the stomach remnant and oesophagus may cause epigastric discomfort, heartburn and vomiting or regurgitation of bile. In the worst cases patients may avoid eating for fear of exacerbating their symptoms. Persistent oesophageal reflux may produce stricturing.

The diagnosis is usually made on clinical grounds. Objective evidence can be obtained with a [99m]technetium-HIDA scan.[76] Gastroscopy is important to confirm whether there is mucosal damage and to exclude any other cause for symptoms.

Treatment is often unsatisfactory and prevention of the problem by a bile diverting reconstruction in the first place is important. Unremitting symptoms are an indication for further surgery to divert the duodenal contents.

Nutritional problems

These can be divided into general malnutrition, reflected by weight loss, and deficits of specific nutrients.

General malnutrition and weight loss

It is important to recognise that malabsorption is a rare cause of malnutrition after a subtotal or total gastrectomy, unless there is bacterial overgrowth.[77] With few exceptions patients who lose weight, or fail to regain their preoperative weight, do so because they fail to ingest sufficient calories. Early satiety and the dumping syndrome are the most common cause of this and correction of these symptoms is usually sufficient to correct malnutrition.

Patients undergoing a subtotal gastrectomy rarely experience serious problems with weight loss. It is a fallacy that patients who have undergone a total gastrectomy invariably lose weight, although most fail to completely regain their pre-illness weight.[72] Women and particularly those over 70, do consistently seem to have difficulty maintaining their weight after total gastrectomy. Although patients will take sufficient calories under close supervision in hospital, their intake usually decreases on first going home.[77] Nutrition then improves over the first 6 months after surgery, by which time more than half the patients are taking their recommended calorie intake.[72] It is advised that all patients are kept under close dietary surveillance for at least 12 months after surgery.

Carbohydrate absorption is nearly complete even after total gastrectomy, but the pattern of absorption is abnormal. Protein absorption is decreased, as reflected by an increase in faecal nitrogen, but this is rarely clinically important. Fat malabsorption is the main cause of inadequate calorie absorption. On average postgastrectomy patients absorb about 80% of ingested fat – easily enough to provide adequate calories provided intake is sufficient. Failure to absorb fat may be due to bacterial overgrowth or relative pancreatic insufficiency due to poor mixing of food with bile and the duodenal juices.

Specific deficiencies

Vitamin B₁₂

Gastric acid is necessary to release B_{12} from foodstuffs and, more importantly, gastric parietal cell intrinsic factor is essential for absorption of this vitamin in the terminal ileum. After total gastrectomy patients absorb virtually no vitamin B_{12} and body stores are gradually depleted, although this may take up to 24 months to become clinically apparent. All patients should receive 1 mg of hydroxycobalamin intramuscularly every three months for life.

Other B vitamins

Deficiency only becomes clinically important if there is intestinal bacterial overgrowth. Treatment of the underlying cause of overgrowth is the priority, but oral B complex supplements should be given during treatment and for several weeks afterwards.

Fat-soluble vitamins

Malabsorption is obviously similar to that of fat. Vitamin A deficiency is detectable but remains a subclinical problem even many years after surgery. There is no evidence of vitamin E or K deficiency. Vitamin D malabsorption is of much more importance and particularly in postmenopausal women and long-term survivors. Osteomalacia may develop at an early stage if there is significant fat malabsorption. In those with apparently normal absorption it is recommended that calcium and alkaline phosphatase levels are measured annually. At 5 years a full assessment for metabolic bone disease should be undertaken in all patients. Postmenopausal women and all patients over 70 should take an oral calcium supplement twice a day for life after a total gastrectomy.

Iron

Absorption is surprisingly normal after total gastrectomy, even if the duodenum has been bypassed. It appears that the jejunum can adapt to absorb iron provided that there are sufficient naturally occurring chelating agents in the food. Iron absorption shows a gradual improvement after gastrectomy and, provided intake is adequate, is near normal 12 months after surgery. An oral iron supplement in combination with vitamin C is given once or twice a day for the first year, but only continued thereafter in those with a poor intake of iron-containing foodstuffs.

Recurrence of cancer

The detection and treatment of recurrent gastric cancer remains a complex issue affected by multiple factors. The mode of recurrence can often be predicted by the stage of the original disease. Cancers that have not penetrated the serosa recur later and usually as liver or distant metastases, whereas those that have invaded through the serosa often recur earlier and within the gastric bed on the peritoneal surfaces.

Although radiotherapy or chemotherapy may occasionally be indicated, the majority of patients with clinical recurrence will simply be treated symptomatically. Further surgery for obstructive symptoms is worthwhile, not least because some patients will be found to have another cause for obstruction that is treatable. Malignant obstruction may be relieved by a bypass procedure, but there are often multiple areas of intestinal involvement and the prognosis is generally very poor. The terminal care of patients with recurrent cancer is a subject in itself and does not fall within the scope of this chapter.

References

1. Heberer G, Teichman RK, Kramling H-J, Gunther B. Results of gastric resection for carcinoma of the stomach; the European experience. World J Surg 1988; 12: 374–81.
2. Hallisey MT, Allum WH, Jewkes AJ, Allis DJ, Fielding JWL. Early detection of gastric cancer. Br Med J 1990; 301: 513–15.
3. Sue-Ling HM, Martin I, Griffiths J *et al.* Early gastric cancer; 46 patients treated in one surgical department. Gut 1992; 33: 1318–22.
4. Hisamichi S. Screening for gastric cancer. World J Surg 1989; 13: 31–7.
5. Maruyama K. Results of surgery correlated with staging. In: Preece PE, Cuschieri A, Wellwood JM (eds) Cancer of the stomach. London: Grune and Stratton, 1986, pp. 145–63.
6. Fielding JWL. Gastric cancer: different diseases. Br J Surg 1989; 76: 1227.
7. Rohde H, Baeuer P, Heitman K, Gebbensleben B and the German Gastric Cancer TNM Study Group. Proximal compared with distal

adenocarcinoma of the stomach: differences and consequences. Br J Surg 1991; 78: 1242–8.

8. Roder JD, Bonenkamp JJ, Craven J et al. Lymphadenectomy for gastric cancer in clinical trials: update. World J Surg 1995; 19: 546–53.

9. Allum WH, Powell DJ, McConkey CC, Fielding JWL. Gastric cancer: a 25 year review. Br J Surg 1989; 76: 535–40.

10. MacIntyre IMC, Akoh JA. Improving survival in gastric cancer. Review of operative mortality in English language publications from 1970. Br J Surg 1991; 78: 773–8.

11. Sue-Ling HM, Johnston D, Martin I et al. Gastric cancer: a curable disease in Britain. Br Med J 1993; 307: 591–6.

12. Averbach AM, Jacquet P. Strategies to decrease the incidence of intra-abdominal recurrence in resectable gastric cancer. Br J Surg 1996; 83: 726–33.

13. Boku T, Nakane Y, Minoura T et al. Prognostic significance of serosal invasion and free intraperitoneal cancer cells in gastric cancer. Br J Surg 1990; 77: 436–9.

14. Iitsuka Y, Kaneshima S, Tanida O, Takeuchi T, Koga S. Intraperitoneal free cancer cells and their viability in gastric cancer. Cancer 1979; 44: 1476–80.

15. Gunderson LL, Sosin H. Adenocarcinoma of the stomach – areas of failure in a reoperation series (second or symptomatic look). Clinicopathological correlation and implications for adjuvant therapy. Int J Radiol Oncol Biol Phys 1982; 8: 1–11.

16. Landry J, Tepper JE, Wood WL, Moulton EO, Keorner F, Sullinger J. Patterns of failure following curative resection of gastric cancer. Int J Radiol Oncol Biol Phys 1990; 19: 1357–62.

17. Douglass HO, Nava MR. Gastric adenocarcinoma: management of the primary disease. Semin Oncol 1985; 12: 32–45.

18. Cunliffe WJ, Sugarbaker PH. Gastrointestinal malignancy: rationale for adjuvant therapy using early postoperative intraperitoneal chemotherapy. Br J Surg 1989; 76: 1082–90.

19. Volpe CM, Koo J, Miloro SM, Driscoll DL, Nava HR, Douglass HO. The effect of extended lymphadenectomy on survival in patients with gastric adenocarcinoma. J Am Coll Surg 1995; 181: 56–64.

20. Jatsko G, Lisborg PH, Klimpfinger M, Denk H. Extended radical surgery against gastric cancer: low implication and high survival rates. Jpn J Clin Oncol 1992; 22: 102–6.

21. Sasako M, McCulloch P, Kinoshita T, Maruyama K. New method to evaluate the therapeutic value of lymph node dissection for gastric cancer. Br J Surg 1995; 82: 346–51.

22. Keller E, Stutzer H, Heitmann K, Bauer P, Gebbensleben B, Rohde H. Lymph node staging in 872 patients with carcinoma of the stomach and the presumed benefit of lymphadenectomy. German Stomach Cancer TNM Study Group. J Am Coll Surg 1994; 1978: 38–46.

23. Hamazoe R, Maeta M, Kaibara N. Intraperitoneal thermochemotherapy for prevention of peritoneal recurrence of gastric cancer. Final results of a randomised controlled study. Cancer 1994; 73: 2048–52.

24. Yonemura Y, Ninomiya I, Kaji M et al. Prophylaxis with intraoperative chemohyperthermia against peritoneal recurrence of serosal-invasion positive gastric cancer. World J Surg 1995; 19: 450–5.

25. Sautner T, Hofbauer F, Depisch D, Schiessel R, Jakesz R. Adjuvant intraperitoneal cisplatin chemotherapy does not improve long-term survival after surgery for advanced gastric cancer. J Clin Oncol 1994; 12: 970–4.

26. Gall FP, Hermanek P. New aspects in the surgical treatment of gastric carcinoma – a comparative study of 1636 patients operated on between 1969 and 1982. Eur J Surg Oncol 1985; 11: 219–25.

27. Hornig D. Hermanek P, Gall FP. The significance of the extent of proximal margins on clearance in gastric cancer surgery. Scand J Gastroenterol 1977; 22 (Suppl. 133): 69–71.

28. Bozzetti F, Bonfanti G, Bufalino R et al. Adequacy of margins of resection in gastrectomy for cancer. Ann Surg 1982; 196: 682–90.

29. Japanese Research Society for Gastric Cancer. The general rules for gastric cancer surgery and pathology. Jpn J Surg 1981; 11: 127–45.

30. Papachristou DN, Fortner JG. Adenocarcinoma of the gastric cardia. The choice of gastrectomy. Ann Surg 1980; 192: 58–64.

31. Bozzetti F. Total versus subtotal gastrectomy in cancer of the distal stomach: facts and fantasy. Eur J Surg Oncol 1992; 18: 572–9.

32. Skandalakis JE, Gray SW, Rowe SJ. Anatomical complications in general surgery. New York: McGraw Hill, 1983, pp. 63–4.

33. Maruyama K, Gunven P, Okabayashi K, Sasako M, Kinoshita T. Lymph node metastases of gastric cancer. General pattern in 1931 patients. Ann Surg 1989; 210: 596–602.
34. Maruyama K, Sadako M, Kinoshita T, Okajima K. Effectiveness of systematic lymph node dissection in gastric cancer surgery. In: Nishi M *et al*. (eds) Gastric cancer. Tokyo: Springer-Verlag, 1993, pp. 293–305.
35. Kodama Y, Sugimachi K, Soejima K, Matsusaka T, Inokuchi K. Evaluation of extensive lymph node dissection for carcinoma of the stomach. World J Surg 1981; 5: 241–8.
36. Soga J, Ohyama S, Miyashita K *et al*. A statistical evaluation of advancement in gastric cancer surgery with special reference to the significance of lymphadenectomy for cure. World J Surg 1988; 12: 398–405.
37. Maruyama K, Okabayashi K, Kinoshita T. Progress in gastric cancer surgery in Japan and its limits of radicality. World J Surg 1987; 11: 418–25.
38. Nakajima T, Nishi M. Surgery and adjuvant chemotherapy for gastric cancer. Hepato-gastroenterology 1989; 36: 79–85.
39. Baba H, Maehara Y, Takeuchi H *et al*. Effect of lymph node dissection on the prognosis in patients with node-negative early gastric cancer. Surgery 1995; 117: 165–9.
40. Siewert JR, Kestlmeier R, Busch R. Benefits of D2 lymph node dissection for patients with gastric cancer and pN0 pN1 lymph node metastases. Br J Surg 1996; 83: 1144–7.
41. Shiu MH, Moore E, Sanders M *et al*. Influence of the extent of resection on survival after curative treatment of gastric carcinoma. Arch Surg 1987; 122: 1347–51.
42. Siewert JR, Bottcher K, Roder JD *et al*. Prognostic relevance of systematic lymph node dissection in gastric carcinoma. Br J Surg 1993; 80: 1015–18.
43. Dent DM, Madden MV, Price SK. Randomised comparison of R1 and R2 gastrectomy for gastric cancer. Br J Surg 1988; 75: 110–12.
44. Robertson CS, Chung SCS, Woods SDS *et al*. A prospective randomised trial comparing R1 subtotal gastrectomy with R3 total gastrectomy for antral cancer. Ann Surg 1994; 220: 176–82.
45. Bonnenkamp JJ, Songun J, Hermans J *et al*. Randomised comparison of morbidity after D1 and D2 dissection for gastric cancer in 996 Dutch patients. Lancet 1995; 345: 745–8.
46. Cuschieri A, Fayers P, Fielding J *et al*. Postoperative morbidity and mortality after D1 and D2 resections for gastric cancer: preliminary results of the MRC randomised controlled surgical trial. Lancet 1996; 347: 995–9.
47. Hayes N, Karat D, Scott DJ, Raimes SA, Griffin SM. Radical lymphadenectomy in the management of early gastric cancer. Br J Surg 1996; 83: 1421–3.
48. Kampschoer GHM, Maruyama K, van de Velde CJH, Sasako M, Kinoshita T, Okabayashi K. Computer analysis in making preoperative decisions: a rational approach to lymph node dissection in gastric cancer patients. Br J Surg 1989; 76: 905–8.
49. Griffith JP, Sue-Ling HM, Martin I *et al*. Preservation of the spleen improves survival after radical surgery for gastric cancer. Gut 1995; 36: 684–90.
50. Fujita T, Matai K, Kohno S, Itsubo K. Impact of splenectomy on circulating immunoglobulin levels and the development of postoperative infection following total gastrectomy for gastric cancer. Br J Surg 1996; 83: 1776–8.
51. Okajima K, Isozaki H. Splenectomy for treatment of gastric cancer: Japanese experience. World J Surg 1995; 19: 537–40.
52. Brady MS, Rogatko A, Dent L, Shui MH. Effect of splenectomy on morbidity and survival following curative gastrectomy for carcinoma. Arch Surg 1991; 126: 359–64.
53. Mishima Y, Kirayama R. The role of lymph node surgery in gastric cancer. World J Surg 1987; 11: 406–11.
54. Sugimachi K, Kodama Y, Kuimashiro R *et al*. Critical evaluation of prophylactic splenectomy in total gastrectomy for stomach cancer. Gann 1985; 71: 704–9.
55. Maruyama K, Sasako M, Kinoshita T, Sano T, Katai H, Okajima K. Pancreas-preserving total gastrectomy for proximal gastric cancer. World J Surg 1995; 19: 532–6.
56. Papachristou DN, Shiu MH. Management by en bloc multiple organ resection of carcinoma of the stomach invading adjacent organs. Surg Gynaecol Obstet 1981; 152: 483–7.
57. Kocherling F, Reck T, Gall FP. Extended gastrectomy: who benefits? World J Surg 1995; 19: 541–5.

58. McNeer G, Bowden L, Booker RJ, McPeak CJ. Elective total gastrectomy for cancer of the stomach: end results. Ann Surg 1974; 108: 252–6.

59. Korenaga D, Okamura T, Baba H, Saito A, Sugimachi K. Results of resection of gastric cancer extending to adjacent organs. Br J Surg 1988; 75: 12–15.

60. Bozzetti F, Regalia E, Bonfanti G, Doci R, Ballarini D, Gennari L. Early and late results of extended surgery for cancer of the stomach. Br J Surg 1990; 77: 53–6.

61. Sawai K, Takahishi T, Suzuki H. New trends in surgery for gastric cancer in Japan. J Surg Oncol 1994; 56: 221–6.

62. Hiki Y, Shimao H, Mieno H, Sakakibara Y, Kobayashi N, Saigenji K. Modified treatment of early gastric cancers: evaluation of endoscopic treatment of early gastric cancers with respect to treatment indications. World J Surg 1995; 19: 517–22.

63. Kodama M, Koyama K. Indications for pylorus-preserving gastrectomy for early gastric cancer located in the middle third of the stomach. World J Surg 1991; 15: 628–34.

64. Goh P, Kum CK. Laparoscopic Billroth II gastrectomy: a review. Surg Oncol 1993; 2 Suppl. 1: 13–18.

65. Yamashita Y, Kurohiji T, Kakeyawa T, Bekki F, Ogata M. Laparoscopy-guided extracorporeal resection of early gastric carcinoma. Endoscopy 1995; 27: 248–52.

66. McCulloch P. Description of the Japanese method of radical gastrectomy. Ann R Coll Surg Engl 1994; 76: 110–14.

67. Craven JL. Radical surgery for gastric cancer. In: Preece PR, Cuschieri A, Wellwood JM (eds) Cancer of the stomach. London: Grune and Stratton, 1986, pp. 165–87.

68. Alderson D, Courtney SP, Kennedy RH. Radical transhiatal oesophagectomy under direct vision. Br J Surg 1994; 81: 404–7.

69. Cuschieri A. Reconstruction after gastric resection for cancer. In: Preece P, Cuschieri A, Wellwood JM (eds) Cancer of the stomach. London: Grune and Stratton, 1986, pp. 209–29.

70. Buhl K, Lehnert T, Schlag P, Herfarth C. Reconstruction after gastrectomy and quality of life. World J Surg 1995; 19: 558–64.

71. Olbe L, Lundell L. Intestinal function after total gastrectomy and possible consequences of gastric replacement. World J Surg 1987; 11: 713–19.

72. Braga M, Zuliani W, Foppa L, Di Carlo V, Cristallo M. Food intake and nutritional status after total gastrectomy: results of a nutritional follow-up. Br J Surg 1988; 75: 477–80.

73. Liedman B, Andersson H, Berglund B et al. Food intake after total gastrectomy for gastric cancer: the role of a gastric reservoir. Br J Surg 1996; 83: 1138–43.

74. Mathias JR, Fernandez A, Sninsky CA et al. Nausea, vomiting and abdominal pain after Roux-en-Y anastomosis, motility of the jejunal limb. Gastroenterology 1985; 88: 101–7.

75. Troidl H. Kusche J, Vertweber K-H et al. Pouch versus oesophagojejunostomy after total gastrectomy: a randomised clinical trial. World J Surg 1987; 11: 699–712.

76. Donovan IA, Fielding JWL, Bradby H et al. Bile diversion after total gastrectomy. Br J Surg 1982; 69: 389–90.

77. Bradley E, Isaacs J, Hersh T et al. Nutritional consequences of total gastrectomy. Ann Surg 1975; 182: 415–29.

7 Radiotherapy and chemotherapy in the treatment of oesophageal and gastric cancer

Thomas N. Walsh

Introduction The role of chemotherapy and radiotherapy, alone or combined, in the management of carcinoma of the oesophagus and stomach is becoming clearer as experience with these modalities increases. That so many issues remain unresolved despite the fact that millions of patients have been treated world-wide with chemotherapy or radiotherapy reflects the fact that only a minute fraction are being treated in the context of a randomised clinical trial. The bulk of the oncology literature adds little to our understanding as the majority of reports are of uncontrolled series, or of non-randomised trials or poorly designed randomised trials with small numbers and therefore insufficient power to support the conclusions drawn. This chapter concentrates primarily on the results of randomised trials, where such exist, or on well-reported large series where randomised trials are not available.

Much of the literature on advanced tumours is even more difficult to interpret, with a wide range of degrees of metastatic involvement, with inaccurate pretreatment staging and with even fewer randomised trials to resolve the issue of effectiveness. Chemotherapy and radiotherapy for advanced disease will only be touched on briefly where randomised trials are available and a definite advantage is demonstrated.

A further confounding issue is that the oesophageal cancer literature to date pools adenocarcinoma and squamous carcinoma assuming similar response rates. No such assumption is supported in the literature. In fact squamous carcinoma seems to be more sensitive to the local effects of these modalities but completely responding adenocarcinomas appear to have a better prognosis than completely responding squamous tumours suggesting different biological behaviour. For these reasons squamous carcinoma and adenocarcinoma of the oesophagus and adenocarcinoma of the stomach are treated separately in the subsequent sections.

A final point of relevance is that these tumours are changing rapidly in their presentation and these changes, outlined below, have implications for management.

Presentation

Oesophageal cancer

A number of important changes have occurred in the presentation of oesophageal cancer over the past two decades which have a bearing on its management and outcome and on the role of multimodality therapy. Whereas the world-wide incidence of oesophageal cancer has remained static, and in some countries has even declined, the incidence along the Western European seaboard has increased. World Health Organisation data show that of 33 countries where the change in incidence was examined Spain, Northern Ireland, Scotland, England/Wales and Ireland ranked 2nd, 3rd, 4th, 5th and 7th, respectively in increasing incidence.[1]

The change is due largely to the dramatic increase in the incidence of adenocarcinoma. In the period between 1976 and 1987 the incidence of adenocarcinoma increased by more than 100% in men in the United States, with an average annual increase of around 10%, whereas the incidence of squamous carcinoma remained unchanged.[2] By 1987 adenocarcinomas accounted for 34% of all oesophageal cancers in white males. Similar trends have been reported from Britain,[3] Germany[4] and Denmark.[5] In most units in the UK and Ireland the incidence of adenocarcinoma and squamous carcinoma is almost equal. Accompanying this change in histological type is an increase in incidence of poorly differentiated tumours and an increase in lymph node involvement.[5]

The reasons for these changes are unclear. Lifestyle factors such as cigarette smoking and a high alcohol intake are regarded as the chief risk factors for the development of squamous carcinoma. The reduction in squamous carcinoma which occurred in some European countries has been linked to an increase in citrus fruit consumption.[1] Little is known about risk factors for adenocarcinoma apart from the link with Barrett's mucosa. Epidemiological data to evaluate trends in the incidence of Barrett's mucosa, however, are lacking but there is a suggestion that its incidence is increasing.

Gastric cancer

The incidence of gastric cancer has fallen progressively and dramatically in the Western world over the past 30 years.[6] This has been linked to improving economic conditions. The cause for this reduction is unclear but it is mainly attributed to a change in food preservation methods and increased ingestion of citrus fruits. Preservation by salting, smoking and pickling lead to nitrosamine production and excess salt may lead to chronic gastritis. Vitamin C blocks the production of N-nitroso carcinogens and retards the progression of transformed clone cells through fibroplasia. β-carotene may protect as a free radical scavenger and through enhanced cell to cell communication.

With this change in incidence has come a proximal migration of cancer and a change in histological type from intestinal to diffuse. The intestinal type is considered to be an environmental tumour and is more common in populations with a high risk. It probably develops in a sequential manner following initial gastritis, through atrophy, intestinal metaplasia and dysplasia to invasive cancer. Several aetiological agents probably act along different points in the chain such as *Helicobacter pylori* and excessive salt, both of which cause inflammation. Another mechanism is through the production or ingestion of nitrosamines which are potent carcinogens.

The diffuse type is becoming relatively more frequent in areas where the incidence is declining. The poorer prognosis of proximal gastric cancers is accepted in the literature and it is probably related to the more advanced stage at presentation and a higher incidence of lymph node involvement. Blot *et al.*[2] reported a drift to proximal gastric lesions of 4.5% per annum between 1976 and 1987. At the end of this period 47% of all gastric tumours occurred in the cardia. This has implications for management. Surgery is more demanding for proximal lesions. The diffuse histological subtype carries a poorer prognosis and a higher incidence of lymph node involvement. The incidence of positive lymph nodes is 75–85% in proximal tumours compared with 60–65% in distal tumours.

This reduction in incidence of gastric cancer is not world-wide as the rates in the developed areas of South America are similar to those seen in the earlier part of this century in Britain and in North America. There the disease has remained distal and of the intestinal subtype. This is attributed to the retention of more traditional food preservation techniques.

The overall 5-year survival rate for gastric cancer has been static for the past 50 years.[7] It is approximately 40% when the nodes are negative but decreases to 10% if the nodes are positive. Only 10–15% of patients have disease confined to the stomach. Approximately 10% of carcinomas are early gastric cancers. This compares with up to 40% of newly diagnosed patients in Japan.[8] Only 30–40% of patients with gastric cancer undergoing exploration have a potentially curative resection. The remaining patients have palliative resection with gross residual tumour or microscopically positive margins or had an unresectable lesion.[9] Most Western series would suggest that no more than 15% of patients are cured by surgery and the commonest cause of death is locoregional failure even after potentially curative resection.

Rationale for various treatment strategies

Radiotherapy

The locoregional failure rate of oesophageal and gastric cancer following surgery is so high that local recurrence can be a significant factor in preventing cure. In about 50% of cases regional lymph node metastases are the only failure after curative resection. Locoregional recurrence may be the main cause of significant symptoms for many of these patients.

Preoperative radiotherapy

The rationale for administering radiotherapy prior to surgery is based on the belief that tumour bulk might be reduced, resectability increased and local control improved. It has often been suggested that oesophageal cancer, with a rich vascular supply to the submucosa, is likely to shed cells at surgery. These cells are well oxygenated and should be more sensitive to radiotherapy. Preoperative radiotherapy might thus reduce the risk of the iatrogenic dissemination of tumour cells and enhance long-term survival. Resection of the diseased and irradiated segment permits intestinal continuity to be restored with healthy, non-irradiated, bowel as a conduit.

Intraoperative radiotherapy

Intraoperative radiation therapy is based on the observation that following initial therapy for tumours such as gastric cancer failure is due to locoregional nodal metastases in about half the cases. Many patients should benefit from more radical attention to this metastatic field.

Postoperative radiotherapy

The rationale for using postoperative radiation therapy is to eradicate gross disease at the resection margins or in the oesophageal bed or to sterilise suspected microscopic residual disease. If gross disease is left behind aggressive radiotherapy focusing on the specific site of residual disease might improve chances of survival. If the aim is to sterilise the tumour bed of microscopic disease there are obvious problems such as accurately mapping the area to be treated. This often requires an extended field approach to embrace all possible foci of residual disease.

The disadvantages of postoperative radiotherapy include the fact that it is impossible to know whether or not irradiation has been successful. As the healthy transposed organ lies in the tumour bed and is subjected to the full irradiation dose it may suffer short- or long-term compromise of its integrity or function.

Chemotherapy

It is suggested that over 70% of patients with oesophageal and gastric cancer have systemic disease at diagnosis. Autopsy studies performed on patients with oesophageal cancer who died a short time after surgery, including patients who died in the perioperative period, revealed metastatic disease in the majority. Systemic therapy is essential, therefore, if we are to hope for cure.

Preoperative chemotherapy

There are a number of theoretical and experimental reasons for providing preoperative chemotherapy. Chemotherapy appears to be as effective as radiation therapy in controlling locoregional disease.[10] When the tumour burden is low preoperative treatment can induce early tumour regression. Treatment before surgery may also reduce the incidence of spontaneous emergence of drug-resistant tumour cell populations.[11] Treatment in the preoperative rather than the postoperative period permits a more accurate assessment of response. This information may subsequently be used to identify more accurately responding patients who may benefit from postoperative chemotherapy. It may also facilitate subsequent surgery and may allow more conservative local measures.

Arguments against neoadjuvant therapy centre on the belief that early use of systemic treatment may allow the emergence of a resistant clone of tumour cells, can delay effective local control and can lead to uncertainty as to the extent of resection required. Responding patients may refuse surgery or irradiation.

Intraperitoneal chemotherapy

Because peritoneal and hepatic recurrences are common the use of intraperitoneal postoperative chemotherapy is being investigated in several centres in Japan and America. The risks of peritoneal implantation and of intra-abdominal tumour spread immediately after laparotomy are high and there is a strong argument for immediate postoperative treatment, especially if intraperitoneal chemotherapy is being used. Preclinical studies have shown that intraperitoneal chemotherapy is capable of treating peritoneal and liver micrometastases in rats.[12] The frequency of tumour formation at sites of surgical trauma in the peritoneum range from 28% to 82% in mice, depending on the type of incision made in the peritoneal cavity, compared with a rate of 33% in non-operated mice.[13]

Although early studies relied on aqueous solutions of chemotherapeutic agents, recent trials have used carbon particles as a vehicle for agents such as mitomycin C.[14] This is because activated carbon particles are taken up selectively by lymphatic tissue and this seems to be a primary site of carcinomatosis in the peritoneal cavity. These sites absorb a large amount of the anticancer agent which is subsequently released slowly and for a protracted period.

Yet another strategy for more effective chemotherapy delivery is as a hyperthermic solution. The rationale for this is that *in vitro* and *in vivo* studies suggest that hyperthermia is tumoricidal once the temperature reaches 42.5°C. DNA replication and RNA and protein synthesis are inhibited. Furthermore, membrane stability and permeability of cancer cells are altered resulting in increased permeability to anticancer drugs. The addition of hyperthermia to anticancer drugs is felt to provide synergistic enhancement of each other's action.

Postoperative chemotherapy

Patients with a T_3 or T_4 lesion and any N stage are at a high risk for recurrence. For example, 50% of patients with stage T_3N_0 lesions will die of their disease within five years of curative resection. Between 80 and 90% of Western patients are felt to be in the high risk group and preoperative identification of the low risk subgroup is difficult with currently available staging modalities. Until adjuvant programmes of proven effectiveness are developed it is important to spare those patients who have an excellent outcome from the potential toxicity of chemotherapy.

It is important to distinguish patients who have undergone potentially curative surgery and who are considered for additional treatment from patients who undergo surgery where the tumour proves unresectable or who only have a palliative procedure, or who had positive margins as therapy in these circumstances cannot be considered adjuvant.

A further issue of importance is the timing of postoperative treatment, which can vary widely. There are several reasons for starting adjuvant therapy soon after resection. Fisher et al.[15] have shown an increased labelling of metastases after resection of the primary tumour, suggesting a potential for increased cell kill and this further suggests that adjuvant treatment should begin immediately before or after resection.

Multimodality therapy with chemotherapy and radiotherapy

The rationale for combining chemotherapy with radiotherapy is based on the belief that chemotherapy can act as a radiosensitiser,[16] enhancing the local effects of radiation and help reduce or eliminate micrometastases. If given preoperatively this should also help decrease the likelihood of spread. It should also reduce the dosage of both modalities thereby reducing toxicity.

The theoretical counterargument is that areas of radionecrosis could become sanctuary sites for treatment-resistant tumour cells and that the combined toxicity may limit the dose of chemotherapy that can be given. This question of sequence has yet to be tested in randomised trials.

Squamous carcinoma of the oesophagus

The role of radiotherapy

Radiotherapy alone

The role of radiotherapy for oesophageal squamous carcinoma is unclear. It has never been compared with surgery in a randomised trial. Early reports generated unwarranted optimism. The best data on response to radiotherapy come from a recent trial which compared high-dose radiotherapy (6400 cGy) with 5500 cGy radiotherapy and chemotherapy.[17] Only 10% of potentially curable patients survive 2 years when treated by radiotherapy alone.

Preoperative radiotherapy

The majority of reports of preoperative radiation therapy have consisted of single arm trials using historical controls. In recent times, however, five randomised trials have compared preoperative radiotherapy with surgery alone. Four have found no survival advantage for preoperative radiotherapy and one has reported a difference between treatment limbs. Launois' group randomised 124 patients to receive either 40 Gy radiotherapy followed by oesophagectomy or oesophagectomy alone.[18] The median survival rates for the combined treatment and control arms were similar at 4.5 and 8 months, respectively. Five-year survival rates, excluding surgical mortality, were 9.5% and 11.5%, respectively. Gignoux *et al.*[19] reported on the EORTC trial of 229 patients randomised to preoperative radiotherapy (3300 cGY) or surgery alone, and found that the resection rates for the treated and control groups were 81% and 75%, respectively. The operative mortality rates were 24% and 19%. It is noteworthy that preoperative radiotherapy did not affect the incidence of lymph node metastases in the resected specimens which were 56% and 57% in the two groups. The mean survival was 12 and 12.3 months with five-year survival rates of 9% and 10% respectively for the groups. In a Beijing trial 360 patients with squamous carcinoma of the mid-thoracic oesophagus were randomised to receive 40 Gy radiotherapy followed by surgery or surgery alone.[20] The survival rates were 47% and 42% at three years and 37% and 33% at five years. Of the patients treated in the surgery limb 61% had lymph node-negative disease suggesting that the majority of these patients had early tumours. Huseman[21] reported on a further large series and found no difference in outcome between patients receiving preoperative irradiation and untreated controls.

Nygaard *et al.*[22] reporting on the second Scandinavian trial described a survival advantage for patients receiving preoperative radiotherapy (3500 cGy) over patients receiving surgery alone and found no additional benefit when preoperative chemotherapy was added. The trial was unsatisfactory, however, because in calculating their results they pooled patients who had preoperative chemotherapy in addition to radiotherapy with those who had radiotherapy only. The numbers in each group were too small for confident subgroup analysis.

Thus, the weight of evidence from randomised trials to date suggests that there is no survival advantage for preoperative radiation therapy and its use should be restricted to the setting of randomised clinical trials.

Postoperative radiotherapy

Three randomised trials have compared the effect of postoperative radiotherapy with surgery alone but no survival advantage was identified in any. Zieran *et al.*[23] reported on 68 patients undergoing curative resection randomised to receive postoperative irradiation (5580 cGy) or surgery alone and found no difference in survival between the groups. The irradiated patients were, however, significantly slower to recover their preoperative quality of life than the control group.

The French University Association for Surgical Research randomised 221 patients, who had undergone potentially curative resection, to postoperative radiotherapy (4500–5500 cGy) and found an overall actuarial 5-year survival of 19% with no survival advantage for postoperative radiation therapy, regardless of lymph node status.[24] There were fewer recurrences, however, in the treated group at a cost of significant complications in 23%.

Fok *et al.*[25] reported on 60 patients undergoing curative resection, and 70 patients undergoing palliative resection randomised separately to receive 4900 cGy (curative) and 5250 cGy (palliative) radiotherapy, respectively, or to surgery alone. There were fewer intrathoracic recurrences in the groups receiving radiotherapy but the median survival for both the treated groups was significantly shorter than the curative group treated by surgery alone. About 37% had complications attributed to radiotherapy of the transposed stomach. A total of 17 patients had gastric ulceration of whom five died from bleeding. They concluded that the role of postoperative radiotherapy was limited to a specific group of patients with residual tumour in the mediastinum after operation for whom radiotherapy could specifically reduce the incidence of local recurrence obstructing the bronchial tree.

Chemotherapy

Chemotherapy alone

No trial has been reported which compared chemotherapy alone with surgery alone for oesophageal carcinoma. Uncontrolled trials of chemotherapy alone in patients with locoregional disease reveal a median survival of 6–8 months.

Preoperative chemotherapy

The majority of preoperative chemotherapy regimes examined to date have been single-arm uncontrolled trials. Only a few randomised trials have been reported and those were confined to small numbers of patients. In one trial preoperative chemotherapy was compared with preoperative radiotherapy.[26] The preoperative radiotherapy group received 5500 cGy and the chemotherapy group received two cycles of cisplatin, vindesine and bleomycin. Objective response, operability rates, resectability and mortality rates were similar and chemotherapy appeared as effective as radiotherapy in controlling locoregional disease.

Postoperative chemotherapy

No reports on the role of postoperative chemotherapy for oesophageal cancer are available for evaluation analysis.

Pre- and postoperative chemotherapy

Trials comparing preoperative and postoperative chemotherapy with surgery alone are few. Roth *et al.*[27] performed a randomised trial on preoperative and postoperative chemotherapy with cisplatin, vindesine and bleomycin in 36 patients and found no difference in actuarial survival between those given chemotherapy and those treated by surgery alone.

In a trial in which patients were randomised to receive preoperative and postoperative chemotherapy (cisplatin, vinblastin and bleomycin) or surgery alone, the operative morbidity was higher in the surgery-alone group (47% compared with 29%), but there was no significant difference in survival between the groups with a mean survival of only nine months for both groups.[28]

Combined chemotherapy and radiotherapy

Chemotherapy and radiotherapy without surgery

Combined chemotherapy and radiotherapy has not been compared with surgery alone in a controlled clinical trial. A number of studies have examined the role of combined chemotherapy and radiotherapy without surgery, but most of these have been uncontrolled phase 2 trials. Three large randomised trials have compared radiotherapy and chemotherapy with radiotherapy alone, two of which showed a survival advantage over radiotherapy alone. Roussel *et al.*[29] reported no survival advantage in 144 patients with advanced carcinoma randomised to single agent chemotherapy (methotrexate) and 5600 cGy radiotherapy over radiotherapy alone. In another study all patients received 4000 cGy initially.[30] Patients not undergoing surgery received an additional 2000–2600 cGy. Patients randomised to combination therapy received 5-fluorouracil (5-FU) and mitomycin C beginning on the second day of radiotherapy. The median survival for patients receiving combined treatment was 14 months compared with 9 months for radiotherapy alone. In, perhaps, the definitive trial in this area potentially curable patients were randomised to receive 6400 cGy of radiation alone, or 5500 cGy given concurrently with two courses of cisplatin and 5-FU and followed by two additional cycles of cisplatin and 5-FU.[17] The trial was closed after 121 patients had been recruited as a significant survival advantage emerged in favour of the chemoradiotherapy limb. The 1- and 2-year survival rates were 55% and 38% for the chemotherapy and radiotherapy group compared with 33% and 10% respectively for the radiation-only group. These trials present a clear case in favour of concurrent chemotherapy and radiotherapy over radiotherapy alone. However, radiotherapy alone is inferior to surgery alone, and the results of chemoradiotherapy are no better than surgery. Longer follow-up is necessary to determine whether these results for chemoradiotherapy alone are sustained.

Chemotherapy and radiotherapy followed by surgery

Because of the encouraging results with concurrent chemotherapy and radiotherapy a number of units have attempted to improve results of surgery by giving combination therapy prior to resection. The majority of trials have been single arm and uncontrolled. In a report of 55 patients treated with mitomycin C, 5-FU and 30 Gy radiotherapy, followed by further chemoradiotherapy postoperatively, five patients had a complete pathological response, and had a median survival of 18 months.[31] A further study from the same unit looked at the results of cisplatin, 5-FU and 30 Gy concurrent radiation therapy. Of 21 patients examined, 15 came to operation of whom five were found to have a complete pathological response.[32] The median survival for complete responders was 24 months compared with 18 months for the group as a whole. Disappointingly, of the five patients with a complete pathological response distant tumour recurred in all between 30 and 60 months and all have subsequently died. A more recent trial examined cisplatin, vinblastin and 5-FU, given by continuous infusion, and radiotherapy given over 21 days to a total dose of 30 Gy.[33] At the time of the last report of these data the median survival had not been reached but the results were encouraging and a controlled trial had been undertaken.

Only three prospective randomised trials comparing preoperative radiotherapy and chemotherapy with surgery alone have thus far been published. LePrise et al.[34] reported on 86 patients randomised to receive chemotherapy (5-FU and cisplatin) plus 2000 cGy radiotherapy prior to surgery or surgery alone.[34] It is noteworthy that the radiotherapy and chemotherapy were given consecutively rather than concurrently denying patients the potential benefit of a radiosensitising effect of the chemotherapeutic agents. The dose of radiotherapy is now considered to be subtherapeutic. Of 39 patients receiving preoperative chemoradiotherapy four (10%) had a complete pathological response. There was no difference in survival, however, between the groups. The second prospective multicentre trial randomised 186 patients into four subgroups to receive either surgery alone, preoperative chemotherapy (cisplatin and bleomycin) and surgery, preoperative irradiation (3500 cGy) and surgery, or preoperative chemotherapy, radiotherapy and surgery.[22] A survival advantage for neoadjuvant radiotherapy over surgery alone was reported but this is refuted by three other studies showing no advantage for preoperative radiotherapy.[18–20]

Walsh et al.[35] have reported an interim analysis of a randomised trial of preoperative chemotherapy (cisplatin and 5-FU) and radiotherapy (4000 cGy) followed by surgery versus surgery alone. A total of 61 patients were randomised. Of 25 patients completing multimodality therapy nine (36%) had a complete pathological response and 79% were node negative versus 42% of surgery patients ($P = 0.01$). Complete responders survived longer than non-responders ($P = 0.05$) but the median survival for the group was 17 months for multimodality therapy versus 13 months for surgery ($P = 0.28$). Chemoradiotherapy resulted in significant downstaging but a survival advantage occurred only in patients with a complete response.

Summary

Surgery remains the gold standard against which other treatment modalities must be compared for oesophageal squamous cell carcinoma. Radiotherapy alone has a very limited role when given preoperatively and has a significant negative impact on quality of life and possibly even on survival when given postoperatively. Neither is there a survival advantage for chemotherapy given preoperatively. Postoperative chemotherapy has received little attention. The combination of chemotherapy and radiotherapy would appear to hold more promise but randomised trials to date have been inconclusive. These have been flawed by ineffective combinations or dosage, or inadequate numbers, or insufficient follow-up. Better trials with longer follow-up will be required to resolve this issue.

Adeno-carcinoma of the oesophagus

Introduction

There are very few trials in the literature which report on the treatment of adenocarcinoma of the oesophagus separate from squamous carcinoma. Two explanations are advanced. There has been a perception that adenocarcinoma, unlike squamous carcinoma, is resistant to chemotherapy or radiotherapy. There has also been a real and dramatic increase in the incidence of oesophageal adenocarcinoma. This increase has outstripped that of all other human tumours. In one study the annual increase in the United States was about 10% per year.[2] This increase suggests that such trials are a matter of considerable urgency.

The role of radiotherapy

Radiotherapy alone

The role of radiotherapy for oesophageal adenocarcinoma has hardly been explored. Many trials which examined the role of radiotherapy for oesophageal carcinoma have pooled adenocarcinomas with squamous tumours. It has never been compared with surgery alone in a randomised trial.

Preoperative radiotherapy

The majority of reports of preoperative radiation therapy have consisted of single arm trials using historical controls. Preoperative radiotherapy has not been compared with surgery alone in a randomised trial.

Postoperative radiotherapy

Postoperative radiotherapy has not been examined in a randomised trial.

The role of chemotherapy

Chemotherapy alone

No trial has been reported which compared chemotherapy alone with surgery alone for oesophageal adenocarcinoma.

Preoperative chemotherapy

The majority of preoperative chemotherapy regimes examined to date have been single-arm uncontrolled trials. Ajani et al.[36] reported on 35 consecutive patients with resectable adenocarcinoma treated preoperatively and postoperatively with etoposide, cisplatin and 5-FU. One patient had a complete pathological response and 37% had negative nodes. The median survival was 24 months. No randomised trial has determined an optimum schedule for chemotherapy alone.

Postoperative chemotherapy

There are no trials on postoperative chemotherapy for oesophageal adenocarcinoma.

Combination chemotherapy and radiotherapy

Concurrent chemotherapy and radiotherapy without surgery

A number of studies have examined the role of combined chemotherapy and radiotherapy without surgery for adenocarcinoma, but most of these have been uncontrolled phase 2 trials.

Chemotherapy and radiotherapy followed by surgery

Because of the encouraging results with concurrent chemotherapy and radiotherapy a number of units have attempted to improve results of surgery by giving combination therapy prior to resection. The majority of trials have been single arm and uncontrolled.

Urba et al.[37] reported an uncontrolled trial of 5-FU as single agent therapy with 4900 cGy radiotherapy followed by transhiatal oesophagectomy in 24 patients. The median survival was only 11 months and it was concluded that there was no survival advantage but considerable toxicity with this regimen. Wolfe et al.[38] reviewed their experience with preoperative multiagent chemotherapy and radiotherapy in 93 patients with adenocarcinoma and reported a 5-year survival among the patients who underwent resection of 25%. Of those who underwent resection 20% had a sterilised specimen and had a 5-year survival of 60% (versus 40% sterilised specimens with a 40% 5-year survival for squamous cell carcinoma). In an uncontrolled trial of cisplatin, 5-FU and leucovorin, and concomitant 30 Gy radiation therapy in 24 patients with adenocarcinoma the median survival was more than 26 months, compared with 8 months for historical controls.[39] Actuarial survival at 24 months was 76% in the multimodality limb compared with 15% in historical controls. Treatment of 39 patients with adenocarcinoma with two cycles of cisplatin, 5-FU, etoposide, leucovorin and 30 Gy radiation therapy followed by resection resulted in a complete response in 19%.[40] Actuarial survival at 12 and 24 months was 72 and 51%. Significantly better survival was associated with adenocarcinoma then squamous carcinoma.

In the first prospective randomised trial comparing preoperative chemotherapy (5-FU and cisplatin) and 4000 cGy radiotherapy with surgery alone in 113 patients[41] the most important finding was the significant downstaging of the tumour in the treated group with 58% of patients in the multimodality therapy limb node negative compared with 18% in the surgery-only limb ($P < 0.001$).[41] A complete pathological response occurred in 13 of 52 patients (25%) who underwent resection following multimodality therapy. Median survival for patients randomised to multimodality therapy was 16 months versus 11 months for surgery alone ($P = 0.01$). At 1, 2 and 3 years 52, 37 and 32%, respectively, of patients randomised to multimodality therapy were alive versus 44, 26 and 6% treated by surgery with a survival advantage at three years favouring multimodality therapy ($P = 0.01$). It was concluded that multimodality treatment was superior to surgery alone for patients with resectable adenocarcinoma of the oesophagus.

Summary

There are few studies on adenocarcinoma of the oesophagus on which to base definite conclusions. Radiotherapy alone has not been examined and chemotherapy alone has a limited role when given preoperatively or postoperatively. When chemotherapy and radiotherapy are combined and given preoperatively up to 25% of patients with adenocarcinoma have a complete pathological response and there appears to be a survival advantage over surgery alone for the group as a whole. Further studies are required to confirm these findings and to optimise treatment regimens.

Gastric cancer

The role of radiotherapy

Radiotherapy alone

No study has compared radiation therapy alone with surgery alone for potentially curable gastric cancer. In patients with advanced gastric cancer Childs et al.[42] reported on a study of patients who were randomised to radiation therapy alone to a dose of 4000 cGy, or radiation therapy combined with 5-FU. There was a significant improvement in the survival with the combination of 5-FU and irradiation compared with irradiation alone.

Preoperative radiotherapy

There are no studies which have examined the role of radiation therapy in a preoperative setting.

Intraoperative radiotherapy

No randomised trial on this approach has yet been reported. Gilly *et al.*[43] treated 20 patients with gastric cancer with intraoperative radiation therapy (IORT). Mortality, morbidity, and average survival rates were compared with a non-randomised control group. Mortality and morbidity rates were similar in the two groups, with or without IORT. The follow-up period was too short for any valid conclusions about IORT in gastric cancer to be reached.

Abe *et al.*[44] reported on 115 patients treated with a single dose of 2800–3500 cGy IORT and compared them with a control group of patients operated on at about the same time with similar disease stage. There appeared to be an improvement in 5-year survival for stage II and stage III disease of the order of 10–20%. Randomised trials are awaited.

Postoperative radiotherapy

Few studies have evaluated radiation therapy alone as an adjuvant to surgical resection. Most studies have evaluated radiation therapy in patients given concomitant chemotherapy, making interpretation difficult. The most important randomised trial of this strategy was carried out by the British Stomach Cancer Group using a postoperative radiation therapy of 4500 cGy in 153 patients and found no survival advantage over surgery alone (145 patients) with a 5-year survival of 12% compared with 20% for surgery alone.[45] Local recurrence rates, however, were decreased by the use of radiation therapy – 54% with surgery alone versus 32% with radiation therapy. In a report on 115 patients who were randomised to receive radiotherapy alone or in a consecutive regimen with various dosage schedules of 5-FU the median survival times were significantly different between the four treatment regimens ($P = 0.04$).[46]

The role of chemotherapy

As the majority of patients presenting with gastric cancer have advanced locoregional or systemic disease it is necessary to consider systemic chemotherapy if any major improvement in survival is to be achieved.

Chemotherapy alone

Trials examining the role of chemotherapy as a sole agent for gastric cancer are largely confined to patients with advanced, unresectable but measurable disease. The median survival of patients with advanced disease left untreated is three to six months. Many single agent regimens have provided a greater than 20% response rate but have not enhanced survival. Multiagent combinations have a higher response rate but in most cases this has not translated to increased survival. Two multiagent trials are of interest. The EORTC group randomised 213 patients to receive 5-FU, doxorubicin, and methotrexate (FAMTx) or

5-FU, doxorubicin and mitomycin C (FAM), and reported a median survival of 10.5 months versus 7.25 months ($P = 0.004$).[47] Kelsen et al.[48] compared FAMTx with etoposide, adriamycin and cisplatin (EAP) and found the response rate and tolerance better for the former.

Preoperative chemotherapy

Results of at least six phase 2 non-randomised trials are available which show a trend towards improved survival compared with historical controls.[49] Only one randomised trial has compared neoadjuvant therapy followed by surgery with surgery alone and this study is ongoing but the survival rate at 2 years is 44%.[50] The authors cautioned that although the available data indicated that this approach was feasible and does not increase postoperative morbidity or mortality it did not show any improvement in patients with resectable tumours. It may have a greater role in patients with more advanced tumours where there appears to be an improved resection rate and a survival advantage for patients who respond and subsequently have a complete tumour resection.

Intraperitoneal chemotherapy

Schiessel et al.[51] in Germany compared intraperitoneal cisplatin and systemic thyrosulphate in 64 patients randomised to receive no additional treatment of the regime but no survival advantage was identified for the treated group. At least three other phase 2 trials are reported which have established the feasibility of this approach and alerted us to the complications which can be considerable.

Using a novel approach Takahashi et al.[14] randomised 113 patients with serosal involvement to intraperitoneal mitomycin C (MMC) bound to activated carbon particles, which are taken up by the lymphatics, or to surgery alone. The 2-year and 3-year survival rates for the MMC group were 42% and 38% compared with 28% and 20% ($P < 0.05$) for the control group. The differences were even more impressive for patients undergoing curative resection with survival rates of 66% and 66% versus 35% and 20% respectively ($P < 0.01$). When macroscopic peritoneal disease was present there was no survival difference.

Intraoperative chemohyperthermia

Yet another bold strategy is the recently reported peroperative instillation into the peritoneal cavity of a hyperthermic (43.5°C) solution of mitomycin C and cisplatin for locally advanced gastric cancer.[52] This non-randomised trial seemed to show a significant survival over surgery-only controls. Randomised trials are awaited with interest.

Postoperative chemotherapy
Single agent chemotherapy

Of six major randomised trials reporting the results of single agent therapy, and comparing outcome with controls, none revealed a significant improvement in overall survival. Subgroup analysis indicated a survival advantage in patients with minimal residual disease. Other studies, however, have indicated increased early mortality or reduced survival as a result of chemotherapy.[53]

One important exception to the poor outcome for single-agent chemotherapy was a trial reported by Estape et al.[54] who investigated the use of high-dose mitomycin C after surgical resection. A total of 33 patients received chemotherapy and 37 were randomised to surgery alone. The 5-year survival was 76% in the treated limb and 30% in the control limb and this difference reached statistical significance. This study has not yet been repeated in a larger number of patients.

Multiagent chemotherapy

The British Stomach Cancer Group recently reported on an important trial in which 436 patients were randomised to surgery alone (145 patients), postoperative radiation therapy of 4500 cGy (153 patients) and postoperative chemotherapy (5-FU, doxorubicin and mitomycin C) (138 patients).[45] They found no survival advantage for adjuvant chemotherapy with a 5-year survival rate of 19% versus 20% for surgery alone.

Two trials have shown a trend towards improved survival. The GITSG trial compared patients treated with methyl-CCNU (Semustine) and 5-FU with controls and found that of 142 patients the median survival was 56 months in the treated group compared with 33 months for controls ($P = 0.06$).[55] Nakajima et al.[56] in a three-limb study compared mitomycin C with mitomycin C, ftorafur ara C and controls and found a trend at 5 years favouring the multiagent limbs.

Hermans et al.[57] carried out a meta-analysis of all of the randomised trials conducted between 1980 and 1991 for adjuvant chemotherapy following curative resection. Only 11 trials, reporting on 2096 patients were suitable for analysis of crude mortality rates. They concluded that adjuvant chemotherapy regimens conferred no survival benefit for patients with a curative resection for gastric cancer. They recommended that further trials of adjuvant chemotherapy should include a no-treatment control arm.

In an analysis of 23 randomised trials, which included many of those in the above meta-analysis, only two of 15 Western trials and four of eight Japanese trials reported a survival advantage for chemotherapy.[58] The regimens with greatest effect contain 5-FU and/or mitomycin C. It is difficult to resolve the difference between the Eastern and Western series but the Japanese tend to initiate treatment immediately post-operatively, when they have a reduced postoperative tumour burden, and include higher doses of mitomycin C. They tend to have higher exclusion rates, however, and engage in subset analysis. Not all investigators have concluded that adjuvant chemotherapy has a role following curative resection and most insist that future studies should retain a surgery-only limb.[58]

Nakajima[59] reviewed 20 randomised trials and found, as others have, that the greatest optimism comes from subset analysis. They also

Figure 7.1 *Results of adjuvant chemotherapy regimens for gastric cancer based on randomised trials, with adjuvant chemotherapy results on the vertical axis and surgery-only controls on the horizontal axis. Reproduced from Nakajima[59] by kind permission from Springer-Verlag.*

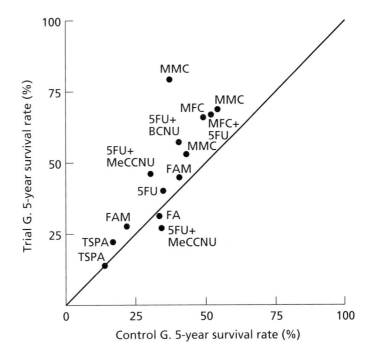

observed that the trials with the poorest responses tended to have surgery-only controls with 5-year survival rates of less than 30% (Fig. 7.1). As a 30% 5-year survival rate is the exception in the West it would appear that only patients with a curative resection and at most, micrometastases will benefit from current regimens.

Immunochemotherapy

Using a novel approach Natazato *et al.*[60] described the use of protein-bound polysaccharide (PSK) in addition to standard chemotherapy for patients undergoing curative resection. They found a significant improvement in 5-year survival rate from 60% to 73% ($P = 0.04$).

Postoperative radiotherapy plus chemotherapy

Postoperative radiotherapy plus chemotherapy

A number of phase 2 single institution trials have shown promise for combination therapy following surgical resection. Gunderson and associates treated 14 patients who had disease extension beyond the gastric wall, or nodal involvement, or both, with 4500–5200 cGy and 5-FU-based chemotherapy. They reported a median survival of 24 months and a 5-year survival of 43%.[61] Regional relapse occurred in only two of the 24 (14%) compared with 35% of patients with similar disease treated in the same hospital.

One prospective randomised trial has been reported from the Mayo Clinic which randomised 62 patients with poor prognosis but completely resected gastric cancer to postoperative chemoradiotherapy (5-FU and 3750 cGy) or surgery alone.[62] When compared by intention to treat, the adjuvant limb had a significantly better relapse-free and overall 5-year survival (23% versus 4% for surgery alone).

The GITSG evaluated 5-FU plus methyl-CCNU with and without 5000 cGy radiation therapy in patients with known residual disease and found a higher 5-year survival with the combined modality treatment of 18% versus 6% treated by surgery alone.[63] Bleiberg *et al.*[46] randomised patients to receive radiotherapy alone or radiotherapy and short-term or long-term 5-FU. The only long-term survivors were in the combined modality limb.

Although chemotherapy and radiotherapy on their own seem to add little to surgery there appears excellent justification for pursuing adjuvant combination chemoradiotherapy, at least in high risk patients. A large US intergroup trial is underway which should provide the definitive answer to this question.

Summary

Surgery remains the gold standard for cure. Extended lymphadenectomy employing the D2 resection is currently under evaluation for Western patients but any advantage that it may have in a subset of patients is offset by the morbidity and mortality associated with resection of the spleen and particularly the pancreas.[64] Radiotherapy improves local control but not survival. There are few confirmed Western trials in which systemic chemotherapy has been of proven benefit. No combination chemotherapy has been shown to be significantly better than 5-FU alone. Mitomycin C shows promise as a useful agent for systemic and intraperitoneal chemotherapy. Most Western studies have allowed a 6–8 week delay before initiating systemic chemotherapy. There are sound theoretical reasons however for giving chemotherapy immediately postoperatively. Preoperative combination chemotherapy and radiotherapy must be compared with surgery alone in a randomised trial. The standard treatment remains observation only after surgical resection, but entrance of high risk patients into carefully designed clinical trials is to be recommended.

Issues for the future

Efficacy, toxicity, cost and long-term complications will ultimately decide the role of multimodality therapy. Optimum regimens await further randomised trials. Most of the current regimens rely on 5-FU or mitomycin-based regimens. Toxicity has been reduced by the introduction of the $5-HT_3$ blockers which have dramatically diminished the nausea of chemotherapy, and by the use of colony stimulating factors to restore leukocyte function. Tumour targeting with non-toxic precursors of potent antitumour agents is a further area of promise.

Since only a certain percentage of tumours will respond to chemoradiotherapy it would be helpful to have an indicator of response.

Tumour growth factor receptor expression holds some promise in this area.[65]

Following successful chemoradiation, surgery is still necessary to resect residual disease. Up to 40% of squamous tumours and 20% of adenocarcinomas have a complete pathological response, yet it is impossible using current modalities, including intraoperative ultrasound, to identify those patients who do not require resection. This may become possible with the development of more sensitive tumour markers or more accurate tumour targeting.

Genetic markers hold promise for future therapy. It should be possible to identify patients at risk in families with a history of oesophageal cancer. Genetic studies may also clarify the aetiology of Barrett's oesophagus. Because of the toxicity of chemotherapy preoperative identification of patients at high risk for recurrence with surgery alone would be invaluable and genetic or molecular markers may hold valuable clues.

The next millennium holds out the wonderful promise of the ultimate demise of the cancer surgeon.

References

1. Cheng KK, Day NE, Davies TW. Oesophageal cancer mortality in Europe: paradoxical time trend in relation to smoking and drinking. Br J Cancer 1992; 65: 613–17.

2. Blot WJ, Devesa SS, Kneller RW, Fraumeni JF. Rising incidence of adenocarcinoma of the oesophagus and gastric cardia. JAMA 1991; 265: 1287–9.

3. Powell J, McConkey CC. The rising trend in oesophageal adenocarcinoma and gastric cardia. Eur J Cancer Prev 1992; 1: 265–9.

4. Husemann B. Cardia carcinoma considered as a distinct clinical entity. Br J Surg 1989; 76: 136–9.

5. Lund O, Kasenkam JM, Aagaard MT, Kimose HH. Time related changes in characteristics of prognostic significance in carcinoma of the oesophagus and cardia. Br J Surg 1989; 76: 1301–7.

6. World Health Statistics Annual 1993. WHO Geneva 1994; D-516.

7. Harrison JD, Fielding JWL. Prognostic factors for gastric cancer influencing clinical practice. World J Surg 1995; 19: 496–500.

8. Yamazaki H, Oshima A, Murakami R et al. A longterm follow-up study of patients with gastric cancer detected by mass screening. Cancer 1989; 63: 613–17.

9. Rohde H, Gebbensleben B, Bauer P et al. Has there been any improvement in the staging of gastric cancer. Findings from the German Gastric Cancer TNM study group. Cancer 1989; 64: 2465–81.

10. Kelsen DP, Minsky B, Smith M et al. Preoperative therapy for esophageal cancer: a randomized comparison of chemotherapy versus radiation therapy. J Clin Oncol 1990; 8: 1352–61.

11. Fisher B, Gunduz N, Saffer EA. Influence of the interval between primary tumour removal and chemotherapy on kinetics and growth of metastases. Cancer Res 1983; 43: 1488–92.

12. Murthy SM, Goldschmidt RA, Rao LN et al. The influence of surgical trauma on experimental metastasis. Cancer 1989; 64: 2035–44.

13. Eggermont AM, Steller EP, Sugarbaker PH. Laparotomy enhances intra-peritoneal tumour growth and aggrogates the antitumour effect of inter-leukin 2 and lymphokine-activated killer cells. Surgery 1987; 102: 71–8.

14. Takahashi T, Hagiwara A, Shimotsuma M, Sawai K, Yamaguchi T. Prophylaxis and treatment of peritoneal carcinomatosis: intraperitoneal chemotherapy with Mitomycin C bound to activated carbon particles. World J Surg 1995; 19: 565–9.

15. Fisher B, Gunduz N, Saffer EA *et al*. Influence of the interval between primary tumour removal and chemotherapy on kinetics and growth of metastases. Cancer Res 1983; 43: 1488–92.

16. Byfield JE. Combined modality infusional chemotherapy with radiation. In: Lokich JJ (ed.) Cancer chemotherapy by infusion, 2nd edn. Chicago: Precept Press, 1990, pp. 521–51.

17. Herskovic A, Martz K, Al-Sharraf M *et al*. Combined chemotherapy and radiotherapy compared with radiotherapy alone in patients with cancer of the esophagus. N Engl J Med 1992; 326: 1593–8.

18. Launois B, Delarue D, Campion JP, Kerbaol M. Preoperative radiotherapy for carcinoma of the oesophagus. Surg Gynecol Obstet 1981; 153: 690–2.

19. Gignoux M, Roussel A, Paillor B *et al*. The value of preoperative radiotherapy in esophageal cancer: results of a study of the EORTC. World J Surg 1987; 11: 426–32.

20. Huang GJ, Gu XZ. Experience with combined preoperative irradiation and surgery for squamous-cell carcinoma of the esophagus. In: Wagner G, Zhang YH (eds) Cancer of the liver, esophagus and nasopharynx. New York: Springer-Verlag, 1987, p. 134.

21. Husemann B. Preoperative radiotherapy or chemotherapy. In: Giuli R (ed.) Cancer of the esophagus in 1984. Paris: Maloine SA. Editeur 1984, pp. 55–58.

22. Nygaard K, Hagen S, Hansen HS *et al*. Preoperative radiotherapy prolongs survival in operable esophageal carcinoma: a randomized, multicenter study of pre-operative radiotherapy and chemotherapy. The Second Scandinavian trial in Esophageal Cancer. World J Surg 1992; 16: 1104–10.

23. Zieren HU, Müller JM, Jacobi CA, Pichlmaier H, Müller R-P, Staar S. Adjuvant postoperative radiation therapy after curative resection of squamous cell carcinoma of the thoracic esophagus: a prospective randomised study. World J Surg 1995; 19: 444–9.

24. French University Association for Surgical Research. Postoperative radiation therapy does not increase survival after curative resection for squamous cell carcinoma of the middle and lower esophagus as shown by a multicenter controlled trial. Surg Gynecol Obstet 1991; 173: 123–30.

25. Fok M, Sham JST, Choy D, Cheng SWK, Wong J. Postoperative radiotherapy for carcinoma of the esophagus: a prospective randomised controlled trial. Surgery 1993; 113: 138–47.

26. Kelsen DP, Minsky B, Smith M *et al*. Preoperative therapy for esophageal cancer: a randomised comparison of chemotherapy versus radiation therapy. J Clin Oncol 1990; 8: 1352–61.

27. Roth JA, Pass HI, Flanagan MM, Graeber GM, Rosenberg JC, Steinberg S. Randomised clinical trial of preoperative and postoperative adjuvant chemotherapy with cisplatin, vindesine and bleomycin for carcinoma of the esophagus. J Thorac Cardiovasc Surg 1988; 96: 242–8.

28. Saltz L, Kelsen D. Combined modality therapy in the treatment of loco-regional esophageal cancer. Ann Oncol 1992: 3: 793–9.

29. Roussel A, Bleiberg H, Dalesio O *et al*. Palliative therapy of inoperable oesophageal carcinoma with radiotherapy and methotrexate: final results of a controlled clinical trial. Int J Radiat Oncol Biol Phys 1988; 16: 67–72.

30. Sischy B, Ryan L, Haller D *et al*. Interim report of EST 1282 phase III protocol for the evaluation of combined modalities in the treatment of patients with carcinoma of the esophagus, stage I and II. Proc Am Soc Clin Oncol 1990; 9: 105–8.

31. Franklin R, Steiger Z, Vaishampayan G *et al*. Combined modality therapy for esophageal squamous cell carcinoma. Cancer 1983; 51: 1062–71.

32. Leichman L, Steiger Z, Seydel HG *et al*. Preoperative chemotherapy and radiation therapy for patients with cancer of the esophagus: a potentially curative approach. J Clin Oncol 1984; 2: 75–9.

33. Forastiere AA, Orringer MB, Perez-Tamayo C *et al*. Concurrent chemotherapy and radiation therapy followed by transhiatal esophagectomy for loco-regional cancer of the esophagus. J Clin Oncol 1990; 8: 119–27.

34. LePrise E, Etienne PL, Meunier B, Maddern G, Ben Hassel M, Gedouin D, Boutin D, Campion JP, Launois B. A randomised study of chemotherapy radiation therapy and surgery versus surgery for localised squamous cell carcinoma of the esophagus. Cancer 1994; 74: 1779–84.

35. Walsh TN, Noonan N, Hollywood D, Kelly A, Keeling N, Hennessy TPJ. Multimodality treatment plus surgery versus surgery alone for oesophageal squamous cell carcinoma. In: Peracchia A, Rosati R, Bonavina L *et al.* (eds) Recent advances in diseases of the esophagus. Milan: Monduzzi Editore, 1995, pp. 451–6.

36. Ajani JA, Roth JA, Ryan B *et al.* Evaluation of per- and post-operative chemotherapy for resectable adenocarcinoma of the esophagus. J Clin Oncol 1990; 8: 1231–8.

37. Urba SG, Orringer MB, Perez-Tamayo C, Bromberg J, Forastiere A. Concurrent pre-operative chemotherapy and radiation therapy in localized esophageal adenocarcinoma. Cancer 1992; 69: 285–91.

38. Wolfe WG, Vaughn AL, Seigler HF *et al.* Survival of patients with carcinoma of the esophagus treated with combined-modality therapy. J Thorac Cardiovasc Surg 1993; 105: 749–55.

39. Stewart JR, Hoff SJ, Johnson DH *et al.* Improved survival with neoadjuvant therapy and resection for adenocarcinoma of the esophagus. Ann Surg 1993; 218: 571–6.

40. Hoff SJ, Stewart JR, Sawyers JL *et al.* Preliminary results with neoadjuvant therapy and resection for esophageal carcinoma. Ann Thorac Surg 1993; 56: 282–6.

41. Walsh TN, Noonan N, Hollywood D, Kelly A, Keeling N, Hennessy TPJ. A comparison of multimodal therapy and surgery for esophageal adenocarcinoma. N Engl J Med 1996; 335: 462–7.

42. Childs D, Moertel CG, Holbrook MA *et al.* Treatment of unresectable adenocarcinoma of the stomach with a combination of 5-Fluorouracil and radiation. Am J Roentgenol Radium Ther Nucl Med 1968; 102: 541–4.

43. Gilly FN, Romestaing PJ, Gerard JP *et al.* Experience of three years with intra-operative radiation therapy using the Lyon intra-operative device. Int Surg 1990; 75: 84–8.

44. Abe M, Nishimura Y, Shibamoto Y. Intraoperative radiation therapy for gastric cancer. World J Surg 1995; 19: 554–7.

45. Hallissey MT, Dunn JA, Ward LC, Allum WH. The second British Stomach Cancer Group trial of adjuvant radiotherapy or chemotherapy in resectable gastric cancer: five year follow-up. Lancet 1994; 343: 1309–12.

46. Bleiberg H, Goffin JC, Dalesio O *et al.* Adjuvant radiotherapy and chemotherapy in resectable gastric cancer. A randomized trial of the gastro-intestinal tract cancer co-operative group of the EORTC. Eur J Surg Oncol 1989; 15: 535–43.

47. Wils JA, Klein HO, Wagener DJT *et al.* Sequential high dose methotrexate and flurouracil combined with doxorubicin – a step ahead in the treatment of advanced gastric cancer: a trial of the European Organisation for Research and Treatment of Cancer. J Clin Oncol 1991; 9: 827–31.

48. Kelsen D, Atiq O, Saltz L *et al.* FAMTx versus etoposide, doxorubicin and cisplatin in advanced gastric cancer. J Clin Oncol 1992; 10: 541–8.

49. Fink U, Stein HJ, Schuhmacher C, Wilke HJ. Neoadjuvant chemotherapy for gastric cancer: update. World J Surg 1995; 19: 509–16.

50. Fink U, Schuhmacher C, Böttcher K *et al.* Neoadjuvant chemotherapy with etopside/ adriamycin and cisplatin (EAP) in locally advanced gastric cancer. In: Salmon SE (ed.) Adjuvant therapy of gastric cancer VII, Philadelphia: Lippincott, 1993, pp. 272–80.

51. Schiessel R, Funovics J, Schick B *et al.* Adjuvant intra-peritoneal cisplatin therapy in patients with operated gastric carcinoma: results of a randomised trial. Acta Medica Austriaca 1989; 16: 68–9.

52. Yonemura Y, Ninomiya I, Kaji M *et al.* Prophylaxis with intraoperative chemohyperthermia against peritoneal recurrence of serosal invasion-positive gastric cancer. World J Surg 1995; 19: 450–4.

53. Koyama Y. The current status of chemotherapy for gastric cancer in Japan with special emphasis on Mitomycin C. Recent Results in Cancer Research 1978; 63: 135–47.

54. Estape J, Grau J, Leobendas F *et al.* Mitomycin C as an adjuvant treatment to resected gastric cancer. A ten year follow up. Ann Surg 1991; 214: 219–21.

55. Gastrointestinal Tumour Study Group. Controlled trial of adjuvant chemotherapy following curative resection for gastric cancer. Cancer 1982; 49: 1116–22.

56. Nakajima T, Takahashi T, Takagi K *et al.* Comparison of 5-fluorouracil with ftorafur in adjuvant chemotherapies would combine

induction and maintenance therapies for gastric cancer. J Clin Oncol 1984; 2: 1366–71.

57. Hermans J, Bonenkamp JJ, Boon MC *et al*. Adjuvant therapy after curative resection for gastric cancer: meta-analysis of randomized trials. J Clin Oncol 1993; 11: 1441–7.

58. Gunderson LL, Donohue JH, Burch PA. Stomach. In: Abeloff MD, Armitage JO, Lichter AS, Niederhuber JE (eds) Clinical oncology. New York: Churchill Livingstone, 1995, pp. 1209–42.

59. Nakajima T. Review of adjuvant chemotherapy for gastric cancer. World J Surg 1995; 19: 570–4.

60. Nakazato H, Koike A, Saji S, Ogawa N, Sakamoto J. Efficacy of immunochemotherapy as adjuvant treatment after curative resection of gastric cancer. Lancet 1994; 343: 1122–6.

61. Gunderson LL, Hoskins B, Cohen AM *et al*. Combined modality treatment of gastric cancer. Int J Radiat Oncol Biol Phys 1983; 9: 965–75.

62. Moertel CG, Childs DS, O'Fallon JR *et al*. Combination 5-fluorouracil and radiation therapy as a surgical adjuvant for poor prognosis gastric carcinoma. J Clin Oncol 1984; 2: 1249–54.

63. Gastrointestinal Tumour Study Group: a comparison of combination of chemotherapy and combined modality therapy for locally advanced gastric carcinoma. Cancer 1982; 49: 1362–6.

64. Cuschieri A, Fayers P, Fielding J *et al*. Postoperative morbidity and mortality after D1 and D2 resections for gastric cancer; preliminary results of the MRC randomised controlled surgical trial. Lancet 1996; 347: 995–9.

65. Hickey K, Grehen D, Reid I, O'Briain S, Walsh TN, Hennessy TPJ. Expression of epidermal growth factor receptor and proliferating cell nuclear antigen predicts response of esphageal squamous cell carcinoma to chemoradiotherapy. Cancer 1994; 74: 1693–8.

8 Palliative treatments of carcinoma of the oesophagus and stomach

Jane M. Blazeby
Derek Alderson

Despite recent improvements in the management of oesophageal and gastric cancer the majority of European and American patients still present with advanced disease. Palliative treatments are aimed at lessening the severity of symptoms with minimum morbidity and mortality and maximum quality of life until death occurs. Palliation, despite not having any curative effect on the disease itself, can prolong life especially where relief of dysphagia or gastric outflow obstruction leads to improved nutrition. This chapter concentrates on treatments designed to alleviate symptoms and improve quality of life in patients with oesophageal and gastric cancer.

Epidemiology

It is difficult to obtain reliable data about patients with advanced disease who eventually undergo only palliative treatment because of lack of standard definitions of the terms 'inoperable', 'unresectable' and 'advanced disease'. Patients may have a resectable tumour but be unfit to withstand surgery or they may be fit but have locally advanced disease. These issues confound many outcomes, in particular in the management of oesophageal cancer where comorbidity strongly determines management. Patients with lymph node involvement have less chance of being cured than those without nodal metastases, but oesophagectomy and adjuvant therapy are frequently performed in patients with Stage IIb cancers. Others define only tumours as advanced if distant lymph node metastases (coeliac axis or para-aortic nodes) or distant organ metastases are present (Stages III and IV). There is also the opinion that advanced disease is present only if resection fails or is incomplete. For patients with gastric cancer the situation differs because total gastrectomy has a lower morbidity and perioperative mortality than oesophagectomy.

Oesophagectomy rates may reflect the number of patients who are given a hope of possible cure. Series published from both the East and West, however, show a wide variation in resection rates, from 13 to 85%.[1,2] In 1990 Müller *et al.*[3] published a critical overview of surgery for oesophageal cancer. The outcomes from 1201 papers on the surgical treatment of oesophageal carcinoma were reviewed using a specially designed scoring system. The resectability rate (69 authors) was just 21%. It was concluded that these numbers indicate that most figures provided do not allow a general statement on resectability of oesophageal carcinoma to be made, but rather that statistics reflect the situation in a particular hospital, the preselection of referrals and the approach of the surgeon. In the United Kingdom at least 50% of patients with oesophageal cancer are considered unsuitable for radical treatment at the time of diagnosis. Figures may be higher as aged, frail patients often never see a surgeon and die without any specific form of treatment. Others are not referred for a surgical opinion despite the fact that many may be reasonable candidates.

In the western hemisphere about 70–80% of patients present with incurable gastric cancer, either due to widespread dissemination or irresectability.[4] This situation contrasts sharply with the East where early gastric tumours account for a much larger proportion of all new patients and 5-year survival rates are above 50%.

Survival

Palliative treatments aim to increase quality of life by relieving symptoms. Serendipitous survival advantages may be gained because of improved nutrition due to relief of dysphagia or gastric outflow obstruction. Most studies, however, demonstrate no significant differences in survival between palliative treatments despite finding differences between relief of symptoms.

Patients with advanced oesophageal cancer have an average life expectancy of 3–4 months after diagnosis and few survive beyond one year. Some authors argue that laser oesophageal recanalisation produces better survival than standard treatment regimens.[5,6] Prospective randomised trials of laser versus intubation have failed to support this suggestion.[7,8] Other evidence suggests that combination chemotherapy may prolong survival in patients with advanced carcinoma of the oesophagus.[9] This finding has yet to be confirmed.

The median survival for patients with gastric cancer undergoing treatment with palliative intent is also poor. About 50% will be dead within six months and the remainder within two years. Most palliative treatments do not change the natural course of advanced gastric cancer although increasing interest has been recently centred around the role of chemotherapy. One phase 3 study comparing best supportive care with combination chemotherapy has found a significant survival difference between the two groups (3 and 12 months, respectively).[10] This small trial has yet to be confirmed in larger studies.

The two factors other than disease stage which appear to influence survival in patients with oesophageal and gastric cancer are severity of dysphagia and performance status at diagnosis. Derodra et al.[11] showed that patients presenting with dysphagia to solid foods and liquids lived significantly longer than those presenting with complete dysphagia (9 weeks and 3 weeks respectively). This retrospective series only included patients referred to a specialist endoscopy unit and thus patients without dysphagia but with haematogenous disease spread (e.g. liver metastases) were not included in the analysis. Pretreatment performance scores may predict outcome but better measures of performance and quality of life which are now available may reveal other important variables.

Selection of patients for palliative treatment

After establishing a diagnosis patients require careful assessment in order to decide whether treatment is directed towards attempting a cure or if palliation of symptoms is more appropriate. Careful patient selection has been shown to significantly influence results.[1,12] Principal factors that influence this judgement are: whether the patient is fit enough to tolerate the procedure; the stage and characteristics of the tumour and consideration of the patient's preferences.

Fitness for treatment

The place of oesophagectomy in many older patients is often quite easily settled because of general debilitation or multiple co-existent medical problems. Age in itself does not preclude octogenarians from surgery but most series of older patients are carefully selected. The role of radical radiotherapy is debatable in patients who are in a poor general state, some report good results and other have found morbidity rates similar to that associated with surgical resection in the elderly.[13] On the whole surgery for gastric tumours is tolerated better by the elderly population than oesophageal surgery but patients still require careful preoperative assessment before undergoing major palliative resections.

Staging investigations

Accurate tumour staging plays a critical part of any therapeutic protocol allowing patients to be assigned appropriately to treatments with either curative or palliative intent. Some investigations may provide clear cut evidence of haematogenous tumour spread or irresectability and thus select patients for palliative treatment. No single investigation is perfect, however, and some patients thought unsuitable for resection still require explorative surgery to settle this point.

Patient preferences

Public demands for new treatments which are based partly on levels of information in the public domain are beginning to influence the provision of health care services in the management of many malignancies. There is an increasing awareness of the variable outcome of treatment for cancer and consequently a growing demand to concentrate care in specialist cancer centres.[14] Although little is known at present about the psychology of patients with oesophageal and gastric cancer, all clinicians will be faced with patients who demand every small chance of cure, despite its risks, and others who wish to receive minimal dignified intervention. In view of this, clinical decisions should be made with the patient and their family having access to as much information as they require.

Symptoms and signs of advanced oesophageal and gastric cancer

Tumours of the oesophagus and gastric cardia

Tumours of the gastric cardia are clinically indistinguishable in their presentation from lower oesophageal cancer. Both produce dysphagia and chest pain in 90% of patients. The progressive nature of malignant dysphagia is usually readily apparent. Initial difficulties in swallowing solid food develops to inability to swallow even saliva. This may lead to persistent coughing, dyspnoea and aspiration pneumonia. Odonyphagia adds to the anxiety already associated with eating and patients rapidly lose weight and become cachexic. Persistent coughing because of food in the bronchial tree leads to bronchial collapse and recurrent chest infections leading to exhaustion and overwhelming sepsis. Oesophagorespiratory fistulas are present in about 5% of patients with oesophageal cancer. They are one of the most distressing and rapidly fatal complications of the disease. Hoarseness and complications of vocal cord palsy because of tumour infiltration of the recurrent laryngeal nerves are frequently present in patients with recurrence or inoperable tumours.

Tumours of the body and distal stomach

Gastric cancer in the mid-stomach commonly has an insidious presentation due to slow blood loss eventually resulting in symptoms of anaemia. By this stage the patient is frequently cachexic with other signs of advanced disease. Patients with a palpable epigastric mass due to carcinoma will usually have locally advanced disease. Carcinomas of the distal stomach produce gastric outlet obstruction. Patients complain of epigastric fullness and discomfort, early satiety and effortless vomiting. Supraclavicular lymphadenopathy, jaundice, ascites, pleural effusion are all evidence of disseminated disease. Less commonly bony pain and symptoms of increased intracranial pressure are seen due to metastatic lesions. Other troublesome symptoms are iatrogenic, e.g. side effects of high dose opiates, constipation, dry mouth and bloating.

The provision of rapid relief of dysphagia or gastric obstruction for patients with advanced oesophageal and gastric malignancies is the main priority of palliative treatment. Patients also require dietary advice from nutrition teams and palliative care physicians who can assist in mobilising multidisciplinary carers.

Palliative treatments for cancer of the oesophagus and gastric cardia

A wide variety of approaches are available to palliate symptoms of advanced tumours of the oesophagus and gastric cardia. There is little place for bypass surgery in the management of oesophageal cancer. As a result of modern preoperative imaging, few patients are selected for surgery who have irresectable tumours. The results of purely palliative resections, i.e. macroscopic tumour left behind, are poor. In the pooled patient study published by Müller et al.[3] palliative resection resulted in 3- and 5-year survival rates of 6% and 2% respectively. Hospital mortality rates were about 10% and 46% had significant post-operative complications. The results of bypass surgery are also poor, with mortality rates in the range 20–35%.[15,16] The only notable exception was the series reported by Mannell et al.[17] in which the hospital mortality was only 11%, with 82% of patients having complete and lasting relief of dysphagia. Although palliative resection can relieve dysphagia and prevent problems such as haemorrhage, aspiration and the risk of aerodigestive fistula, all of these can usually be addressed by other approaches. Patients not only suffer the in-hospital morbidity and mortality but they also take several months to recover from major surgery; time taken from a short life expectancy. Nowadays with far better, safer methods of alleviating the obstructed oesophageal or gastric lumen there seems little place for this approach.

The following section will concentrate on the non-resectional palliative means for treating oesophageal cancer. It is divided into four categories: methods of replacing the obstructed lumen, treatment of aerodigestive fistulas; management of recurrent laryngeal nerve palsy and the management of chronic bleeding.

Methods of replacing the obstructed lumen

Malignant dysphagia may be relieved by repeated dilatations, endoscopic or open insertion of a stent, tumour ablation with laser, heat or diathermy or injection of cytotoxic substances. Many modalities can be viewed as complementary.

Oesophageal dilatation

This is essentially of historic interest and its role nowadays is reduced to that of a temporary measure prior to definitive management of dysphagia. Results are short lived and dysphagia returns rapidly within a few days. One series of 38 patients undergoing dilatation, reported a 14% failure rate.[18] It was impossible to safely position the guide wire in three patients and after the first dilatation two tracheo-oesophageal fistulas occurred. Dilatation before intubation, laser treatment or tumour necrosis with ethanol or diathermy is safest with dilators passed over a prepositioned guidewire.[19]

Intubation

In the United Kingdom this is the most commonly used palliative treatment for malignant dysphagia.[20] Prostheses should be placed endoscopically, there is little place for insertion of the tube at laparotomy with its attendant high morbidity and mortality.[12,20] There are still a few indications for an open intubation. After a failed endoscopic attempt because of extreme angulation of the tumour or if the tumour is found to be inoperable at resection, then traction intubation at laparotomy may be indicated if relief cannot be obtained by other means. Insertion of a prosthesis with a flexible endoscope should be performed under intravenous sedation and analgesia (midazolam and pethidine), although many endoscopists continue to use general anaesthesia. Intravenous sedation still requires continual attention to the airway. Saliva and regurgitated fluids should be constantly sucked from the patient to prevent aspiration during the procedure.

It is contraindicated to place a plastic prosthesis less than 2 cm from the upper oesophageal sphincter. There is risk of proximal migration into the hypopharynx and laryngeal compression or an unpleasant sensation of a foreign body can occur. Relative contraindications are more dependent on operator expertise, but total luminal obstruction, non-circumferential tumour growth prohibiting proper anchoring of the prosthesis, almost horizontal orientation of the malignant lumen, prior chemoradiation and multi-angulated lesions, particularly with tumours at the gastro-oesophageal junction, make preliminary dilatation hazardous.[21,22] There are two types of stents available: non-expandable plastic prostheses and expandable metal prostheses.

Non-expandable plastic endoprostheses

There are several types of plastic endoprosthesis available.

1. Custom made polyvinyl prosthesis (Tygon). These are purpose built to match the individual anatomical needs of the patient's tumour. Tubing with an outer diameter of 15.7 mm, an internal diameter of 12.5 mm and a wall of 1.6 mm is the preferred choice. It should be cut 5–6 cm longer than the stricture. The proximal end may be expanded to form a flange.

2. The KeyMed Atkinson prosthesis (KeyMed Ltd, Southend, UK) (Fig. 8.1) is made of silicone rubber tubing. It has an internal diameter of 11–11.7 mm and external diameter of 14–16 mm. A nylon spring is incorporated into its wall to prevent kinking. A shoulder is attached to the distal end to prevent migration. Lengths of 7–19 cm are available.

3. The Medoc–Celestin tube (Medoc Ltd, Tetbury, UK) (Fig. 8.1) is made of latex rubber with a nylon spiral incorporated into the wall.[24] Celestin tubes may be inserted either with the traction or pulsion technique. A proximal inkwell funnel is designed to collect food and prevent distal migration. A non-traumatic collapsible umbrella-shaped flange attached at the distal end prevents proximal migration. They are available in four lengths: 9.5, 12.5, 15 and 21 cm with internal diameters of 11.5–15 mm.

4. The Procter–Livingstone tube is made of armoured soft latex with an internal diameter of 12 mm and external diameter of 18 mm. The tube is available in 10, 15 and 19 cm lengths and is inserted endoscopically.[25]

5. The Wilson–Cook prosthesis Wilson–Cook Medical, Winston-Salem, NC, USA) (Fig. 8.1) is made of silicone rubber reinforced with a metal spiral; outer diameter 16mm, inner diameter 12 mm, available in lengths ranging from 4.4 to 16.4 cm. A prosthesis with a short proximal funnel for placement close to the cricopharyngeus is also available.[26]

6. The ESKA–Buess oesophageal tube (ESKA, Lubeck, Germany) is made of medical grade silicone with a metal spiral embedded in the wall. It has an oval-shaped proximal funnel to prevent upper airway compression. The distal funnel collapses completely when passed through a stenosis. Metal hooks integrated in the proximal funnel can be snared if repositioning of the tube is required.[27]

Figure 8.1 *Three of the most frequently used plastic oesophageal stents (left to right): Wilson–Cook, Atkinson and Medoc Celestin.*

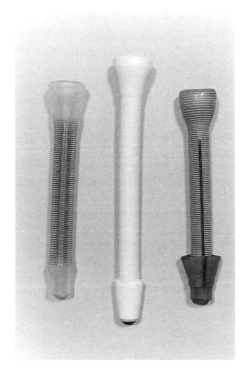

7. The Mousseau–Barbin tube, although now rarely used, was designed to be pulled through at laparotomy.[28]

Method of insertion

There are many methods of endoscopic insertion of a non-expandable plastic endoprosthesis. They are all based on the same principles. The most important step is dilatation of the stricture before insertion of the stent. Dilatation may be performed gradually a few days before intubation or just prior to intubation. The number of dilators of increasing diameter depends on the length of the stricture, the degree of narrowing and the tortuosity of the lesion. In all situations endoscopic guidewire placement should be performed using fluoroscopy. Recent advances in radiological equipment now ensure that safe guidewire placement is nearly always possible. A luminal diameter of at least 15 mm is required to accommodate a prosthesis. Some scirrhous malignancies require dilatation to 18 or 20 mm. After adequate dilatation the exact measurement of the tumour from the incisors is determined endoscopically and the location point for the proximal funnel edge is marked on the introducer tube. Proximal and distal extents of the tumour may also be marked with radio-opaque skin markers or the tumour limitations injected with contrast.[29,30] The selected tube is then placed onto a supporting device. This device can be a dilator shaft (the Eder–Puestow dilator[31]), over a bougie (Savary–Gilliard type[32]), over a balloon catheter, over a commercially available device (Wilson–Cook, KeyMed[33], Celestin or the Amsterdam Metal introducing devices[21]) or over a small-calibre endoscope itself.[33] In addition to the introducing device a pusher tube may be used. The pusher tube slides over the introducing device and rests against the proximal end of the stent. The pusher and the introducing device carrying the well-lubricated endoprosthesis are then passed over the guidewire to the predetermined position. This should be confirmed with screening. The prosthesis should now be seated properly with its funnel located above the proximal margin of the tumour. With the tube in position the operator holds the pusher tube steady as the introducing device is withdrawn. The endoscope is then reinserted to check the position of the prosthesis. Care must be taken not to dislodge the tube upon withdrawal of the endoscope.

Postoperative management

After stent insertion the patient must be instructed to sit bolt upright. Clinical and radiological examination must be checked for evidence of perforation before oral fluids are commenced. Patients should receive written dietary information with advice to chew food carefully and to drink regularly during and after meals. Daily intake of 10 ml of hydrogen peroxide 20 vol. is sometimes recommended. Table 8.1 summarises this care.

Table 8.1 *Management of patients after intubation*

Postprocedure care
Sit bolt upright
Chest radiograph
Dietary advice

Complications

Even in experienced hands endoscopic intubation has a high morbidity and mortality. Most series report 30–40% morbidity rates and procedure-related mortality rates of 3–16%.[12,20] Complications are listed in Table 8.2. Successful placement should be obtained in at least 90% of patients. Malposition requires immediate removal and repositioning. Chest pain lasting for several days is not uncommon although it is important to ensure it does not represent a small perforation. Predisposing factors to oesophageal perforation are previous radiotherapy, sharp angulation, extensive tumour encasing the oesophagus and involvement of the cardia. Rapid development of subcutaneous emphysema, severe pain or radiological evidence of pneumomediastinum, air under the diaphragm or a pleural effusion should raise suspicion. Diagnosis is confirmed with contrast radiography. The most appropriate form of therapy depends on the time of detection. If recognised at endoscopy the insertion of a prosthesis may seal off the perforation and prevent mediastinitis. Alternatively the procedure may be abandoned and conservative treatment started. Conservative measures include administration of broad spectrum antibiotics, cessation of oral intake and feeding either parenterally or by jejunostomy. An intercostal drain may need to be inserted if there is evidence of pleural contamination. Survival rates following conservative management are 70–80%, the key to success being early diagnosis to avoid mediastinal contamination.[34] Early migration occurs in about 1% of patients. Tubes may be left in the stomach although obstruction of the pyloric channel or intestinal perforation necessitates removal at

Table 8.2 *Complications of stent insertion*

Early complications	Late complications
Malposition	Migration
Incomplete expansion[a]	Tumour ingrowth[a]
Pain	Tumour overgrowth
Perforation	Food bolus obstruction
Bleeding	Reflux
Migration	Late perforation
Aspiration pneumonia	Disintegration of prosthesis

[a]Specific to metal stents.

laparotomy.[35] Occasionally tubes pass per anus. Between 3 and 13% of patients aspirate during tube insertion and may develop pneumonia. Severe upper gastrointestinal haemorrhage occasionally occurs.

Late complications

Late complications occur in at least 20% of patients. They require hospital admission, repeat endoscopic manoeuvres and occasionally replacement of the prosthesis. Late distal stent migration has been reported to occur in about 7–14%. Patients present with recurrent dysphagia and a new prosthesis is required. Food bolus obstruction also leads to recurrent dysphagia. Atkinson tubes, which have a narrower diameter, may be more prone to this problem. It is easily dealt with by passage of a paediatric endoscope up and down the tube displacing the impacted food bolus on into the stomach. Ogilvie et al.[20] found that food blockage tended to occur more often in tubes over 10 cm in length. Prostheses may also block because of tumour overgrowth. This can be treated with laser or insertion of another tube within the prosthesis.[36] Diathermy and alcohol injection are often ineffective at ablating the tumour overgrowth because of its bulky nature. The use of an endoscopic sphincterotomy knife to resect recurrent tumour has been described.[37] Reflux of gastric acid occurs in all patients whenever the tube crosses the gastro-oesophageal junction. It may lead to oesophagitis and occasionally benign stricture formation above the tube. This can be controlled with conservative measures, dilatation and acid suppressive therapy.[21] Pressure necrosis and late oesophageal perforation can occur at the funnel edge of the tube in an area either invaded by tumour or previously irradiated. It is made worse by marked angulation between the oesophagus and prothesis. It causes pain and may lead to the formation of a mediastinal fistula. Prostheses may deteriorate, disintegrate and migrate causing obstruction. This is rare as most patients do not live long enough. Celestin latex tubes are, theoretically, more prone to structural deterioration when exposed to hydrochloric acid, bile and radiation than non-degradeable silicone rubber Atkinson tubes.[38] If this occurs the prosthesis needs to be changed to prevent potentially serious complications of disintegration and fracture of the prosthetic tube which may lead to small bowel ulceration and perforation.[35] Endoscopic removal may be achieved by inserting a through-the-scope balloon inside the tube, inflating it and then pulling it out. Other methods have been described, using rat-toothed forceps, polypectomy snares or with the distal end of the scope sharply bent to act as a hook.[21,39] Operative removal of some tubes is only rarely required.

Relief of dysphagia

Once a prosthesis is in place the quality of swallowing is similar for several months, but all food must pass through a rigid tube. Most prostheses allow 10–15% of patients to eat virtually normally, 50–60% to eat a semi-solid diet and the remainder only to drink liquids.[20]

The immediate relief of dysphagia in one endoscopy session at low cost makes plastic endoprostheses an attractive simple palliative treatment. The high mortality and morbidity rates make conventional intubation an unsatisfactory method of relieving malignant dysphagia. The procedure is uncomfortable and results are far from perfect. It is hoped that the introduction of expanding metallic stents which do not require wide preliminary oesophageal dilatation will overcome the limitations of plastic tubes.

Expandable metal stents

Expanding metal stents have been used in the bile duct, the urinary tract, the arterial and bronchial tree and are now available for the treatment of malignant dysphagia. It is claimed that they have numerous advantages compared to plastic tubes although they cost about 10 times more. Theoretically, they are easy to insert on a slim delivery system and this requires intravenous sedation only. They are expected to improve dysphagia significantly because the fully expanded stent lumen is 18–25 mm and they may be better tolerated than plastic tubes in high oesophageal strictures.[40] Early results of randomised trials have not completely confirmed this and because of the considerable expense of metal stents, evidence of both clinical and cost-effectiveness is still needed before their routine introduction into clinical practice.[41]

Commercially available metal prostheses

There are four systems available for deployment in the oesophagus (Fig 8.2).

1. The Wallstent (Schneider, Bulach, Switzerland) is woven in the form of a tubular mesh configuration from surgical-grade stainless super

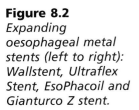

Figure 8.2
Expanding oesophageal metal stents (left to right): Wallstent, Ultraflex Stent, EsoPhacoil and Gianturco Z stent.

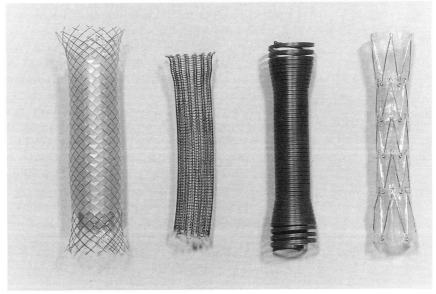

alloy monofilament wires. The stent is pliable, self-expanding and flexible in the longitudinal axis. It is loaded in a small diameter delivery catheter, constrained in a compressed form by a double plastic membrane. During expansion the stent shrinks by approximately one-third. The change in length and diameter is dependent on the nature of the malignant stricture. It is available with or without a surrounding silicone membrane. The partially covered stent has 2 cm bare at either end to allow epithelialisation and prevent stent migration.

2. The Ultraflex stent (Boston Scientific, Watertown, Massachusetts, USA) is knitted from nitinol wire, a single-stranded alloy of nickel and titanium. Nitinol has a shape 'memory' as well as super elastic behaviour. The design incorporates a proximal flare for secure placement. A covered stent has just become available. It is available in three length: 7, 10 and 15 cm.

3   The Gianturco Z stent (Wilson–Cook Medical, Winston-Salem, North Carolina, USA) is made of 0.5 mm latticed stainless-steel wire constructed in a cylindrical fashion. It is fully covered with a polyethylene film and has 3 mm-long wire hooks at its mid portion to facilitate anchoring. Unlike the Ultraflex and Wallstents it does not shrink on release.

4. The EsoPhacoil (Instent, Eden Prairie, Minnesota, USA) is a tightly wound coiled spring that shortens and widens on release. The stent is robust and external compression by a tumour is unlikely. Theoretically, kinking due to tumour angulation should be less with this design than the other types.

Implantation

The principles of metal stent implantation are similar to those of plastic stent insertion, requiring intravenous sedation and analgesia and precise radiological measurement. Certain details differ and deployment techniques of the compressed stents vary between commercially available prostheses. The stricture is measured and its exact location identified with skin markers or submucosal injection of radio-opaque contrast. Preinsertion dilatation may be required if an endoscope with an outer diameter of 12 mm is unable to negotiate the stricture. A guidewire is passed and the slim delivery device advanced over the guide wire until the radio-opaque markers of the compressed stent are correctly aligned. Once in position the stent is deployed. It is possible to reposition the Wallstent after partial deployment. Other stents require balloon dilatation to fully expand the prosthesis. Post-stent insertion patients should be examined and observed for signs of perforation and other clinical care is similar to that received by patients with traditional plastic prostheses.

Complications

Expanding metal stents are subject to similar complications associated with plastic tubes and problems specific to their particular design

(Table 8.2). Combined case series report a procedure-related mortality of about 2% and morbidity rates of about 20%.[42,43] Successful deployment can almost always be achieved but more than one stent may be required to adequately cover the tumour. Incomplete stent expansion most frequently occurs with the Ultraflex oesophageal stent; it has been reported in up to 40% of procedures.[43] Balloon dilatation may improve expansion and can be performed up to several days later. Malposition of the stent above or below a stricture will occur less as technical skill increases. It is hoped that stent designs will be improved to diminish this difficulty. About 10% of stents migrate distally.[42] Stents crossing the gastro-oesophageal junction seem to be more prone to this complication than those that have both ends anchored within the oesophagus. Endoscopic retrieval has been described but it is not routinely advocated by stent manufacturers. Like their plastic counterparts metal stents may be left in the stomach unless they obstruct the pylorus or cause further complications. Rates of oesophageal perforation seem to be lower with metal stents than those associated with plastic prostheses.[44,45] It is hypothesised that less perforation occurs because of the slim delivery system used to introduce metal stents, thus avoiding the need for the forceful insertion required for large diameter plastic tubes. Of 119 consecutive patients undergoing implantation of Gianturco stents no perforations were reported.[42]

Late complications

There are reports of oesophageal wall necrosis resulting in bleeding related to stent erosion or late perforation. Previous chemotherapy or radiotherapy may increase such a problem.[22,46] Obstruction due to impaction of food in or above the stent seems to occur in 5–30% of patients and appears to be more frequent if the stent is uncovered.[42,43,47] Tumour ingrowth or overgrowth can be managed by a variety of endoscopic methods: balloon trawling, laser treatment, diathermy, ethanol injections, intraluminal radiotherapy, dilatation or placement of a standard plastic stent through the metal stent.[47] It is not yet established if metallic stents reduce the number of other symptoms such as reflux and pain from an indwelling prosthesis. Reports indicate that about 20% of patients complain of heartburn. Results of randomised trials which contain validated patient outcome measures are awaited.[42]

Trials comparing expandable with non-expandable stents

There is currently only one published randomised trial comparing Wallstent with plastic endoprostheses.[41] A lower rate of immediate complications was reported in the metal stent group although no difference was seen in the 30-day mortality. The Wallstents were uncovered and a number of design problems occurred in the small study. Patients receiving conventional tubes were treated under general anaesthetic whereas those receiving metal stents had only intravenous sedation. Technical complications encountered with the plastic tube were substantial but most oesophageal surgeons consider it unnecessarily aggressive to use a 20 mm balloon dilator before inserting a prosthesis. Recurrent dysphagia was equally common in both groups and most frequently resulted from tumour ingrowth in the group treated with metal stents and tube migration in the plastic endoprosthesis group. Despite their higher costs, the metal stents proved cost effective because of the decreased complication rate and shorter hospital stay. The question of whether ease of placement and versatility offsets the high cost of metal stents remains unanswered. Manufacturers are currently tackling new improved designs to prevent distal migration and tumour ingrowth.

Laser treatment

The most widely used laser is based on the solid crystal neodymium yttrium aluminium garnet (Nd:YAG). This has a wavelength of 1064 nm, is in the near infrared part of the spectrum and therefore invisible to the naked eye. A low power helium–neon laser is incorporated in the system to provide a visible red aiming beam. It has been used to alleviate obstruction and arrest haemorrhage secondary to metastatic or locally unresectable carcinomas of the oesophagus and stomach. It can also be employed as a temporary measure before definitive operative management of malignant dysphagia. Laser light may be absorbed, scattered, transmitted or reflected by living tissue. Absorption leads to dissipation of light energy and generation of heat. Scatter leads to a larger volume of tissue absorbing the incident light. Different laser systems are currently available and each has varied effects on tumours. The Nd:YAG laser is poorly absorbed by living tissue but significantly scattered, which produces a uniform light distribution. Thermal contraction occurs when this laser is used in normal tissue. Continued exposure with a significantly powerful source leads to tissue necrosis with eventual vaporisation. Its effect on the tissue depends on the power output selected, the duration of application, the distance between the fibre tip and target, the aim of the application and the colour of the tissue. Hence only approximate predictions can be made about the effect of the laser on a particular tumour. The first tissue reaction is a white circular burn. If the beam is continuously focused on the same site, cavitation may occur at close distances (< 0.5 cm) and high power (90–100 W). When applied to bleeding areas a blacked charred appearance develops. Treatment continues until the target is vaporised. In view of these varied responses it is not surprising that conflicting results have been reported in the response to treatment between squamous cell and adenocarcinoma of the upper gastrointestinal tract. Some have found no differences in sensitivity, others claim that adenocarcinoma is more susceptible to laser light destruction due to its texture, than the whiter, less vascular squamous epithelium.[48] Each laser treatment session may recanalise the whole or just 2–3 cm of stricture. Some recommend routine endoscopic review at 48–72 h, when oedema has subsided and accurate assessment of the overall effect can be made. The treated area should be whitish-yellow, soft and necrotic. The destroyed tumour may then be evacuated with forceps, polyp graspers, lavage or pushed distally with the endoscope. Others administer treatment as dictated by need.

Endoscopic technique

If the malignant stricture is negotiable the laser is first applied to the distal end of the tumour. The scope is then withdrawn in a circular fashion onto the more proximal tumour. If complete obstruction is encountered, tumours can be vaporised in the prograde direction or first dilated to allow passage of the endoscope. Prograde therapy may be more dangerous because information about the luminal axis is lacking, and the areas first treated rapidly become oedematous which impairs access to more distal parts. Pretreatment dilatation also introduces risks. Retrograde treatment may be more efficient than prograde tumour necrosis because recanalisation can be achieved in one session and thus allow reduced hospitalisation and early enteral feeding.[49] Laser treatment requires only intravenous sedation and often pharyngeal anaesthesia although some continue to use a rigid endoscope, general anaesthesia and endotracheal intubation. Those in favour of a rigid scope believe its advantages are that is allows better suction of fluid, smoke and debris, with improved visualisation of the tumour.[50] A few clinicians recommend the routine use of prophylactic antibiotics because of bacteraemia induced by endoscopy.[51] Most endoscopists only administer antibiotics to those known to be at risk of endocarditis.

High or medium power non-contact therapy

The laser energy is conveyed through a single quartz flexible monofibre which is enclosed in a Teflon sheath (diameter 1.6–2.5 mm). This readily passes down the biopsy channel of a conventional endoscope. At the tip of the light guide a metal jet encloses the end of the fibre to support the system. The average power setting of the non-contact Nd:YAG is 60–120 W. At an irradiation distance of 5–10 mm multiple pulses for a duration of about 0.5–1 s are given. Coaxial gas (usually CO_2 or NO_2) is administered around the quartz fibre, to cool the probe tip and clear the debris. Gas is removed with the suction channel of the endoscope. A nasogastric tube next to the endoscope can be used to vent the insufflated carbon dioxide and smoke produced by vaporisation and minimise over distension.[48]

Low power contact Nd:YAG therapy

A contact laser synthetic sapphire probe was developed in 1985 which may be attached to the end of a standard quartz fibre using a universal metal connector.[52] Coaxial water is used to cool the tip, remove debris and reduce adherence of the contact probe. Power settings are lower than used for the non-contact system, about 10–40 W on a pulsed duration of 1–5 s. Essentially the sapphire laser tip acts like a hot knife. Tips with a variety of shapes have been developed: hemispherical, cylindrical, wedge-shaped and spiked. A newer ceramic probe made from aluminium hydroxide powder has also been developed which can be used with the universal metal connector.[53] Theoretically, the lower power settings mean that the chances of perforation by excessive laser energy are reduced. Tissue damage only occurs up to 0.5 mm beyond the treatment site. Some find that the tactile feedback of the contact laser probe helps the endoscopist to destroy the tumour with greater precision and safety.

Complications

The incidence of major complications and mortality is usually lower for YAG laser destruction than for endoscopic intubation, in the region of 1–5%.[54] Some report 100% technical success, but patients with long circumferential tumours often have less good functional results. The response in this type of tumour usually lasts only 4–6 weeks.[55] Early complications are listed in Table 8.3. Chest pain which may result from extensive mucosal burning in patients who have had large sub-mucosal tumours treated is quite common but not severe. Non-contact laser treatment may cause more pain than contact therapy due to heat build up on the mucosal surface. It is possible to inject local anaesthetic using a sclerotherapy needle to reduce mucosal pain. Pain may be a symptom of oesophageal perforation although this is less common following laser recanalisation then intubation. The perforation risk is about 5% and is said to be a result of oesophageal dilatation rather than a direct complication of laser treatment.[56] Perforation rates are higher after radiotherapy, or if there is acute angulation of the tumour at the cardia. A benign pneumoperitoneum or pneumomediastinum may be produced after laser treatment. This is thought to be related to a jet of coaxial gas passing through abnormal, often necrotic, tumour tissue. Patients rarely have symptoms. It is detected on routine chest radiography.[57] Contrast studies do not show a leak and patients usually make an uneventful recovery. Gastric distension as a result of carbon dioxide infusion can be quite uncomfortable despite using good decompression probes through the stenosis to avoid symptoms due to bloating.[58] The pain is visceral in nature and may be confused with chest pain from excessive mucosal burning. Haemorrhage after laser treatment is rare, occurring in about 1% of patients.[59] Aspiration

Table 8.3 *Complications of laser treatment*

Early complications	Late complications
Pain	Repeated hospital admissions
Perforation	Tumour recurrence
Pneumoperitoneum	Benign strictures
Pneumomediastinum	Functional swallowing problems
Gastric distension	
Bleeding	
Aspiration pneumonia	

pneumonia is less frequently encountered during laser treatment than during intubation, but high oesophageal tumours may predispose to aspiration because there is little room to manoeuvre the endoscope.

Late complications

Late complications frequently occur following laser treatment. The main problem is tumour recurrence needing further laser therapy. Patients have to remain closely tied to the hospital for repeated endoscopic follow-up. Most require about monthly sessions leading on average to four or five treatments. It is perceived by the medical profession that this is burdensome and disruptive. However, there have been few studies objectively measuring patients' views about this matter and some may like the continued hospital contact. Delayed laser-associated benign strictures can occur in up to 20% of patients.[60] They require repeated dilatation and occasionally stent insertion. The pathogenesis of these strictures is unclear but may be related to deep thermal injury to the submucosal layer or muscle, followed by subsequent collagen deposition, shrinkage and scarring.

Relief of dysphagia

Laser treatment may recanalise 90% of all stenoses but the clinical results obtained do not always come up to expectations. There appears to be a motility disturbance together with progressive cachexia that may make it impossible for some patients to take solid foods again. Other factors that affect functional outcome appear to be the general health of the patient, previous treatments and complications. Overall, about one-third of patients have normal swallowing after laser treatment, one-third can eat some solids (comparable to having a tube) and the remainder struggle. In view of these varied responses, means of improving the efficacy of laser treatment by increasing the period between laser treatment and symptomatic relapse have been explored largely through combination treatments.

Combination laser treatment

Laser therapy can be combined with external or internal beam radiotherapy to try to prolong the interval between treatments. Sargeant et al.[61] performed a pilot study in 22 patients receiving laser and radiotherapy with fractions of either 30 or 40 Gy. Patients receiving fractions of 30 Gy had a longer dysphagia-free interval than historical controls, but 40 Gy was very poorly tolerated. The advantage of additional intraluminal radiotherapy is to treat mural invasion after debulking of the tumour. Several reports of the combined effectiveness of laser and brachytherapy have been published.[50,54,62] Bader et al.[54] reported a pilot study of 40 patients receiving laser treatment followed by therapy with iridium-192; 80% of patients remained free of re-stenosis irrespective of their tumour histology. A randomised trial comparing laser treatment alone and laser treatment plus therapy with iridium-192, reported a significantly prolonged first dysphagia-free interval after recanalisation of the stricture in patients with squamous cell tumours receiving combined treatment.[62] The patients, however, had a shorter dysphagia-free interval from re-stenosis onwards and patients required significantly more endoscopic procedures, since after-loading therapy also needs endoscopy. They also found that patients with a good Karnofsky score seemed to benefit more, with a shorter inpatient stay than those with poor Karnofsky indices of 30–40. The authors concluded that only in the case of squamous cell tumours in patients with a high Karnofsky score would after-loading treatment appear helpful.

Laser palliation is probably better than intubation with regards to incidence of complications and achievement of normal swallowing. It seems to be preferable for non-circumferential, polypoid or exophytic tumours although this has not been demonstrated conclusively. The main drawback of laser palliation is the need to attend hospital on a regular basis and the capital cost of the equipment. Laser treatment also has nothing to offer patients with an extrinsic lesion causing oesophageal compression, patients with a fistula or patients with a diffuse subepithelial tumour. If laser is used as a first line treatment then salvage intubation can still be used as a final resort.

Photodynamic therapy

Photodynamic therapy is a modification of conventional laser treatment. It is an investigational treatment of which the role in clinical practice has not been established. It essentially has three elements: light, a photosensitising drug (a haematoporphyrin derivative) and oxygen. The drug acting as a photosensitiser is injected intravenously three to four days before irradiation of the tumour. Laser light (administered endoscopically) then activates the drug within the tissue. Once stimulated, the photosensitiser interacts with oxygen to create a high reactive singlet state. This reacts with cell membranes and organelles and is cytotoxic. Retention of the photosensitiser is longer in dysplastic or frankly neoplastic than normal tissues, at a ratio of about two to one. Damage to normal tissues heals by regeneration.

Clinical indications

Photodynamic (PDT) therapy may be best suited to treat patients with small mucosal tumours (uT_1, N_0) who are unfit or who do not wish to undergo major surgery. Its role in palliative treatments of upper gastrointestinal malignancies is yet to be determined.[63] A number of specific complications have been recognised. The activated photosensitiser creates an iatrogenic porphyria which may persist for up to six weeks after injection of the drug. Patients are all advised to avoid sunlight because of reports of minor erythema, cutaneous oedema and even blistering of the skin.[64] Oesophagitis and stricture formation is a worrying complication, which may require repeated dilatations.[64] There is also a considerable risk of delayed haemorrhage. This occurs in patients with large lesions when partial necrosis may occur. Experimental work indicates that the most likely cause of these delayed bleeds is the presence of raw tumour surfaces with large vessels following sloughing of the necrosed tumour.[65] Until more selective tumour photosensitisers can be developed it is likely that PDT will remain largely experimental.

Bipolar electrocoagulation

Electrocoagulation, a thermal method of tumour destruction, has always suffered from the problem of adhesion between the tissue and probe tip. Recently, to overcome this difficulty probes that deliver bipolar electrocoagulation energy (BICAP®) have been developed.[66] BICAP has the potential advantage of being able to treat a large area, therefore producing rapid relief of dysphagia. It is portable and relatively cheap.[60,67] Bipolar tumour probes can be used to destroy long tight submucosal tumours, but they must be circumferential. Where there is marked tumour angulation they are less effective, because the probes are rigid and difficult to direct.

Endoscopic technique

BICAP® treatment is performed under intravenous sedation and analgesia. Probes must be tested before treatment. The continuity of the metallic strips should be inspected. The probes should then be connected to the generator and tested with the generator dials set at two or three for 1 s duration. A drop of saline is put on each of the metallic strips and by stepping on the foot pedal, boiling of the saline should be observed. If the probe fails the test, it should not be used. Endoscopy is carried out to define the tumour geography and length (dilatation being performed if necessary). The scope is then removed and the BICAP® probes inserted over a guide wire to the stricture at the proximal end (centimetres are marked on their handles). Placement of the probe may be checked with direct endoscopic vision by passing a small scope down next to the probe or with fluoroscopy. With a dial setting of 10 and a pulse duration of 2 s, five pulses are delivered. The probe is then advanced to the next position and the process repeated. The standard kit consists of five probes and a 50 W bipolar generator. Probes are similar to metal olive dilators with bipolar radiant electrode strips in the central portion. Four probes have 360° circumferential coagulation configuration, 6, 9, 12 and 15 mm in diameter. The fifth probe has a 180° hemicircumferential figuration and is 15 mm in diameter. The depth of coagulated tissue depends on forces applied radially by the probe.[68] Usually 2–4 mm of coagulation occurs. Once this has sloughed the luminal diameter can increase by 4–8 mm. Generally one or two treatment sessions are required to treat the entire tumour.

Complications

Electrocoagulation is usually carried out under fluoroscopy and not direct endoscopic vision. Adequate care must, therefore, be taken to avoid damage to normal or less thickened oesophageal wall. This will result in perforation, possible fistula formation or strictures. The reported incidence of perforation is similar to that of laser treatment.

Strictures have been reported in up to 13% of patients.[69] These are thought to be due to thermally induced fibrosis. Fistulas have been reported in up to 15% of patients although these may have occurred as part of the natural history of oesophageal cancer.[67] Such problems may be decreased by precise three-dimensional tumour mapping with endoluminal ultrasound. This would provide anatomical information that could then inform the endoscopist if the tumour is near the trachea or only superficial. Others have suggested careful use of asymmetrical bipolar probes or reduced treatment times.[67] Immediate and delayed haemorrhage has also been reported following BICAP treatment.[67]

Relief of dysphagia
Like laser treatment, reported technical success is about 90%, but functional relief of dysphagia is only achieved in about 70% of patients. Others have reported about 85% improvement in dysphagia grade, lasting four to ten weeks.[60]

Bipolar electrocoagulation therapy versus laser treatment
In view of the preliminary efficacy reported by Johnston et al.[66] with the BICAP tumour probe, several authors have sought to compare it with YAG laser recanalisation.[60] Jensen performed a non-randomised prospective study in which the first 14 patients with inoperable malignant dysphagia received laser treatment and the second 14, bipolar electrocoagulation therapy.[60] During the 16-week follow-up no statistically significant results were found between the two groups. Dysphagia was equally relieved in 86% of patients. Minor complications of pain and transient oedema were seen more frequently in the laser group, 21% of whom developed treatment-related oesophageal strictures. One patient in the BICAP group developed a fistula. It was concluded that advantages of the BICAP system were portability, lower-cost equipment and the ability to treat long submucosal tumours in any part of the oesophagus in one session.[60] More data are needed before firm conclusions can be reached. The machine costs less than laser equipment, but costs to the patients must be further evaluated.

Ethanol induced tumour necrosis
The use of ethanol to induce tumour necrosis in inoperable oesophago-gastric tumours was first reported by Spiller and Misiewicz in 1987.[70]

Endoscopic technique
Patients require intravenous sedation and flexible endoscopy. Using a sclerotherapy needle, 0.5–1 ml aliquots of absolute alcohol are injected into the protuberant part of the tumour. Resistance is felt and blanching and swelling of the tumour observed. In patients with long tumours the injections are started distally so that oedema induced should not impede the passage of the endoscope. There is no limit to the total volume injected in one session (1–20 ml reported). Polidocanol may be used (instead of ethanol).[71] Dilatation is needed if the endoscope is unable to transverse the stricture.

Relief of dysphagia and complications

Chung studied 36 patients with inoperable cancers of the oesophagus or gastric cardia. Endoscopy was repeated three to five days later to observe necrosis and thereafter until the endoscope could be passed without resistance.[72] Of the 36 patients 29 reported an improvement in dysphagia grade, but this relapsed at a mean of 35 days later. Dysphagia was occasionally made temporarily worse because of tumour oedema and swelling. Retrosternal chest pain and a low-grade pyrexia were reported by all patients. One perforation and one tracheo-oesophageal fistula occurred following injection of quite large volumes of alcohol (13 and 36 ml). Others have reported better results with few or no complications.[73,74]

Injection of absolute alcohol to relieve malignant dysphagia has all the hallmarks of a good technique, being safe, inexpensive and readily available. No particular specialist equipment or expertise are required. The technique is less precise than laser treatment because it is difficult to be sure just where the alcohol is going once it enters the tissue. One group tried to combat this risk by adding 0.5% methylene blue to the alcohol to allow clear observation of the alcohol diffusion.[74] As yet few comparative studies have been reported and until further information is available it is recommended only as an adjunct to more conventional methods for relieving dysphagia.

Radiotherapy

Radiotherapy aims to recanalise the oesophagus and inhibit local tumour progression. It may be given by external beam or an intra-luminal source (brachytherapy). The role of palliative external beam radiotherapy is difficult to delineate because many series include unfit patients with small tumours who would not be considered for surgery on the basis of their general health. Prior to external beam therapy a form of endoscopic recanalisation is often recommended because oedema and swelling of the tumour can cause complete dysphagia. Ten or more treatment fractions may be required and the optimum dose is unknown. Side effects are common and often serious: pulmonary fibrosis, fistula and benign stricture formation. Acceptable palliation of dysphagia occurs in less than 40% of patients of whom at least 25% get recurrent dysphagia due to cicatricial narrowing of the oesophagus.[75] Some reports of increased survival exist but these have not been easily reproduced.[76]

Brachytherapy (intracavitary irradiation)

The development of the Selectron (Nucleotron, Zeersum, Holland) remote-control after-loading machine has generated considerable interest in recent years. It is a simple and safe procedure. There is no radiation exposure to staff and personnel. The brachytherapy applicator, only 8 mm in diameter is passed over an endoscopically placed guidewire and positioned with fluoroscopy into the tumour. This is immobilised at the mouth or nose. The patient is then transferred to a protected treatment room and connected to the Selectron machine. A microprocessor controls the pneumatic transfer of caesium-137 pellets down a flexible tube inserted into the applicator. The optimal dose is at present unknown and varies between 15 and 20 Gy to a depth of 1 cm in single or multiple fractions. Some suggest that doses in excess of 66 Gy are needed in the cervical oesophagus, but others argue that these doses cause an accumulation of complications.[77,78] Treatment may be repeated on alternate days, leaving the nasogastric tube *in situ* or replacing it as necessary.[79] The great merit of brachytherapy is that the radiation dose is highest to the tumour while adjacent normal tissues are relatively spared. It can also be used in combination with laser treatment as discussed above.

Relief of dysphagia

Fast relief of dysphagia is obtained in 70% of patients with squamous cell tumours and 60% of those with adenocarcinoma.[54,80] All patients suffer a varying degree of radiation oesophagitis which leads to painful oesophageal ulceration in up to 30% of patients as well as the development of postirradiation strictures or tracheo-oesophageal fistula.[78,81] In a randomised trial, Low and Pagliero[82] compared the efficacy of brachytherapy with laser treatment in 23 patients. No significant differences were found between the two groups but re-treatments were three times more common with laser therapy.[82]

Brachytherapy seems an attractive new development although the cost of an Nd:YAG laser is significantly less than the Selectron unit. Brachytherapy also requires an expensive specially fitted treatment area separate from the endoscopy suite and close liaison with radiotherapist colleagues. The endoscopic techniques required for brachytherapy are straightforward whereas laser delivery has a steep learning curve. Brachytherapy should be subject to the scrutiny of a large randomised trial to discover whether single or combination treatment provides the best palliation of malignant dysphagia.

Aerodigestive fistulae

Aerodigestive fistulae cause paroxysmal coughing fits, aspiration and eventually death from recurrent chest infection. They occur in about 5% of patients with oesophageal cancer either because of invasion and spontaneous necrosis of the tumour into the bronchial tree or as a sequel of irradiation, laser therapy or intubation. They are difficult to treat and patients usually die within a month.[83] The creation of a cervical oesophagostomy and gastrostomy is pointless because of the patient's poor prognosis. Palliative bypass surgery with stomach or colon for interposition is highly invasive and the abject general health of the patient produces at least a 50% perioperative morbidity and mortality.[84] Endoscopic insertion of a prosthesis is the treatment of choice although results following the use of rigid prostheses have not been encouraging.[83] Many modifications have been developed. Wilson–Cook produce a fistula prosthesis carrying a circumferential foam-rubber sponge contained in a silicone sheath which expands and closes the fistula once the vacuum is released. A modified Celestin prosthesis is also available. An Atkinson tube may be wrapped in a circumferential polyvinyl alcohol (Ivalon) sponge which swells into the fistula and may fill a defect up to 30 mm in diameter. A specially designed ESKA-Buess wide fistula funnel is supplied as a separate part, designed to fit over the proximal end of the standard prosthesis. The use of covered metal stents to seal aerodigestive fistulas seems to be promising although no randomised trials have been performed.[40,85,86] Fistulas close to the cricopharyngeus are particularly difficult to manage. In this situation simultaneous tracheal and oesophageal stenting has been described although there is currently little experience of this novel technique.[87] There is also one report of the use of primary chemotherapy in four patients with tracheo-oesophageal fistulae. Two patients healed during treatment.[88] At present the role of chemotherapy in this regard needs further evaluation.

Recurrent laryngeal nerve palsy

Recurrent laryngeal nerve palsy caused by tumour infiltration results in eating difficulties, hoarseness and repeated chest infections because of aspiration pneumonia. It has been reported in up to 20% of patients at least three months after oesophagectomy.[89] Nerve damage at the time of surgery usually causes a temporary paralysis that resolves within six weeks. Patients classically are hoarse, may complain of dysphagia and choking problems when eating and drinking. The diagnosis is confirmed with barium swallow, endoscopy and laryngoscopy. Characteristically, aspiration is seen during the pharyngeal phase of swallowing on barium studies and endoscopy demonstrates no mechanical obstruction to food passage. Other causes of swallowing difficulties such as muscular incoordination in the pharynx may be assessed with manometry but this is not usually necessary. The left nerve is predominantly involved because of its largely intrathoracic course, but patients with bilateral palsies may have palpable supra-clavicular nodes. Teflon injection to re-establish glottic competence should help swallowing, speech and problems with coughing. In a series of 15 patients these improved in all but one, who developed stridor and required emergency tracheostomy.[89]

Bleeding

Bleeding from inoperable oesophageal and cardia tumours causes problems with refractory anaemia and occasionally acute upper gastrointestinal haemorrhage. It is often difficult to completely eradicate because of the advanced nature of the tumour, but symptoms may be controlled by a variety of endoscopic means. Palliative laser therapy can achieve haemostasis by coagulating the exposed bleeding tissues. Injection sclerotherapy is also effective although it may need to be repeated. Electrocoagulation can also control upper gastrointestinal haemorrhage due to controlled tissue heating. In general this problem may be relieved temporarily, but is usually a sign of very advanced disease.

Palliative treatment of tumours of the gastric body and antrum

Patients in whom potentially curative radical surgery for gastric cancer is not suitable require adequate palliation of symptoms of pain, vomiting, bleeding and malaise. The treatment of gastric outflow obstruction and chronic bleeding will be discussed separately.

Gastric outlet obstruction

Obstruction associated with cancer of the gastric corpus or antrum is difficult to manage regardless of the therapeutic modality. Such tumours generally involve extensive segments of the stomach and result in interference with both reservoir function and normal motility patterns. The endoscopic management of malignant gastric outflow obstruction is particularly hazardous and there is little doubt that whenever possible, resection of the primary tumour as a means of providing symptomatic relief, provides better palliation than bypass surgery provided the patient's general health will allow this. Opinions are divided, however, as to the best type of palliative gastrectomy (subtotal or total). Total gastrectomy for advanced gastric cancer, may be worthwhile but often at the expense of a higher complication rate. Despite a successful palliative gastrectomy, however, many patients subsequently become anorexic because of the widespread nature of their disease. The role of gastric resection in linitis plastica remains controversial. It probably has little to offer for those patients who additionally have peritoneal or liver metastasis or contiguous organ involvement, where life expectancy is around four months.[90] Patients with linitis plastica who have disease limited to the stomach or regional lymph nodes may, however, survive beyond 12 months and thus be appropriately palliated by total gastrectomy.[91] Although it is accepted that many operations undertaken with curative intent, turn out to be entirely palliative procedures, with modern approaches to preoperative staging, this is becoming less of a problem.

Patients with non-resectable distal lesions should have an antecolic gastrojejunostomy performed. The loop of jejunum is anastomosed as high as possible to the greater curve of the stomach. Posterior jejunal loops are not recommended because tumour tends to quickly reach the margins causing recurrent obstruction. The Devine exclusion bypass operation for inoperable antral tumours was thought to increase survival by preventing recurrent tumour obstructing the gastro-jejunostomy.[92] Very poor results mean that is it now seldom performed.

Patients with advanced tumours of the body of the stomach causing problems with bleeding and/or obstruction may undergo palliative total gastrectomy. The morbidity is much higher than for segmental gastrectomy and therefore opinions remain divided as to its benefits.[91] Total gastrectomy should not be performed if the patient has liver or peritoneal disease spread or if the tumour has extension into the pancreas or diaphragm. Monson *et al.*[91] concluded that total gastrectomy in selected patients when technically feasible is recommended, but should be performed by an appropriately qualified surgeon.

A variety of approaches are under investigation to expand the role and benefits of palliative surgery. Chemotherapy and radiotherapy are being used by a number of centres. Major drawbacks of chemoradiotherapy for advanced cancer are inevitably toxicity and undesired side effects, which make these treatments unattractive options for many patients if the objective is simply to relieve symptoms. Palliative adjuvant treatment may render some inoperable patients candidates for a palliative gastrectomy. Up to 50% of patients with metastatic and locally advanced gastric adenocarcinomas receiving epirubicin, cisplatin and 5-fluorouracil have been shown to have at least a partial response, without a significant decrease in quality of life.[93] On the whole the regimen was well tolerated. Definitive conclusions are still awaited as these phase 2 studies have not been confirmed in randomised clinical trials. At present there is still an overwhelming opinion that toxic chemotherapy is not standard treatment for patients with advanced gastric cancer.

Placement of a conventional plastic endoprosthesis in the gastric antrum often results in deviation of the tube due to the unfavourable anatomic conditions. Case reports of expanding metallic stents for recanalisation of the pyloric channel exist, but larger series are needed to confirm this finding.[94] Metal stents may be more successfully placed across recurrent tumour at oesophagojejunal anastomoses following total gastrectomy although results have been mediocre so far.[95] Treatment of recurrent anastomotic tumours because of their exophytic luminal projections can often be effective with laser.[96] Some report effective treatment of gastric outflow obstruction with laser treatment alone, but other studies have not confirmed this.[97]

The insertion of nasogastric tubes and percutaneous endoscopically placed feeding tubes will enable nutritional support in patients with inoperable tumours of the oesophagus and stomach. This manoeuvre alone, however, will fail to palliate the patient's principal complaints. Many believe that such palliation merely perpetuates suffering except in situations where they may be used to buy time before definitive recanalisation or for the patient's personal wishes.

Chronic bleeding

Surgery is again recommended wherever possible to palliate the symptoms of chronic blood loss from gastric tumours. Laser therapy can successfully achieve haemostasis in bleeding gastric malignancies but this is not always available and requires repeated admissions.[98]

Conclusions and future research

The number of therapeutic options available for the palliation of patients with oesophageal and gastric cancer has significantly increased over the past decade. Yet, no one treatment completely relieves all symptoms without notable side effects. Common clinical situations such as management of fistulas, high oesophageal tumours and bleeding inoperable gastric lesions still present formidable problems. The introduction of expanding metal stents, brachytherapy, laser coagulation and combination treatment offers some new hopes. These new therapies still require careful evaluation before they become widely available. Referral of suitable patients should be encouraged so that large prospective trials focusing on palliative treatments can be completed expeditiously. Few controlled trials have so far been undertaken (Table 8.4). Whether public pressure to centralise cancer services in order to provide high technology specialised care will be realised is unknown, but evidence of improved outcomes for patients attending this type of tertiary referral centre is accumulating.[14,99] There is also a need to define outcomes for patients with inoperable malignancies of the upper gastrointestinal tract. Dysphagia scores should be standardised and future palliative trials should include an objective assessment of quality of life of patients as well as cost effectiveness during the follow-up period.[100,101] This ideal

Table 8.4 *Prospective randomised controlled trials of the palliation of oesophageal and gastric cancer*

Author	n	Group 1	Group 2	Group 3	Outcomes	
					Dysphagia score	**Morbidity**
Alderson[102]	40	Laser alone	Plastic tube		No difference	No difference
Barr[7]	40	Laser alone	Laser and plastic tube		No difference	Morbidity higher in Grp 2
Low[82]	23	Laser alone	Brachytherapy		No difference	Re-treatment more frequent in Grp 1
Reed[103]	27	Plastic tube	Plastic tube and DXT	Laser and DXT	No difference	Inpatient stay longer Grp 3 than Grp 1 Morbidity higher Grp 1 than Grp 3
Angelini[71]	34	Laser alone	Polidocanol		No difference	No difference
Fuchs[104]	40	Laser, DXT and brachy	Plastic tube		No difference	No difference
Sander[62]	39	Laser alone	Laser and brachy		Grp 2 squamous cell better	No difference
Carter[105]	40	Laser alone	Plastic tube		Dysphagia worse in Grp 2	No difference
Knyrim[41]	42	Plastic tube	Wallstent		No difference	Morbidity and inpatient stay worse in Grp 1

NB No differences in 30-day mortality were reported in all of the above trials.

approach, however, is not without disadvantages. Severely debilitated patients with a limited life expectancy may be compelled to travel long distances to a centre with specialised endoscopic facilities only to find that treatment has to be performed more than once. Genuine efforts should be made to see if patients with very short survival times (less than four weeks) can be identified and perhaps spared unnecessarily aggressive attempts at palliation.

Making a decision on the selection of palliation for patients with advanced disease is difficult. Every patient is unique with regard to tumour histology, stricture location, clinical stage, premorbid state and emotional requirements. Choosing one technique over another must be justifiable on the grounds of treatment efficacy, as well as its ease of application, overall adaptability to other therapeutic areas and the patient's acceptance while minimising both complications and cost. Skilled clinicians with a thorough understanding of all the available palliative treatments should also be aware of the other needs of the patient with advanced malignancy. Close liaison with multidisciplinary teams including oncologists, dieticians and palliative care nurses is essential to minimise suffering.

References

1. Hennessy TPJ, O'Connell R. Carcinoma of the hypopharynx, oesophagus and cardia. Surg Gynecel Obstet 1986; 162: 243–7.
2. Huang GJ, Wang LJ, Liu JS *et al.* Surgery of oesophageal carcinoma. Semin Surg Oncol 1985; 1: 74–83.
3. Müller JM, Erasmi H, Stelzner M, Zieren U, Pichlmaier H. Surgical therapy of oesophageal carcinoma. Br J Surg 1990; 77: 845–57.
4. Irvin TT, Bridger JE. Gastric cancer: an audit of 122 consecutive cases and the results of R1 gastrectomy. Br J Surg 1988; 75: 106–90.
5. Karlin DA, Fisher RS, Krevsky B. Prolonged survival and effective palliation in patients with squamous cell carcinoma of the oesophagus following endoscopic laser therapy. Cancer 1987; 59: 1969–72.
6. Siegel HI, Laskin KJ, Dabezies MA, Fisher RS, Krevsky B. The effect of endoscopic laser therapy on survival in patients with squamous cell carcinoma of the oesophagus. J Clin Gastroenterol 1991; 13: 142–6.
7. Barr H, Krasner N, Raouf A, Walker RJ. Prospective randomised trial of laser therapy only and laser therapy followed by endoscopic intubation for the palliation of malignant dysphagia. Gut 1990; 31: 252–8.
8. Loizou LA, Rampton D, Atkinson M, Robertson C, Bown SG. A prospective assessment of quality of life after endoscopic intubation and laser therapy for malignant dysphagia. Cancer 1992; 70: 386–91.
9. Highley MS, Parnis FX, Trotter GA *et al.* Combination chemotherapy with epirubicin, cisplatin and 5-fluorouracil for the palliation of advanced gastric and oesophageal adenocarcinoma. Br J Surg 1994; 81: 1763–5.
10. Pyrhonen S, Kuitunen T, Nyandoto P, Kouri M. Randomised comparison of fluorouracil, epidoxorubicin and methotrexate (FEMTX) plus supportive care with supportive care alone in patients with non-resectable gastric cancer. Br J Cancer 1995; 71: 587–91.
11. Derodra JK, Hale PC, Mason RC. Inoperable oesophageal cancer: factors affecting outcome. Gullet 1992; 2: 163–6.
12. Watson A. A study of the quality and duration of survival following resection, endoscopic intubation and surgical intubation in oesophageal carcinoma. Br J Surg 1982; 69: 585–8.
13. Pearson JG. The present status and future potential of radiotherapy in the management of oesophageal cancer. Cancer 1977; 39: 882–90.

14. Matthews HR, Powell DJ, McConkey CC. Effect of surgical experience on the results of resection for oesophageal carcinoma. Br J Surg 1986; 73: 621–3.

15. Abe S, Tachibana M, Shimokawa T, Shiraishi M, Nakamura T. Surgical treatment of advanced carcinoma of the oesophagus. Surg Gynecol Obstet 1989; 168: 115–20.

16. Orringer MB. Sub-sternal bypass of the excluded oesophagus – results of an ill advised operation. Surgery 1984; 96: 467–71.

17. Mannell A, Becker PJ, Nissembaum M. Bypass surgery for unresectable oesophageal cancer: early and late results in 124 cases. Br J Surg 1988; 75: 283–6.

18. Aste H, Munizzi F, Martines H, Pugliese V. Oesophageal dilation in malignant dysphagia. Cancer 1985; 56: 2713–15.

19. Tulman AB, Boyce HWJ. Complications of oesophageal dilatation and guidelines for their prevention. Gastrointest Endosc 1981; 27: 229–34.

20. Ogilivie AL, Dronfield MW, Ferguson R, Atkinson M. Palliative intubation of oesophagogastric neoplasms at fibreoptic endoscopy. Gut 1982; 23: 1060–7.

21. Tytgat GNJ, den Hartog Jager FCA, Bartelsman JFWM. Endoscopic prosthesis for advanced oesophageal cancer. Endoscopy 1986; 18 (Suppl 3): 32–9.

22. Kinsman KJ, DeGregorio BT, Katon RM et al. Prior radiation and chemotherapy increase the risk of life-threatening complications after insertion of metallic stents for oesophagogastric malignancy. Gastrointest Endosc 1996; 43: 196–203.

23. Den Hartog Jager FCA, Bartelsman JFWM, Tytgat GNJ. Palliative treatment of obstructing oesophagogastric malignancy by endoscopic positioning of a plastic prosthesis. Gastroenterology 1979; 77: 1008–14.

24. Celestin LR. Permanent intubation in inoperable cancer of the oesophagus and cardia: a new tube. Ann R Coll Surg Engl 1959; 25: 165–70.

25. Procter DS. Carcinoma of the oesophagus. A review of 523 cases. S Afr J Surg 1968; 6: 137–59.

26. Lux G, Wilson D, Wilson J, Demling L. A cuffed tube for the treatment of oesophagobronchial fistulae. Endoscopy 1987; 19: 28–30.

27. Buess G, Schellong H, Kometz B, Grussner R, Junginger TH. A modified prosthesis for the treatment of malignant oesophagotracheal fistula. Cancer 1988; 61: 1679–84.

28. Ammann JF, Collis JL. Palliative intubation of the oesophagus: analysis of 59 cases. J Thorac Cardiovasc Surg 1971; 61: 863–9.

29. Raijman I, Kortan P, Haber GB, Marcon NE. Contrast injection to identify tumour margins during oesophageal stent placement. Gastrointest Endosc 1994; 40: 222–4.

30. Chan AC, Leong HT, Chung SS, Li AK. Lipiodal as a reliable marker for stenting in malignant oesophageal stricture. Gastrointest Endosc 1994; 40: 520–1.

31. Boyce HW. Medical management of oesophageal obstruction and oesophagealpulmonary fistula. Cancer 1982; 50: 2597–600.

32. Monnier P, Hsieh V, Savary M. Endoscopic treatment of oesophageal sterosis using Savary–Gillard bougies: technical innovations. Acta Endosc 1985; 15: 119.

33. Atkinson M, Ferguson R, Parker CG. Tube introducer and modified Celestin tube for use in palliative intubation of oesophagogastric neoplasms at fibreoptic endoscopy. Gut 1978; 19: 669–71.

34. Sarr MG, Pemberton JH, Payne WS. Management of instrumental perforations of the oesophagus. J Thorac Cardiovasc Surg 1982; 84: 211–18.

35. Shaw JFL, Coombes GB. Multiple intestinal perforation due to Celestin tube. Br J Surg 1979; 66: 807–8.

36. Sargeant IR, Loizou LA, Tulloch M, Thorpe S, Bown SG. Recanalisation of tube overgrowth: a useful new indication for laser in palliation of malignant dysphagia. Gastrointest Endosc 1992; 38: 165–9.

37. Sharpstone D, Colin-Jones DG. A novel approach to the management of oesophageal tube overgrowth by tumour. Endoscopy 1994; 26: 630.

38. Branicki FJ, Ogilivie AL, Willis MR, Atkinson M. Structural deterioration of prosthetic oesophageal tubes – an in vitro comparison of latex rubber and silicone rubber tubes. Br J Surg 1981; 68: 861–4.

39. Tampieri I, Triossi O, Melandri G, Michieletti G, Casetti T. Distal migration of an oesophageal prosthesis: a new technique for endoscopic retrieval. Endoscopy 1994; 26: 268.

40. Nicholson AA, Royston CMS, Wedgewood K, Milkins R, Taylor AD. Palliation of malignant

oesophageal perforation and proximal oesophageal malignant dysphagia with covered metal stents. Clin Radiol 1995; 50: 11–14.

41. Knyrim K, Wagner HJ, Bethge N, Keymling M, Vakil N. A controlled trial of an expansile metal stent for palliation of oesophageal obstruction due to inoperable cancer. N Engl J Med 1993; 329: 1302–7.

42. Song HY, Do YS, Han YM *et al.* Covered, expandable oesophageal metallic stent tubes: experiences in 119 patients. Radiology 1994; 193: 689–95.

43. May A, Selmaier M, Hochberger J *et al.* Memory metal stents for palliation of malignant obstruction of the oesophagus and cardia. Gut 1995; 37: 309–13.

44. Kozarek R, Ball T, Patterson D. Metallic self-expanding stent application in the upper gastrointestinal tract: caveats and concerns. Gastrointest Endosc 1992; 38: 1–6.

45. Lindberg CG, Cwikiel W, Lundstedt C, Stridbeck H, Tranberg KG. Laser therapy and insertion of Wallstents for palliative treatment of oesophageal carcinoma. Acta Radiol 1991; 32: 345–8.

46. Vermeijden RJ, Bartelsman JFWM, Fackers P, Meijer RCA, Tygat GNT. Self-expanding metal stents for palliation of oesophageal malignancies. Gastrointest Endosc 1995; 41: 58–63.

47. Neuhaus H, Hoffmann W, Dittler HJ, Niedermeyer HP, Classen M. Implantation of self expanding oesophageal metal stents for palliation of malignant dysphagia. Endoscopy 1992; 24: 405–10.

48. Krasner N, Barr H, Skidmore C, Morris AI. Palliative laser therapy for malignant dysphagia. Gut 1987; 28: 792–8.

49. Pietrafitta JJ, Dwyer RM. New laser technique for the treatment of malignant oesophageal obstruction. J Surg Oncol 1987; 35: 157–62.

50. Renwick P, Whitton V, Moghissi K. Combined endoscopic laser therapy and brachytherapy for palliation of oesophageal carcinoma, a pilot study. Gut 1992; 33: 435–8.

51. Wolf D, Fleischer D, Sivak MJ. Incidence of bacteremia with elective upper gastrointestinal endoscopic laser therapy. Gastrointest Endosc 1985; 31: 247–50.

52. Joffe SN, Daikuzono N, Sarkar MY. Contact probes for the Nd: YAG laser. SPIE. Optical

fibres in Medicine and Biology 1985; 576: 42–50.

53. Suzuki S, Aoki J, Shiina T, Nomiyama T, Miwa T. New ceramic endoprobes for endoscopic contact irradiation with Nd:YAG laser: experimental and clinical applications. Gastrointest Endosc 1986; 32: 282–6.

54. Bader M, Dittler HJ, Ultsch B, Ries G, Siewart JR. Palliative treatment of malignant stenoses of the upper gastrointestinal tract using a combination of laser and after loading therapy. Endoscopy 1986; 18(Suppl): 27–31.

55. Marcon NE. The endoscopic management of oesophageal cancer. Acta Gastroenterol Belg 1994; 57: 143–54.

56. Tyrrell MR, Trotter GA, Adam A, Mason RC. Incidence and management of laser-associated oesophageal perforation. Br J Surg 1995; 82: 1257–8.

57. Brooks PT, Troop AC, Barr H, Krasner N. Massive pneumoperitoneum following laser treatment of inoperable oesophageal carcinoma. Clin Radiol 1988; 39: 305–7.

58. Sander RR, Poesl H. Cancer of the oesophagus – Palliation – Laser treatment and combined procedures. Endoscopy 1993; 25 (Suppl): 679–82.

59. Bown SG. Endoscopic laser therapy for oesophageal cancer. Endoscopy 1986; 18 (Suppl 3): 26–31.

60. Jensen DM, Machicado G, Randall G, Tung LA, English-Zych S. Comparison of low power YAG laser and BICAP tumour probe for palliation of oesophageal cancer strictures. Gastroenterology 1988; 94: 1263–70.

61. Sargeant IR, Loizou LA, Tobias JS, Blackman G, Thorpe S, Bown SG. Radiation enhancement of laser palliation for malignant dysphagia: a pilot study. Gut 1992; 33: 1597–601.

62. Sander R, Hagenmueller F, Sander C, Riess G, Classen M. Laser versus laser plus after loading with iridium-192 in the palliative treatment of malignant stenosis of the oesophagus: a prospective, randomised and controlled study. Gastrointest Endosc 1991; 37: 433–40.

63. Thomas RJ, Abbott M, Bhathal PS, St John DJB, Morstyn G. High-dose photo irradiation of oesophageal cancer. Ann Surg 1987; 206: 193–9.

64. McCaughan JS, Nims TA, Guy JT, Hicks WJ, Williams TE, Laufman LR. Photodynamic therapy for oesophageal tumours. Arch Surg 1989; 124: 74–80.

65. Barr H, Chatlani P, Tralau CJ, MacRobert AJ, Boulos PB, Bown SG. Local eradication of rat colon cancer with photodynamic therapy: correlation of distribution of photosensitiser with biological effects in normal and tumour tissue. Gut 1991; 32: 517–23.

66. Johnston J, Quint R, Petruzzi C, Namihira Y. Development and experimental testing of a large BICAP probe for treatment of obstructing oesophageal and rectal malignancy. Gastrointest Endosc 1985; 31: 156 [abstract].

67. Johnston JH, Fleischer D, Petrini J, Nord HJ. Palliative bipolar electrocoagulation therapy of obstructing oesophageal cancer. Gastrointest Endosc 1987; 33: 349–53.

68. Laine L. Determination of the optimal technique for bipolar electrocoagulation treatment. Gastroenterology 1991; 100: 107–12.

69. Fleischer D, Ranard R, Kamarth R, Bitterman P, Benjamin S. Stricture formation following BICAP tumour probe therapy for oesophageal cancer. Clinical observation and experimental studies. Gastrintest Endosc 1987; 33: 183.

70. Spiller RC, Misiewicz JJ. Ethanol induced tumour necrosis for palliation of malignant dysphagia. Lancet 1987; ii: 792.

71. Angelini G, Pasini AF, Ederle A, Castagnini A, Talamini G, Bulighin G. Nd:YAG laser versus pilodocanol injection for palliation of oesophageal malignancy: a prospective randomised study. Gastrointest Endosc 1991; 37: 607–10.

72. Chung SCS, Leong HT, Choi CYC, Leung JWC, Li AKC. Palliation of malignant oesophageal obstruction by endoscopic alcohol injection. Endoscopy 1994; 26: 275–7.

73. Nwokolo CU, Payne-James JJ, Silk DBA, Misiewicz JJ, Loft DE. Palliation of malignant dysphagia by ethanol induced tumour necrosis. Gut 1994; 35: 299–303.

74. Moreira LS, Coelho RCL, Sadala RU, Dani R. The use of ethanol injection under endoscopic control to palliate dysphagia caused by oesophagogastric cancer. Endoscopy 1994; 26: 311–14.

75. Earlam R, Cunha-Melo JR. Oesophageal squamous cell carcinoma: II. A critical view of radiotherapy. Br J Surg 1980; 67: 457–61.

76. Pearson JG. Radiotherapy for oesophageal carcinoma. World J Surg 1981; 5: 489–97.

77. Mendenhall WM, Parsons JT, Vogel SB, Cassisi NJ, Million RR. Carcinoma of the cervical oesophagus treated with radiation therapy. Laryngoscope 1988; 98: 769–71.

78. Hishikawa Y, Tanaka S, Miura T. Oesophageal ulceration induced by intracavitary irradiation for oesophageal carcinoma. Am J Radiol 1984; 143: 269–73.

79. Fleischman EH, Kagan AR, Bellotti JE, Streeter OE, Harvey JC. Effective palliation for inoperable oesophageal cancer using intensive intracavitary radiation. J Surg Oncol 1990; 44: 234–7.

80. Rowland CG, Pagliero KM. Intracavitary radiation in palliation of carcinoma of oesophagus and cardia. Lancet 1985; ii: 981–2.

81. Hishikawa Y, Kurisu K, Taniguchi M, Kamikonya N, Miura T. high-dose-rate intraluminal brachytherapy for oesophageal cancer: 10 years experience in Hyogo College of Medicine. Radiol Oncol 1991; 21: 107–14.

82. Low DE, Pagliero KM. Prospective randomised clinical trial comparing brachytherapy and laser photoablation for palliation of oesophageal cancer. J Thorac Cardiovasc Surg 1992; 104: 173–9.

83. Burt M, Diehl W, Martini N et al. Malignant oesophago-respiratory fistula: management options and survival. Ann Thorac Surg 1991; 52: 1222–8.

84. Duranceau A, Jamieson CG. Malignant tracheoesophageal fistula. Ann Thorac Surg 1984; 37: 346–54.

85. Brown TH, Nicholson DA, Irving MH, Bancewicz J. Use of a self-expanding metal stent for oesophagogastric fistulation. Br J Surg 1995; 82: 663–4.

86. Wu WC, Katon RM, Saxon RR et al. Silicone-covered self-expanding metallic stents for the palliation of malignant oesophageal obstruction and oesophagorespiratory fistulas: experience in 32 patients and a review of the literature. Gastrointest Endosc 1994; 40: 22–33.

87. Ellul JPM, Morgan R, Gold D, Dussek J, Mason RC, Adam A. Parallel self-expanding covered metal stents in the trachea and oesophagus for the palliation of complex high tracheo-oesophageal fistula. Br J Surg 1996; 83: 1767–8.

88. Malik SM, Krasnow SH, Wadleigh RG. Closure of tracheoesophageal fistulas with primary chemotherapy in patients with oesophageal cancer. Cancer 1994; 73: 1321–3.

89. Griffin SM, Chung SCS, van Hasselt CA, Li AKC. Late swallowing and aspiration problems after oesophagectomy for cancer: malignant infiltration of the recurrent laryngeal nerves and its management. Surgery 1992; 112: 533–5.

90. Aranha GV, Georgen R. Gastric linitis plastica is not a surgical disease. Surgery 1989; 106: 758–63.

91. Monson JRT, Donohue JH, McIlrath DC, Farnell MB, Ilstrup DM. Total gastrectomy for advanced cancer. A worthwhile palliative procedure. Cancer 1991; 68: 1863–8.

92. Kwok S, Chung SCS, Griffin SM, Li AKC. Devine exclusion for unresectable carcinoma of the stomach. Br J Surg 1991; 78: 684–5.

93. Bamias A, Hill ME, Cunningham D *et al.* Epirubicin, cisplatin, and protracted venous infusion of 5-fluorouracil for oesophago-gastric adenocarcinoma. Cancer 1996; 77: 1978–85.

94. Truong S, Bohndorf V, Geller H, Schumpelick V, Gunther RW. Self-expanding metal stents for palliation of malignant gastric outlet obstruction. Endoscopy 1992; 24: 433–5.

95. Iguchi H, Kimura Y, Yanada J, Murasawa M. Treatment of a malignant stricture after oesophagojejunostomy by a self-expanding metallic stent. Cardiovasc Int Radiol 1993; 16: 102–4.

96. Swain C, Bown S, Edwards D, Kirkham JS, Salmon PR, Clark CG. Laser recanalisation of obstructing forgut cancer. Br J Surg 1984; 71: 112–15.

97. Stange EF, Dylla J, Fleig WE. Laser treatment of upper gastrointestinal tract carcinoma: determinants of survival. Endoscopy 1989; 21: 254–7.

98. Schwesinger WH, Chumley DL. Laser palliation for gastrointestinal malignancy. Am Surg 1988; 54 (2): 100–4.

99. Sagar PM, Gauperaa T, Sue-Ling H, McMahon MJ, Johnston D. An audit of the treatment of cancer of the oesophagus. Gut 1994; 35: 941–5.

100. Blazeby JM, Alderson D, Winstone K *et al.* Development of a EORTC questionnaire module to be used in quality of life assessments for patients with oesophageal cancer. Eur J Cancer 1996; 32: 1912–17.

101. Griffin SM, Robertson CS. Non-surgical treatment of cancer of the oesophagus. Br J Surg 1993; 80: 412–13.

102. Alderson D, Wright PD. Laser recanalisation versus endoscopic intubation in the palliation of malignant dysphagia. Br J Surg 1990; 77: 1151–3.

103. Reed CE, Marsh WH, Carlson LS, Seymore CH, Kratz JM. Prospective, randomised trial of palliative treatment for unresectable cancer of the oesophagus. Ann Thorac Surg 1991; 51: 552–6.

104. Fuchs KH, Freys SM, Schaube H, Eckstein AK, Selch A, Hamelmann H. Randomised comparison of endoscopic palliation of malignant oesophageal stenoses. Surg Endosc 1991; 5: 63–7.

105. Carter R, Smith JS, Anderson JR. Laser recanalisation versus endoscopic intubation in the palliation of malignant dysphagia: a randomised prospective study. Br J Surg 1992; 79: 1167–70.

9 Management of other oesophageal and gastric neoplasms

Deirdre M. O'Hanlon
S. Michael Griffin

Oesophageal neoplasms

The majority of oesophageal tumours world wide (over 90%) are squamous cell carcinomas and the next most common are adenocarcinomas occurring in association with Barrett's oesophagus. In western countries, including the UK, adenocarcinomas form a larger proportion of oesophageal tumours than is found world wide. Both of these tumours are outside the remit of this chapter.

Leiomyomas

Leiomyomas, which account for 50–70% of benign oesophageal tumours, are relatively common in the oesophagus, may be multiple, and occur in up to 50% of adults.[1-4] Although most are small and asymptomatic, larger lesions may produce symptoms. Over half are found in the lower third and 30% in the middle third of the oesophagus corresponding to the relative amount of smooth muscle in the muscularis propria, from which most of these arise. Patients are usually in their 40s and males are affected twice as often as females. Over 90% of leiomyomas are intramural–extramucosal, whereas subserosal and polypoid intraluminal lesions are less common. They grow slowly and lesions greater than 1 kg have been described. Patients present with a long history of intermittent dysphagia, vague retrosternal discomfort or pressure. Pain and features of bronchial compression are less common. Cystic degeneration may occur but is less common than in other sites and malignant transformation is rare. Some may calcify but this is also uncommon. An association between hypertrophic osteoarthropathy and oesophageal leiomyoma has been reported.[5] Barium swallow may demonstrate a smooth defect in the contour of the oesophagus; proximal dilatation with retention of contrast is uncommon (Fig. 9.1). Endoscopy may reveal a polypoid

Figure 9.1 *Barium swallow showing intraluminal mass of oesophageal leiomyoma.*

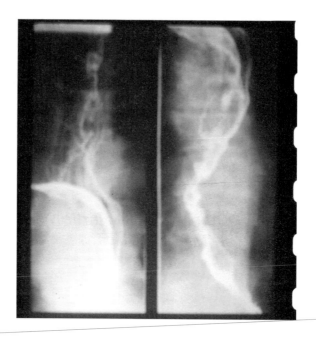

mass which bulges into the lumen. There is usually no obstruction and the overlying intact mucosa should not be biopsied as this may interfere with surgical removal. If lesions are symptomatic, large, pedunculated or at the gastro-oesophageal junction, surgical removal is indicated, while small lesions may be observed. The approach to removal is determined by the site and size of the lesion. Endoscopic removal is suitable for small pedunculated tumours. Enucleation may be possible for larger lesions unless the overlying mucosa is inflamed or damaged by endoscopic biopsy and oesophageal resection may be required for large or annular lesions, for those adherent to the mucosa or for lesions crossing the gastro-oesophageal junction.

Diffuse leiomyomatosis of the oesophagus is a rare disorder, usually affecting young women, and may result in irregular thickening and narrowing of a segment of the oesophagus and sometimes of the stomach leading to dysphagia. It may represent hypertrophy of the oesophageal wall in response to diffuse oesophageal spasm and must be differentiated from multiple leiomyomas which occur in less than 3% of patients.[6]

Sarcomatous lesions

Sarcomatous lesions of the oesophagus are rare, nodal or distant metastases are uncommon and these tumours generally have a favourable prognosis following successful surgical resection. Leiomyosarcoma may in many cases represent a pseudosarcoma, and although rare, is the most common malignant non-epithelial tumour of the oesophagus.[2,7] Lesions are found equally distributed throughout the oesophagus and commonly present as polypoid lesions with a broad base which may infiltrate adjacent organs and which can metastasise to viscera, most commonly the liver.[8] Treatment is resection and palliative irradiation is often of benefit. Leiomyoblastoma has been recorded in the oesophagus.[9] Rhabdomyosarcoma has been described but again is very rare and may represent a poorly differentiated leiomyosarcoma especially when found in the distal oesophagus.[8] Treatment is resection, radiotherapy is ineffective and the prognosis is poor. Fibrosarcoma is equally rare and some cases have followed thyroid irradiation. Treatment is again resection. Chondrosarcoma is very uncommon. Liposarcoma, osteosarcoma, malignant schwannoma, synovial sarcoma, malignant granular cell tumour and malignant fibrous histiocytomas have all been described as case reports.[10] Kaposi's sarcoma is usually found in associated with AIDS or immunosuppression.[11] The literature contains isolated case reports of other rare tumours which may occur in the oesophagus, including reticulum cell sarcomas, lymphosarcomas and plasmacytomas.

Lymphomas

Both Hodgkin's and non-Hodgkin's lymphomas as well as primary extramedullary plasmacytomas have been reported in the oesophagus and are being increasingly reported in immunocompromised patients.[12,13] Although many patients are asymptomatic, obstruction and perforation have been described. A barium meal may reveal diffuse nodularity resulting from lymphomatous infiltration. Radiotherapy or chemotherapy should be considered.

Metastases

Metastases to the oesophagus are present in 3–4% of all carcinomas. They most commonly result from direct invasion of tumours in the mediastinum or mediastinal lymph nodes or from tumours of the hypopharynx or stomach but they may also be blood borne. Direct extension from a lung primary and spread from a lymphoma are the most commonly observed form of secondary involvement whereas 9% of women dying from breast cancer have oesophageal metastases giving rise to a syndrome of postmastectomy dysphagia. The tumours are usually submucosal but intraluminal extension or ulceration may occur. Metastases may also arise from leukaemias, renal, pancreatic, cervical and bladder primaries. Treatment is radiotherapy with or without chemotherapy or hormone therapy. Dilatation is contraindicated because of the high risk of perforation.

Adenocarcinoma

Primary adenocarcinoma of the oesophagus, other than tumours occurring in association with Barrett's epithelium, are uncommon and comprise approximately 3% of all oesophageal neoplasms. They are separated from the cardiac mucosa by a variable amount of normal oesophageal squamous epithelium, and submucosal infiltration from a primary gastric neoplasm can be excluded. The presenting signs and symptoms as well as demographic criteria are similar to patients with primary squamous cell carcinoma and biopsy is required to distinguish these lesions. Four sources of columnar epithelium which may give rise to these tumours are recognised in the oesophagus: superficial submucosal glands; deep submucosal glands; heterotopic islands of gastric mucosa and columnar epithelial lining of the lower oesophagus.[8]

Small-cell carcinoma

Small-cell (oat cell) carcinoma (argyrophil cell carcinoma, apudoma, small cell undifferentiated carcinoma) of the oesophagus, which was first reported by McKeown,[14] is identical to oat cell carcinoma of the lung in ultrastructure, histological characteristics, staining and behaviour and it is important to exclude spread from a lung primary. It compromises 0.05–7.6% of all oesophageal carcinomas and probably arises from argyrophil cells which are found in the basal layer of the oesophageal epithelium.[15,16] Two thirds of tumours are pure oat cell carcinomas whereas the remainder may have squamous, adenocarcinomatous, or rarely carcinoid elements. These tumours may produce a variety of hormonally active compounds including calcitonin, vasoactive intestinal peptide, ADH or somatostatin.[17] ACTH activity is often present, but Cushing's syndrome has not been reported. The tumours are usually located in the distal oesophagus, have a 3:2 male preponderance and occur in patients aged 50–70 years. The tumours are usually fungating or ulcerating, may cause strictures, are rarely polypoid and may be multiple. The lesions are anaplastic, highly malignant, difficult to control and have a poor prognosis. There are no reports of disease-free long-term survivors. It is important to have an accurate histological diagnosis because multiagent chemotherapy and radiotherapy rather than surgery are the first line of therapy.[17,18] Non-oat cell small cell carcinoma refers to a lesion which does not demonstrate an argyrophilic reaction but is clinically similar to oat cell carcinoma.

Malignant melanoma

Malignant melanoma of the oesophagus accounts for 0.1–0.4% of oesophageal malignancies,[19] and may arise from melanocytes, which are found in the epithelium in 2.5–11.5% of patients, from metaplasia of normal basal epithelial cells or from ectopic melanoblast containing epithelium.[20] Melanomas occurring in the oesophagus are more likely to be secondary than primary but both are rare. A primary melanoma may be diagnosed when the cells contain melanin or show ultra-

Figure 9.2
Oesophageal metastatic malignant melanoma.

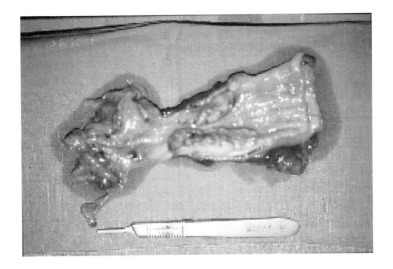

structural evidence of melanomacytic differentiation in a patient without history or evidence of another lesion. Primary melanomas were previously diagnosed by the presence of junctional change at the interface with squamous epithelium, but this is present in less than 50% of cases.[21] The tumours are often large, are usually single but may be multiple or have satellite lesions (Fig. 9.2). They frequently affect the lower oesophagus and are often polypoid with a wide pedicle and melanosis of the adjacent oesophageal mucosa may be seen on endoscopy. The melanomas are often ulcerated and friable and bleed readily on contact. Pigmentation is often striking but may be absent and special techniques such as the Mason–Fontana stain may be required to identify melanin.[20] There is a 2:1 male preponderance and although all ages may be affected patients are most commonly in their sixth and seventh decade. Melanomas often grow to a considerable size before presenting and wide lateral growth is common. Obstructive symptoms and odynophagia are frequent presenting complaints. Lymphatic and haematologic metastases are common at presentation. Barium swallow may demonstrate a shaggy polypoid lesion. Treatment is resection, which offers the best palliation and the only hope for cure. Radio-chemotherapy may have a role.[22] The prognosis is poor with a five-year survival of 2–4% and an average survival of 13.4 months.[19]

Carcinoid tumours

Carcinoid tumours of the oesophagus are rare with only six cases reported to 1980. They are normally a locally spreading and relatively benign neoplasm of neuroendocrine origin.[23]

Carcinosarcomas

Carcinosarcomas are characterised by the presence of both superficial polyhedral carcinomatous elements and deep sarcoma-like spindle cells in the same tumour and account for 1% of primary oesophageal tumours in China. The carcinoma cells are of squamous origin. The spindle cells are also of epithelial origin but very occasionally appear to be fibroblasts, resulting from metaplasia of mesenchymal cells.[8,24,25] The metastases are usually composed of carcinomatous elements, less commonly of sarcomatous elements or both. Aneuploidy is found more frequently with the squamous element suggesting an explanation for the more frequent occurrence of carcinomatous metastases. The tumours are usually polypoid, occasionally with a narrow stalk and have been termed polypoid carcinomas. However, only a small number of polypoidal tumours are carcinosarcomas. They are often large when diagnosed, measuring up to 12 cm. Gross ulcerative, infiltrative or stenosing tumours are rare. Although the lumen may be distended, obstructive symptoms occur late. Lymph node metastases are often present. The age and sex distribution as well as the location is similar to squamous cell carcinoma. A barium meal frequently demonstrates a large polypoid mass in the middle or lower third of the oesophagus. Survival is dependent on the depth of invasion and tumours are potentially curable with wide surgical resection when diagnosed early.[9,26] Prognosis is similar to squamous cell carcinoma when advanced. The overall prognosis is poor with a 2–6% 5-year survival but survival rates of 71% have been reported for some polypoid tumours.[26]

When the carcinomatous elements are limited to the surface without intermingling with the more deeply seated sarcomatous elements the tumour is termed a pseudosarcoma. The metastases from these lesions were formerly believed to contain only carcinomatous cells but more recently sarcomatous elements have been described and the term pseudosarcoma is now best avoided.[8,27]

Verrucous carcinoma

Verrucous (varicoid) carcinoma is rare and has been described in association with achalasia and oesophageal diverticula. It is more frequently found in the oral cavity. The tumour is usually well differentiated, often papillary or warty and may show acanthosis and hyperkeratosis. It may be associated with leukoplakia, although less commonly than at other sites. The natural history is of a slow growing but invasive neoplasm and the tumour may become quite large.[28] Nodal involvement tends to be due to direct extension of the tumour and distant metastases have not been reported. Diagnosis may be difficult due to the well-differentiated nature of the tumour and it may be difficult to distinguish from squamous cell papilloma. The radiological appearance may be similar to that of varices. Treatment should be by en bloc surgical resection. Radiotherapy is not advised; although the tumour may regress it may also be transformed into an anaplastic lesion. The outlook should be more favourable than for patients with the usual type of squamous cell carcinoma. However, most patients with this lesion die from their disease.

Adenoid cystic carcinomas

Adenoid cystic carcinomas (cylindroma) probably arise in the deep oesophageal submucosal glands. Although a common tumour of the major salivary glands and the oropharyngeal region, they are rare in the oesophagus. Oesophageal lesions are histologically similar to tumours of the salivary glands but are more aggressive with a poorer prognosis.[8] They are located submucosally but may become polypoid or ulcerated. The overlying squamous mucosa may have focal areas of dysplasia and *in situ* carcinoma. They are usually found in the mid-third of oesophagus, have an equal sex distribution or a male preponderance, and affect patients in their 60s.

Oesophageal tumours tend to have widespread metastases and a low survival rate. Treatment is resection and combination radiochemotherapy may be of some benefit.[29]

Mucoepidermoid tumours

Mucoepidermoid tumours are uncommon in the oesophagus and share similarities with analogous tumours of the major salivary glands. They exhibit distinct epidermoid features with histological evidence of mucus secretion and must be distinguished from adenoacanthoma. They probably arise from secretory ducts of the deep submucosal glands or from aberrant gastric epithelium.[8] They are located primarily in the submucosa and often present as an intramural mass with intact mucosa, making diagnosis difficult. They may occur anywhere in the oesophagus but are most commonly found in the mid or lower thirds. They usually affect males in their 60s. Although most are resectable, they are aggressive tumours, metastases are common and, as a result, prognosis is poor.

Oesophageal polyps

Oesophageal polyps (fibrous or fibrovascular polyps), composed of vascular fibroblastic tissue are the second most common benign tumour of the oesophagus and account for less than 5–21% of benign oesophageal neoplasms. They commonly occur in the upper third and are covered by squamous mucosa which often shows patchy ulceration. They may be large with long pedicles and regurgitation with the polyp obstructing the trachea or hanging outside the mouth has been described. Other presenting complaints include dysphagia, weight loss, haemorrhage and pain. They may be missed on endoscopy, even when large, because the surface is similar to normal mucosa but should be visible on barium swallow. Polyps may also be composed of fat, eosinophilic granulomatous material or glandular hamartomatous material. Inflammatory polyps have also been described. Treatment is polypectomy or formal excision.

Benign epithelial tumours

Benign epithelial tumours of the oesophagus may be classified according to the tissue of origin. Squamous cell papillomas are sessile and account for 2.7% of benign oesophageal tumours with an incidence at endoscopy of 0.04%. They are usually single, multilobulated with a granular or warty surface and are found in the distal oesophagus. They are commonly only a few millimetres but may be up to 6 cm in size. There is a possible link with papillomavirus infection and there is no evidence of malignant potential in man.[30,31] Adenomas have been described in association with Barrett's oesophagus, but are uncommon.[32]

Haemangiomas

Haemangiomas are rare and arise from submucosal blood vessels. Most cases are asymptomatic and are discovered incidentally. The main presenting complaint is minor, rarely major, haematemesis. On endoscopy, a sessile red granular lesion, a nodule or a collection of dilated submucosal blood vessels may be seen. Biopsy is not recommended. Treatment is indicated in all symptomatic cases and includes sclerotherapy or laser coagulation for small lesions and formal excision of larger lesions.

Granular cell tumours

Granular cell tumours or granular cell myoblastomas[33] arise from Schwann cells and, although rare, the oesophagus represents the commonest site of occurrence in the gastrointestinal tract. They affect middle-aged women, are usually found in the distal oesophagus and range in size from 0.5–4 cm. Patients present with dysphagia, nausea and retrosternal discomfort. Endoscopy demonstrates small well-circumscribed firm yellow plaques. Less than 5% are malignant. Treatment is conservative or with endoscopic resection. Surgical excision is only recommended for larger lesions causing severe symptoms.

Neurofibromas

Neurofibromas are rare submucosal tumours. They may be multiple and many occur as a manifestation of von Recklinghausen's neurofibromatosis.

Table 9.1 *Rare variants of squamous cell carcinoma and adenocarcinoma in the oesophagus.*

Squamous cell carcinoma	Adenocarcinoma
Carcinosarcoma	Primary adenocarcinoma
Polypoid carcinoma	Adenoid cystic carcinoma
Pseudosarcoma	Adenosquamous carcinoma
Spindle cell carcinoma	Adenoacanthoma
Verrucous carcinoma	Mucoepidermoid tumours
SCC with pseudoglandular differentiation	Choriocarcinoma

Rare forms

There are many rare variants of squamous cell carcinoma and adenocarcinoma described in the oesophagus (Table 9.1). Unfortunately many of these malignant tumours share the same biological behaviour of the more typical oesophageal carcinomas. Spindle cell carcinoma is a variant of squamous cell carcinoma characterised by spindle-shaped cells which resemble fibroblasts. It is poorly differentiated and may resemble a sarcoma. It is postulated that they originate from mesenchymal metaplasia of squamous cells. Squamous cell carcinoma with pseudoglandular differentiation is characterised by glandular differentiation without evidence of mucous secretion. Adenosquamous carcinoma is rare and is a squamous cell carcinoma in which there are occasional aggressive glandular as well as epidermoid elements. Adenoacanthoma is a well-differentiated adenocarcinoma with focal squamous metaplasia and exhibits groups of squamous cells surrounded by glandular tumour. It probably arises from islands of gastric mucosa.[34] Choriocarcinoma is an uncommon lesion of the oesophagus and may arise due to metaplasia of an oesophageal adenocarcinoma to produce a hormonally active tumour, producing gonadotropins. Surgical resection is the treatment of choice.

Gastric neoplasms

The majority of gastric carcinomas are adenocarcinomas and these are outside the remit of this chapter. Lymphoma is the next most common tumour affecting the stomach.

Primary gastric lymphoma

Primary gastric lymphoma is the commonest extranodal non-Hodgkin's lymphoma and accounts for between 0.4 and 9% of all gastric neoplasms.[35,36] The incidence appears to be increasing. They arise from lymphoid tissue in the submucosa and thickened rugae and plaques are characteristic of early disease. Later these patches extend to form single ulcers or polypoid tumours and may give rise to diffuse infiltration of the gastric wall. The mean age of patients is in the 60s but these may occur in the young and the sexes are affected equally. The majority of non-Hodgkin's lymphomas are derived from B cells and light chain restriction indicative of a monoclonal B cell proliferation is often demonstrated by immunohistochemistry.

The organised lymphoid tissue present in mucosal sites is referred to as mucosa-associated lymphoid tissue (MALT) and forms part of a distinctive gut-associated lymphoid tissue (GALT). The majority of gastrointestinal lymphomas are B cell MALT tumours and arise from the 'centrocyte-like' cells that surround the B cell follicles.[37] A minority are derived from other GALT lymphocytes, including T cells. All lymphomas arising in MALT share certain clinical and biological features. The cells may infiltrate epithelium, forming characteristic lympho-epithelial lesions. Low-grade B cell lymphoma of MALT can occur anywhere in the gastrointestinal tract but the stomach is the commonest site. MALT lymphomas are often preceded by autoimmune disease of the involved organ. The lymphoid nodules found in the stomach are almost always associated with chronic gastritis caused by *Helicobacter* infection. A relationship between chronic gastritis, *Helicobacter pylori* infection and lymphoma has been postulated.[38] MALT lymphomas may remain localised for long periods of time and when they do disseminate it is often to other mucosal organs. These lymphomas have a good prognosis and can often be treated conservatively using local measures alone. High-grade B cell lymphoma of MALT is sometimes associated with low-grade MALT lymphoma but often occurs independently and a relationship with *Helicobacter* is not as well defined.[38] When no low-grade component is present it is difficult to determine whether these are of MALT origin, since they have no distinctive features.

The presentation of gastric lymphomas is similar to that of adenocarcinomas of the stomach, i.e. pain often ulcer-like, bleeding (massive bleeding is rare), fever, anorexia, weight loss nausea, vomiting and rarely perforation. Physical examination may reveal an abdominal mass in 30% of patients and the presence of hepatomegaly or splenomegaly suggests a diffuse process as does generalised lymphadenopathy (50% of patients ultimately develop disseminated disease).[39]

Barium meal usually reveals abnormalities but these are non-specific and peristalsis often persists throughout the lesion in spite of its suspicious nature. Radiological abnormalities include: subserosal nodules, plaque-like thickening of the wall, polypoid lesions with ulceration at the tip, multiple shallow large ulcerations or diffuse giant rugae (Fig. 9.3). Endoscopy may demonstrate ulcers and masses. Biopsies should be performed, but in view of the submucosal location biopsies may be negative in up to 70% of patients. The positivity of biopsies is related to the number of biopsies and the areas from which they are taken. A snare biopsy has been suggested but in many cases adequate tissue is obtained only at laparotomy. Computed tomography is increasingly used to define spread and stage. Bone marrow aspirate and biopsy may demonstrate diffuse disease.

Figure 9.3 *Barium meal of primary gastric lymphoma.*

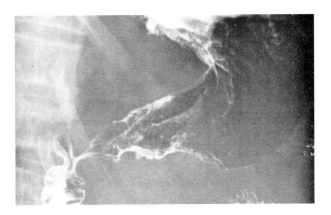

Numerous attempts have been made to classify gastric lymphomas based on the immunologic nature of the lymphocytes from which the tumour is derived. Monoclonal antibodies allow subclassification in terms of cell lineage. The most common classification was that of Rappaport[40] in which tumours were divided into nodular or diffuse and subdivided on the basis of grade and cell characteristics. The working formulation[41] for clinical use and the Kiel classification are now more commonly used. Diffuse histiocytic lymphoma, most commonly composed of B cells, is the commonest type followed by nodular lymphoma.

The TNM classification has been used for staging but the Ann Arbor system[42] is the most commonly used. In stage III and IV disease it may not be possible to distinguish primary from secondary lymphoma of the stomach. A primary site in the stomach may be inferred from extensive involvement of the stomach with any involved lymph nodes related to the stomach, a normal chest radiograph and white cell count, no demonstrable superficial lymphadenopathy and lack of hepatic or splenic involvement.

Treatment

In patients with stage IE disease surgery offers the best results. Radiotherapy is used in patients who are unfit for surgery or who refuse surgery. Adjuvant chemotherapy has also been used. Combination radiotherapy and chemotherapy have been used as primary treatment for stage IIE disease. However, it has been argued that surgery should be the first line of therapy because of the potential risks of fatal bleeding or of perforation as a result of rapid tumour lysis following radiochemotherapy.[43] Frequently radical surgery followed by radiochemotherapy is employed for stage II1E disease and stage II2E disease is treated primarily by radiochemotherapy. In patients presenting with stage IIIE and stage IV disease the primary treatment should be combination chemotherapy. The chemotherapeutic regimens most commonly employed utilise multiagent chemotherapy and commonly include cyclophosphamide, vincristine and prednisolone often in combination with other agents. Other authors have reported that low-grade gastric MALT lymphomas may regress after eradication of *Helicobacter pylori*.[44]

Survival is correlated with the depth of invasion and involvement of perigastric lymph nodes.[45] Histological features also appear to play a role with the nodular form of lymphoma doing better. Patients with stage IE disease have a 5-year survival approaching 100% whereas stage IIE patients have a 50% 5-year survival.

Secondary lymphoma frequently involves several sections of the gastrointestinal tract. The stomach is the organ most frequently involved after the pancreas.

Hodgkin's lymphoma

Hodgkin's lymphoma is an uncommon malignancy of the stomach accounting for 5–10% of gastric lymphomas and may represent a pleomorphic histiocytic lymphoma.

Pseudolymphoma

Pseudolymphoma (lymphoid hyperplasia) is the result of an exaggerated lymphocyte infiltration in response to chronic inflammation such as in the presence of benign peptic ulcer disease. Although many workers believe this to be benign others have postulated a progression to lymphoma and some have suggested that these be reclassified as lymphomas.[46] Pseudolymphomas must be distinguished from lymphoma proper and immunological studies may be required. A monoclonal pattern of immunoglobulins in cells is consistent with lymphoma.[47] Lymphoma is also suggested by regional node involvement, invasion through vessels, serosa or invasion with destruction of the muscular wall of the stomach.

Gastric carcinoids

Gastric carcinoids are uncommon tumours accounting for 3% of all GI carcinoids and 0.3% of all gastric neoplasms in the US.[48,49] They affect the sexes equally. They appear to be more common in Japan and may account for 41% of all GI carcinoids. Gastric carcinoids arise from enterochromaffin cells of the GI tract and are more common in patients with atrophic gastritis and pernicious anaemia. It has been suggested that achlorhydria and the resulting hypergastrinaemia may have an aetiological role[50] but this theory has been disputed by others.

Carcinoids arising from the foregut are composed microscopically of uniform round or polygonal cells with monotonous-appearing round and centrally located nuclei. They typically demonstrate an argyrophil reaction and are only rarely argentaffin positive.[51] The majority are located in the body and fundus of the stomach and there may be single or more commonly multiple lesions present. The tumours are frequently submucosal and endoscopic biopsies may be negative. Multiple 'button-hole' biopsies and biopsies in areas of ulceration may be required for diagnosis. If polypoid, polypectomy makes accurate histological diagnosis more likely.

The patients usually present with non-specific symptoms such as dyspepsia or abdominal pain; gastrointestinal (GI) bleeding is not uncommon. Usually these lesions are endocrinologically silent but occasionally the development of metastases may give rise to the carcinoid syndrome. The carcinoid syndrome produced by gastric lesions may be atypical with blotchy bright red geographic blushing, attributable to the release of 5-hydroxytryptophan and histamine rather than 5-hydroxytryptamine (serotonin).

Typically gastric carcinoids have an indolent course and conservative treatment may be adopted for small lesions. However, all are potentially malignant and may metastasise (20% have metastasised by the time of laparotomy. This figure is higher in series).[49] Small carcinoids can sometimes be treated by endoscopic removal or limited surgical resection. For larger lesions more extensive resection is advised. If regional nodal metastases are found these should be excised and if metastases are present an attempt should be made to resect these. Chemotherapy has been employed in patients who are not suitable for resection; doxorubicin is first-line therapy and 5-fluorouracil and imidazole carboxamide have also been used. Combination chemotherapy regimens have been used but the response rates are not significantly different from single agent chemotherapy.

Gastric polyps

Gastric polyps are present in 0.1–0.8% of autopsies and in 4–5% of symptomatic patients undergoing endoscopy (with a higher incidence in older patients).[52] Hyperplastic polyps account for 75–95% of these lesions and arise following regenerative hyperplasia after mucosal damage.[53,54] They are sometimes termed regenerative polyps. They may be multiple, occur in any part of the stomach, are usually small and average 1 cm in size. They are oval in shape often with a central dimple, have a smooth contour without crevices and may be sessile or the base may be well defined with a discrete pedicle. Hyperplastic polyps frequently remain stable and spontaneous regression has been observed. Malignant changes occurs in 0–4.5% (average 0.5%) of these polyps and tends to occur in the larger polyps (over 2 cm). These polyps may be associated with an independent carcinoma (6.5–25%) elsewhere in the stomach.

Adenomatous polyps

Adenomatous polyps represent the second most common type of polyp in the stomach (10–20%). They occur in 1% of the population in pathological studies and 0.23% in endoscopic studies. These polyps are often an incidental finding at endoscopy but rarely may be responsible for an intussusception. They may be distinguished macroscopically from hyperplastic polyps because they most commonly occur in the antrum, are single, tend to be larger (4 cm), have a papillary or villous pattern with an irregular contour, there are crevices present on the surface and the base is ill defined with a broad pedicle (Fig. 9.4). They are often associated with intestinal metaplasia and approximately 85% of patients have achlorhydria. True villous adenomas of the stomach have been reported but are rare. Malignant change may occur within these polyps with a reported frequency of 6–75%, with an average of 40% and is related to the size of the polyp.[53,54] During a follow-up period of 4 years 11% of patients with adenomatous polyps developed foci of carcinoma.[55] Ming[53] stated that adenomatous polyps, although not a frequent precursor of gastric cancer, were an important one. Treatment of these polyps is resection. This may be achieved by endoscopic polypectomy or by surgical resection. Endoscopic polypectomy must be combined with prophylactic antiulcer treatment because of the risks of bleeding or peptic ulceration at the excision site. It is important to examine the entire polyp because of the risk of harbouring a focus of carcinoma (13–22%). A high recurrence rate has been reported (over 40%) after endoscopic excision and gastric carcinoma may develop in 3.4% of patients following polypectomy for adenoma (compared to 1.4% of patients undergoing resection for hyperplastic polyps).[53,55,56] Thorough examination of the remainder of the stomach to rule out a separate concurrent carcinoma (present in 20% or more of patients) plus biopsies from the mucosa around an adenoma to check for dysplasia are an important part of the management of these lesions.

Fundic gland polyps

Fundic gland polyps are believed to be hamartomas; they are small (1–5 mm), with a sessile glassy appearance on endoscopy. They may

Figure 9.4
Endoscopic photograph of adenomatous polyp.

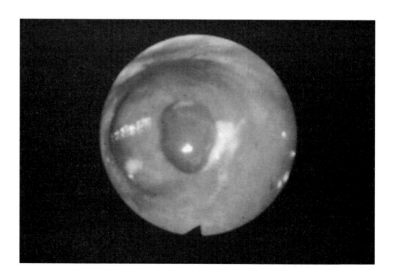

be single or multiple, are restricted to the body and fundus of the stomach and are found in middle-aged women and in patients with familial adenomatous polyposis. The term diffuse polyposis is used when all or a large part of the gastric mucosa is covered with polyps.[57]

Polyposis syndromes

Polyps, which may be adenomas, fundic gland polyps or hyperplastic polyps are found in 11–66% of patients with familial adenomatous polyposis.[58] Gastroduodenal polyps are found in 40% of patients with Peutz–Jegher's syndrome and are usually hamartomas. Hamartomatous polyps are also found in the stomach in Gardner's syndrome[59] and in juvenile polyposis. In Cronkhite–Canada syndrome (gastrointestinal polyposis, alopecia, onychodystrophy and hyperpigmentation) retention type gastric cysts occur and Cowden's disease is associated with hyperplastic polyps.[53]

Depressed gastric adenomas

Depressed gastric adenomas refer to depressions in the mucosa filled with atypical columnar type intestinal cells. Severe atypia or carcinoma *in situ* is commonly seen and malignant change is probably more common than in polypoid adenomas. Adenomyoma (myoepithelioma) composed of smooth muscle and ducts is an uncommon benign tumour of the stomach.

Squamous cell carcinoma

Squamous cell carcinoma of the stomach is an uncommon tumour (0.04–0.7% of all cancers) and is four times more common in men. It is frequently associated with areas of adenocarcinomatous change and the term 'adenosquamous carcinoma' or 'adenoacanthoma' is applied to the lesion.[60,61] Several pathogenic mechanisms have been postulated: (1) local extension or metastases from squamous cell carcinoma in neighbouring organs and in particular the oesophagus; (2) heterotropic squamous epithelium; (3) squamous cell metaplasia; (4) differentiation from totipotent stem cells or more likely (5) overgrowth of squamous components of existing adenocarcinoma. They have been described following ingestion of corrosive acids and following gastric involvement by tertiary syphilis. They are often large and ulcerated and more than half are found in the antrum. The prognosis is poor and long-term survival uncommon. Mucoepidermoid carcinoma is another tumour with both squamous and glandular elements and is very uncommon.

Hepatoid carcinoma

Hepatoid carcinoma is a rare adenocarcinoma which contains distinct foci of hepatic differentiation. The cells secrete substances produced by normal liver cells such as α-fetoprotein. This tumour is believed to reflect the common embryonic origin of liver and stomach from the primitive foregut.

Carcinosarcoma

Carcinosarcoma is composed of adenocarcinoma and spindle cell sarcoma and may result from growth of different cell lines within a tumour with the sarcomatous tissue probably originating from carcinoma cells.

Neurogenic tumours

Neurogenic tumours such as schwannomas, neuromas or neurofibromas may occur as isolated tumours in the stomach. Neurofibromas may also occur as part of a generalised neurofibromatosis. Neurofibromas demonstrate sarcomatous change in up to 10% of patients. Other tumours such as paragangliomas, neurogangliomas and sympathoblastomas may occur but are rare.[62]

Leiomyomas

Leiomyomas which may arise from stomach muscle tissue are the most common benign non-epithelial tumour of the stomach and are most frequently found in the body.[63] They are composed mostly of undifferentiated cells which may demonstrate features of smooth muscle or Schwann cell differentiation or other stromal cell features.[64] They enlarge from submucosal sites to form intraluminal polypoid lesions which may have multiple small ulcers on the surface. Less commonly they grow out from the serosal surface of the stomach and occasionally are 'dumb-bell' in appearance. Although most are clinically silent and are found incidentally, larger tumours (> 2 cm) may be symptomatic. Asymptomatic small leiomyomas may be present in 50% of people over 50 years[65] and in 50% of post mortems and may be multiple. They may present with GI bleeding, abdominal pain and occasionally pyloric obstruction; intussusception is rare; necrosis and calcification may occur. Biopsy is usually not diagnostic unless the lesion is ulcerated (Fig. 9.5). Local surgical resection, i.e. polypectomy or excision with a cuff of normal tissue is curative. Microscopically they may be divided into a cellular and epitheloid variant. Cellular leiomyomas are lesions with a higher mitotic count and more densely packed cells than ordinary leiomyomas.

Leiomyosarcoma

Leiomyosarcoma is the malignant counterpart of leiomyoma and it can be difficult to distinguish between the two unless there is evidence of local extension or metastases. The number of mitotic figures is the

Figure 9.5
Endoscopic photo-graph of gastric leiomyoma with central ulceration.

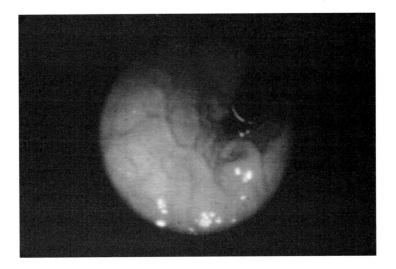

most important criterion for making this distinction However some clinically malignant lesions may show few mitoses. In some patients leiomyosarcoma is only diagnosed following recurrence after resection of a 'leiomyoma'.[64,66,67] An increased tumour DNA has also been associated with malignancy. Leiomyosarcomas account for 1–3% of gastric malignant tumours. The presenting symptoms are similar to those of leiomyoma but bleeding is common (75%) and weight loss is often present. Gastric leiomyosarcomas may present as part of Carney's triad, which also includes pulmonary chondroma and extra-adrenal paraganglioma.[68] Leiomyosarcomas are often larger than leiomyomas and 30–60% of patients have a palpable abdominal mass. Macroscopically these lesions may be bulky and vascular with areas of ulceration. Tumours greater than 8 cm are more likely to be associated with disseminated disease. Extragastric extension is found in two-thirds of patients at operation. Treatment is surgical resection and the five-year survival is 37–54%. Neither palliative or adjuvant radiotherapy nor chemotherapy has been shown to be of benefit.

Leiomyoblastoma

Leiomyoblastomas are smooth muscle tumours composed predominantly of epithelioid cells and are clinically similar to, but pathologically distinct from, leiomyoma or leiomyosarcoma.[69] Up to 10% ultimately become malignant. They run a relatively benign course even in the presence of metastases.

Lipomas

Lipomas of the stomach are rare and arise from submucosal fat. They are usually solitary and are found in the distal stomach. Symptoms are commonly due to bleeding and ulceration. One-third of patients have lipomas in other locations. Liposarcomas are very uncommon. In one series they represented one in 1192 cases of gastric malignancy over a 30-year period. They usually present with bleeding.

Other tumours

Kaposi's sarcoma may involve the stomach especially in patients with AIDS. Fibromas, granular cell tumours (myoblastoma) rhabdomyoma, myxomas, osteomas and chondromas have all been described in the stomach. Vascular tumours including glomus tumours (arterioangio-myoneuroma), lymphangiomas, haemangioendotheliomas, haemangio-pericytomas and haemangiomas affecting the stomach have been described but are rare. Teratomas have been described, are rare, and most commonly occur in infants. Choriocarcinomas have also been described and have a poor prognosis. Small-cell carcinomas similar to those in the lung have been described and frequently show foci of adenocarcinoma or squamous cell differentiation. The prognosis is very poor.

Metastases

Metastases to the stomach from extragastric carcinoma are uncommon (0.2% of autopsies) and one quarter of these are malignant melanomas.[8] These are followed in frequency by breast and pancreatic and lung carcinoma. Malignant melanoma may be mucosal or submucosal. At endoscopy a slightly elevated or polypoid black nodule may be seen. Some lesions however do not contain pigment and may not be recognised as melanomas. On X-ray a characteristic 'bull's eye' or 'target' lesion may be seen which represent a circumscribed defect with central ulceration. These lesions often remain silent for some time but bleed frequently and sometimes massively. Metastases from breast carcinoma are found in 5–10% of patients and are frequently noted on post mortem examination.[70] On radiological examination, a thickened rigid stomach wall with sluggish or absent peristalsis may be demonstrated and polypoid defects and ulceration may also be present. It may be difficult to distinguish from primary gastric carcinoma and laparotomy may be necessary to make the diagnosis. Cancer of the lung, ovary, testes, liver, colon and parotid gland as well as leukaemias may also spread to the stomach and spread from a squamous cell carcinoma of the head and neck has been described following placement of a PEG tube.

References

1. Seremetis MG, Lyons WS, de Guzman VC, Peabody JW. Leiomyomata of the oesophagus. Cancer 1976: 38: 2166–77.
2. Appleman HD. Stromal tumours of the esophagus, stomach and duodenum. In: Appleman HD (ed.) Pathology of the esophagus, stomach and duodenum. New York: Churchill Livingstone, 1984.
3. Deverall PB. Smooth muscle tumours of the esophagus. Br J Surg 1968; 55: 457–61.
4. Game PA, Jamieson GG. Benign tumours of the oesophagus. In: Jamieson GG (ed) Surgery of the oesophagus. New York: Churchill Livingstone, 1988, pp.893–8.
5. Ullal SR. Hypertrophic osteoarthropathy and leiomyoma of the esophagus. Am J Surg 1972; 123: 356–8.
6. Heald J, Moussalli H, Hasleton PS. Diffuse leiomyomatosis of the oesophagus. Histopathology 1986; 10: 755–9.
7. Choh JH, Khazei AH, Ihm HJ. Leiomyosarcoma of the esophagus: report of a case and review of the literature. J Surg Oncol 1986; 32: 223–6.
8. Ming SC. Tumours of the esophagus and stomach. In: Atlas of tumour pathology. Second Series, Fascicle 7. Washington DC: Armed Forces Institute of Pathology, 1973.
9. DeMeester TR, Skinner DB. Polypoid sarcomas of the oesophagus: a rare but potentially curable neoplasm. Ann Thorac Surg 1975; 20: 405–17.
10. Perch SJ, Soffen EM, Whittington R, Brooks JJ. Esophageal sarcomas. J Surg Oncol 1991; 48: 194–8.
11. Friedman-Kien AE, Laubenstein LJ, Rubinstein P et al. Disseminated Kaposi's sarcoma in homosexual men. Ann Intern Med 1982; 96: 693–700.
12. Stein HA, Murray D, Warner HA. Primary Hodgkin's disease of the esophagus. Dig Dis Sci 1981; 26: 457–61.
13. Givler RL. Esophageal lesions in leukaemia and lymphoma. Am J Dig Dis 1970; 15: 31–6.
14. McKeown F. Oat-cell carcinoma of the oesophagus. J Path Bact 1952; 64: 889–91.
15. Briggs JC, Ibrahim NBM. Oat cell carcinoma of the oesophagus: a clinico-pathological study of 23 cases. Histopathology 1983; 7: 261–77.
16. Nichols GL, Kelsen DP. Small cell carcinoma of the esophagus. The Memorial Hospital experience 1970 to 1987. Cancer 1989; 64: 1531–3.
17. Johnson FE, Clawson MC, Bashiti HM, Silverberg AB, Brown GO. Small cell undifferentiated carcinoma of the esophagus. Cancer 1984; 53: 1746–51.
18. Kelsen DP, Weston E, Kurtz R, Cvitkvoic E, Lieberman P, Golbey RB. Small cell carcinoma of the esophagus: treatment by chemotherapy alone. Cancer 1980; 45: 1558–61.
19. Chalkiadokis G, Wihlm JM, Morand G, Weil-Bousson M, Witz JP. Primary malignant melanoma of the esophagus. Ann Thorac Surg 1985; 39: 472–5.
20. de la Pava S, Nogogosyan E, Pickren JN, Caberra A. Melanosis of the oesophagus. Cancer 1963; 16: 48–50.
21. Isaacs JL, Quirke P. Two cases of primary malignant melanoma of the oesophagus. Clin Radiol 1988; 39: 455–7.
22. Ludwig ME, Shaw R, De Suto-Nagy G. Primary malignant melanoma of the esophagus. Cancer 1981; 48: 2528–34.
23. Siegal A, Swartz A. Malignant carcinoid of the oesophagus. Histopathology 1986; 10: 761–5.
24. Morson BC, Dawson IMP. Gastrointestinal Pathology. Oxford: Blackwell, 1979.
25. Gal AA, Martin SE, Kernen JA, Patterson MJ. Spindle cell carcinoma of the esophagus. An Immunohistochemical study. Cancer 1987; 60: 2244–50.
26. Sasajima K, Takai A, Taniguchi Y et al. Polypoid squamous cell carcinoma of the esophagus. Cancer 1989; 64: 94–7.
27. Matsusaka T, Watanabe H, Enjoji H. Pseudosarcoma and carcinoma of the esophagus. Cancer 1976; 37: 1546–55.
28. Meyerowitz BR, Shea LT. The natural history of squamous verrucose carcinoma of the esophagus. J Thorac Cardiovasc Surg 1971; 61: 646–9.
29. Petersson SR. Adenoid cystic carcinoma of the esophagus. Complete response to combination chemotherapy. Cancer 1986; 57: 1464–7.
30. Schmidt HW, Claggett OT, Harrison EG. Benign tumours and cysts of the esophagus. J Thorac Cardiovasc Surg 1961; 41: 717–32.
31. Fernandez-Rodriguez CM, Badia-Figuerola

N, Ruiz del Arbol L *et al.* Squamous cell papilloma of the esophagus: report of six cases with long term follow-up in four patients. Am J Gastroenterol 1986; 81: 1059–62.

32. McDonald GB, Brand DL, Thorning DR. Multiple adenomatous neoplasms arising in a columnar lined (Barrett's) esophagus. Gastroenterology 1977; 72: 1317–21.

33. Lack EE, Worsham GF, Calliham MO *et al.* Granular cell tumours, a clinicopathological study of 110 patients. J Surg Oncol 1980; 13: 301–16.

34. Smith RRL, Hamilton SR, Boitnott JK, Rogers EL. Spectrum of carcinoma arising in Barrett's esophagus. A clinicopathological study of 26 patients. Am J Surg Pathol 1984; 8: 563–73.

35. Isaacson PG, Spencer J, Wright DH. Classifying primary gut lymphomas. Lancet 1988; ii: 1148–9.

36. Hayes J, Dunn E. Has the incidence of primary gastric lymphoma increased? Cancer 1989; 63: 2073–6.

37. Isaacson PG, Wright DH. Malignant lymphoma of the mucosa associated lymphoid tissue. Cancer 1983; 52: 1410–16.

38. Karat D, O'Hanlon DM, Raimes S, Scott D, Griffin SM. A prospective study questioning the aetiological role of *H. pylori* in primary gastric lymphoma. Br J Surg 1995; 82: 1369–70.

39. Isaacson P, Wright D, Judd M, Mephan B. Primary gastrointestinal lymphomas. Cancer 1979; 43: 1805–19.

40. Rappaport H. Tumours of the hematopoietic system. In: Atlas of tumour pathology. Washington DC: Armed Forces Institute of Pathology, 1966.

41. National Cancer Institute. National Cancer Institute sponsored study of classification of non-Hodgkin's lymphomas. Summary and description of a working formulation for clinical usage. Lymphoma Pathologic Classification Project. Cancer 1982; 49: 2112–35.

42. Carbone PP, Kaplan HS, Musshoff K, Smithers DW, Tubiana M. Report of a committee of Hodgkin's disease staging classification. Cancer Res 1971; 31: 1860–1.

43. Fleming ID, Mitchell S, Ali Dilawari RA. The role of surgery in the management of gastric lymphoma. Cancer 1982; 49: 1135–41.

44. Wotherspoon AC, Doglioni C, Diss TC *et al.* Regression of primary low-grade B-cell gastric lymphoma of mucosa-associated tissue type after eradication of *Helicobacter pylori*. Lancet 1993; 342: 575–7.

45. Weingrad DN, Decosse JJ, Sherlock P, Straus D, Lieberman PH, Fillipa DA. Primary gastrointestinal lymphoma. A 30-year review. Cancer 1982; 49: 1258–65.

46. Schwarz MS, Sherman H, Smith T *et al.* Gastric pseudolymphoma and its relationship to malignant gastric lymphoma. Am J Gastroenterol 1989; 84: 1555–9.

47 Villar HV, Wong R, Paz B *et al.* Immunotyping in the management of gastric lymphoma. Am J Surg 1991; 161: 171–5.

48. Muller J, Kirchner T, Muller-Hermelink HK. Gastric endocrine cell hyperplasia and carcinoid tumours in atrophic gastritis type A. Am J Surg Pathol 1987; 11: 909–17.

49. Hajdu SI, Winawer SJ, Laird Myers WP. Carcinoid tumours. A study of 204 cases. Am J Clin Pathol 1974; 61: 521–8.

50. Borch K, Renvall H, Leidberg G. Gastric endocrine cell hyperplasia and carcinoid tumours in pernicious anemia. Gastroenterology 1985; 88: 638–48.

51. Wilander E, El-Salhy M, Pitkanen P. Histopathology of gastric carcinoids: a survey of 42 cases. Histopathology 1984; 8: 183–93.

52. Neimark S, Rogers AI. Gastric polyps: a review. Am J Gastroenterol 1982; 77: 585–7.

53. Ming SC. The classification and significance of gastric polyps. In: International Academy of Pathology Monograph: The Gastrointestinal Tract, 1977.

54. Nakamura T, Nakano G. Histopathological classification and malignant change in gastric polyps. J Clin Pathol 1985; 38: 754–64.

55. Kamiya T, Morishita T, Asakura H *et al.* Long-term follow-up study on gastric adenoma and its relation to gastric protruded carcinoma. Cancer 1982; 50: 2496–503.

56. Seifert E, Gail K, Weismuller J. Gastric polypectomy. Long term results (survey of 23 centres in Germany). Endoscopy 1983; 15: 8–11.

57. Sipponen P, Laxen F, Seppala K. Cystic 'hamartomous' gastric polyps: a disorder to oxyntic glands. Histopathology 1983; 7: 729–37.

58. Jagelman DG, DeCosse JJ, Bussey HJR. Upper gastrointestinal cancer in familial adenomatous polyposis. Lancet 1988; i: 1149–51.

59. Eichenberger P, Hammer B, Gloor F *et al.* Gardner's syndrome with glandular cysts of the fundic mucosa. Endoscopy 1980; 12: 63–7.
60. Callery CD, Sanders MM, Pratt S, Turnbull AD. Squamous cell carcinoma of the stomach. A study on four patients with comments on histogenesis. J Surg Oncol 1985; 29: 166–172.
61 Boswell JT, Helwig EB. Squamous cell carcinoma and adenoacanthoma of the stomach. A clinicopathological study. Cancer 1965; 18: 181–92.
62. Shivshanker K, Bennetts R. Neurogenic sarcoma of the gastrointestinal tract. Am J Gastroenterol 1981; 75: 214–17.
63. Appelman HD (ed.) Stromal tumours of the esophagus, stomach and duodenum. Edinburgh: Churchill Livingstone, 1984.
64. Appelman HD. Smooth muscle tumours of the gastrointestinal tract. What we know now that Stout didn't know. Am J Surg Pathol 1986; 10(S1): 83–99.
65. Morson BC, Dawson IMP. Nonepithelial tumours. In: Gastrointestinal pathology. Oxford and St Louis: Blackwell Scientific Publications, 1979.
66. Shiu MH, Farr GH, Papachristou DN, Hajdu SI. Myosarcomas of the stomach: natural history, prognostic factors and management. Cancer 1982: 49: 177–87.
67. Appleman HD, Helwig BE. Gastric epitheloid leiomyoma and leiomyosarcoma (leiomyoblastoma). Cancer 1976; 38: 708–28.
68. Carney JA. The triad of gastric epitheloid leiomyosarcoma, pulmonary chondroma and functioning extra-adrenal para-ganglioma. A five year review. Medicine 1983; 62: 159–69.
69. Stout AP. Bizarre smooth muscle tumours of the stomach. Cancer 1962; 15: 400–6.
70. Asch MJ, Wiedel PD, Habif DB. Gastrointestinal metastases from carcinoma of the breast: autopsy study and 18 cases requiring operative intervention. Arch Surg 1968; 96: 840–3.

10 Pathophysiology and investigation of GORD and motility disorders

David F. Evans
Charles S. Robertson

Introduction

Structure

The oesophagus is a muscular tube approximately 25 cm long connecting the pharynx to the stomach and lies in loose connective tissue in the posterior mediastinum. The distal 1–3 cm is normally intra-abdominal having passed through the diaphragmatic hiatus in the left hemidiaphragm formed by the crura, just anterior to the aorta and posterior to the left lobe of the liver. The oesophagus joins the stomach at the gastro-oesophageal junction (GOJ) or cardia. The oesophagus is usually lined with squamous epithelium which terminates close to the GOJ where it joins the columnar-lined epithelium of the stomach at the squamocolumnar junction (SCJ or Z line) (Fig. 10.1).

Figure 10.1
Important anatomical and functional structures in the human oesophagus.

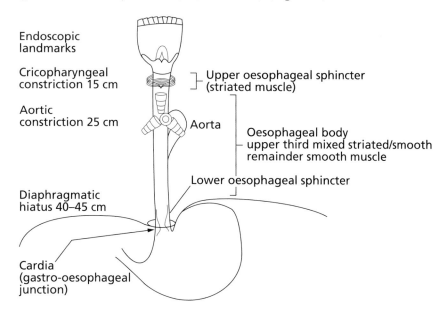

Endoscopic landmarks

Cricopharyngeal constriction 15 cm

Aortic constriction 25 cm

Diaphragmatic hiatus 40–45 cm

Cardia (gastro-oesophageal junction)

Upper oesophageal sphincter (striated muscle)

Aorta

Oesophageal body upper third mixed striated/smooth remainder smooth muscle

Lower oesophageal sphincter

The blood supply to the oesophagus in the neck is principally from the inferior thyroid arteries and in the thorax is from branches directly off the aorta and bronchial arteries. Venous drainage is into the azygos vein. Lymphatic drainage is to paraoesophageal nodes and then into the thoracic duct which lies to the right of the oesophagus and vertebral column.

Histologically, the oesophagus can be separated into the following layers:

1. The mucosa consists of non-keratinised stratified squamous epithelium, lamina propria and muscularis mucosae. Mucous secreting glands are also present, close to GOJ.
2. The submucosa contains connective tissue, blood vessels, lymphatics and mucous glands.
3. The muscularis layer (circular and longitudinal) is composed of striated muscle in the most proximal 5–10% of the oesophageal body, immediately distal to the upper sphincter. The next 35–40% is mixed striated and smooth muscle, with an increasing proportion of smooth to striated muscle moving distally. The most distal 35–40% is composed entirely of smooth muscle fibres.[1,2] The outer adventitial layer is composed of connective tissue which merges with adjacent structures within the thorax.

Extrinsic innervation of the oesophagus is via sympathetic and parasympathetic pathways with differing innervation depending on the type of muscle (proximal striated, distal smooth). Parasympathetic innervation is via the vagus nerves[3,4] which form a plexus of nerve fibres on the outer surface of the oesophagus which coalesce in the distal third to form the anterior and posterior vagal trunks. Sympathetic innervation is via the postganglionic fibres of the superior cervical ganglion and ganglia from the thoracic sympathetic chain. There appears to be no important sympathetic function in the striated oesophagus and most axons terminate in the myenteric and submucosal plexuses.

Intrinsic innervation is controlled by two ganglionated neural plexuses.[5-7] The submucosal or Meissners' plexus lies between the submucosal and circular muscle layer and the myenteric or Auerbachs' plexus lies between the circular and longitudinal muscle layers. The function of the submucosal plexus is mainly control of secretion and blood flow in the epithelium and submucosa. The myenteric plexus controls motor function including sphincter activity during deglutition. Extrinsic neural modulation is also via these nerve plexuses and this is important in the control of swallowing.[8,9]

The oesophageal sphincters

The upper sphincter
The upper sphincter (UOS) separates the pharynx and oesophagus and is met at about 15 cm from the incisor teeth at endoscopy. It lies behind

the hyoid bone and is formed by the cricopharyngeus muscle. Manometrically, it is approximately 3–4 cm long, having a high pressure (50–100 mmHg) and is asymmetrical forming a slit, predominantly in the anterior and posterior orientation, with lower pressures laterally. Functionally the UOS prevents pulmonary aspiration of gastrointestinal (GI) contents and aerophagia.

The lower oesophageal sphincter

The lower oesophageal sphincter (LOS) is found in the GOJ and usually lies across the hiatus. Anatomically, no major distinction is found with the remainder of the muscle layers. Functionally, a high pressure zone exists in the most distal 2–5 cm of the circular smooth muscle. The LOS exhibits both radial and axial asymmetry from extrinsic and intrinsic influence and also shows diurnal, postural and prandial variations in pressure. Many external factors have been demonstrated to affect the overall pressure in the LOS (Table 10.1). The LOS acts as a two-way valve using the flutter valve principle and is a weak sphincter with an intrinsic pressure of only 10–25 mmHg. The LOS is a major component of the antireflux mechanism and is under both neural and hormonal control. The intrinsic basal tone has to resist reflux of gastric contents under the challenge of a wide range

Table 10.1 *Factors affecting the LOS*

	Decrease LOS activity	Increase LOS activity
Hormones and peptides	Glucagon	Gastrin
	Secretin	Motilin
	Cholecystokinin	Bombesin
	VIP	Histamine (H_1 receptors)
	GIP	Serotonin (M receptors)
	Progesterone	
	Oestrogens	
	Serotonin	
	Histamines	
	Enkephalins	
Prostoglandins	E_1, E_2, A_2	F_2
Drugs	Atropine	Metoclopramide
	Ca^{2+} inhibitors	Domperidone
	Ganglion inhibitors	Cisapride
	Tricyclic antidepressants	Cholinergic drugs
		Anticholinesterases
Foods	Caffeine	Protein meal
	Fats	
	Chocolate	
	Alcohol	
Other	Smoking	

of intrathoracic (± 60 mmHg) and intra-abdominal pressures (up to 100 mmHg). Not surprisingly, LOS dysfunction is very common.

Normal swallowing

Swallowing can be initiated voluntarily or as part of a reflex following stimulation of the mouth and pharynx. However, once initiated, the act of swallowing becomes an involuntary reflex. The sensory nerves for this reflex are the glossopharyngeal and superior laryngeal branches of the vagus. Stimuli reach the swallowing centre in the medulla and pons where swallowing is coordinated. Efferent impulses travel via the 5th, 7th, 10th, 11th and 12th cranial nerves as well as the motor neurons from C1–C3. There are three phases to normal swallowing.

Oral phase

Ingested food is broken down into smaller particles by the action of the teeth and muscles of the mouth and jaws and lubricated with saliva by mastication. The bolus is moved into the posterior oropharynx by the tongue and forced into the hypopharynx.

Pharyngeal phase

Simultaneously with the posterior movement of the tongue, the soft palate is raised to close off the nasopharynx to prevent nasal regurgitation. The hyoid is pulled upwards elevating the larynx to bring the epiglottis under the tongue. This backward tilt of the epiglottis covers the opening of the larynx and with adduction of the vocal cords and the inhibition of respiration, prevents the passage of food into the airway. The pressure in the hypopharynx rises abruptly during swallowing to reach at least 60 mmHg. A pressure differential develops between the pharynx and the subatmospheric pressure of the intrathoracic oesophagus which results in movement of the bolus into the oesophagus when the cricopharyngeus relaxes. Once the bolus enters the oesophagus proper, the cricopharyngeus closes with the immediate closing pressure of double the resting pressure (100 mmHg). The peristaltic wave in the proximal oesophageal body is initiated at the time of the highest cricopharyngeal pressure to prevent reflux into the pharynx. Once the peristaltic wave progresses distally, the UOS returns to its resting pressure.

Oesophageal phase

The pharyngeal activity in swallowing initiates the oesophageal phase. The transmission of the food bolus from the distal oesophagus into the stomach is accomplished over a pressure gradient of 5 mmHg below atmospheric pressure in the thorax to 5 mmHg above atmospheric pressure in the abdomen. A primary peristaltic wave is initiated by a pharyngeal swallow and consists of an occlusive pressure varying from 30 to 160 mmHg. The peak wave of contraction moves down the oesophagus at a velocity of 2–5 cm/s and reaches the distal oeso-phagus 4–10 s after the initial pharyngeal stimulus. Once the bolus reaches the lower oesophagus, a further peristaltic wave may be initi-ated by a reflex secondary to lower oesophageal distension and this is termed secondary peristalsis. At the time the bolus is approaching the stomach and after the initial pharyngeal stimulus, the LOS relaxes com-pletely to the level of the gastric baseline pressure to allow passage of the content. The relaxation phase is present for up to 4 s. The LOS under-goes an after-contraction with a pressure rise of up to 50–100 mmHg in some cases before returning to its basal tone of 15–20 mmHg. The func-tion of the after contraction is suggested to be a clearing contraction to ensure that any remaining content is moved into the stomach.

The third type of contraction in the oesophageal body is termed a tertiary contraction. These contractions may be seen as isolated contractions at any site in the oesophageal body and are not preceded by a voluntary swallow or oesophageal distension. Whether tertiary contractions have a function is unclear but they are considered to be pathological in significant amounts.

The antireflux mechanism

Infrequent, short-lived periods of gastro-oesophageal reflux (GOR) are common and are regarded as a physiological phenomenon. Physio-logical GOR is often associated with eating and is most commonly experienced in the postprandial period, sometimes in conjunction with eructation (belching). It is rarely seen during sleep unless a meal has been taken shortly before retiring or there has been a degree of dietary abuse (large volume intake, high fat content, alcohol excess, hot spices etc.). Pathological GOR is associated with symptoms and is usually caused by more frequent reflux episodes including some at night. This type of GOR can give rise to oesophageal damage (oesophagitis) by gastric juice.

The majority of episodes of GOR occur during transient periods of LOS relaxation. Transient relaxations of the LOS (TLOSRs) were first described by Dent et al.[10] and are termed 'inappropriate' as they are not preceded by a corresponding primary peristaltic wave in the oesophageal body initiated by a voluntary swallow.

Although the LOS in itself is an important barrier to GOR, it is only one of a number of factors that are likely to be important in the overall antireflux mechanism (ARM). Failure of one or more of these factors may result in reflux, which, when also giving rise to symp-toms, precipitates the disease entity of gastro-oesophageal reflux disease (GORD). The following factors have been proposed as being important in maintaining an effective reflux barrier. Although some have been unequivocally proven as being important in the reflux control of others, although based on sound physiological principles, have not been sufficiently well defined, or the order of their impor-tance classified. Fig. 10.2 summarises the major factors contributing to the ARM.

Figure 10.2
Anatomical and functional mechanisms contributing to the antireflux mechanism (ARM).

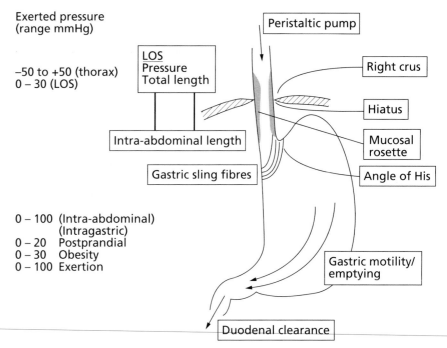

Exerted pressure
(range mmHg)

−50 to +50 (thorax)
0 – 30 (LOS)

LOS
Pressure
Total length

Peristaltic pump

Right crus

Hiatus

Intra-abdominal length

Mucosal rosette

Gastric sling fibres

Angle of His

0 – 100 (Intra-abdominal)
(Intragastric)
0 – 20 Postprandial
0 – 30 Obesity
0 – 100 Exertion

Gastric motility/ emptying

Duodenal clearance

Oesophageal factors

Lower oesophageal sphincter

LOS intrinsic pressure
The LOS is naturally a low pressure valve (10–25 mmHg) and hypotension is a logical cause of failure of the ARM. However, in clinical terms, many studies have demonstrated that there is no correlation between LOS pressure and GORD. Patients with GORD may have a normotensive LOS or asymptomatic subjects may have low sphincter pressure and no GORD.

LOS total length
An important physical factor relating to valve competence is the length of the valve closure. The LOS is normally 2–4 cm in length and total lengths of less than 2 cm are regarded as a significant factor in the failure of the ARM.

Intra-abdominal length
Because of pressure differences across the diaphragm (positive pressure in the abdomen, negative pressure in the thorax), the greater the LOS length in the abdomen, the greater the augmentation of LOS pressure with any progressive rise in intra-abdominal pressure (IAP). For example, in the case of a sliding hiatus hernia, by definition, the LOS lies in the thorax so no intra-abdominal segment exists. In

this case, no augmentation of LOSP by abdominal pressure is possible. In spite of this, there remains no absolute correlation with the existence of hiatus hernia and GORD with only approximately 50% of patients with a hernia having GORD and 50% with GORD without a hernia.

Oesophageal motility

Oesophageal passage of swallowed food is normally effected by coordinated contraction of the oesophageal smooth muscle to propel the food bolus distally and is termed peristalsis. This mechanism is essential in quadrupeds, where the stomach is usually higher than the mouth during feeding (e.g. horse, cow, zebra), but also desirable in bipeds such as man, even though gravity helps the passage of the bolus into the stomach. Any dysfunction of normal oesophageal motility may give rise to, or worsen GOR by impaired oesophageal clearance of refluxate.[11] Other important motility factors in the efficiency of oesophageal contractility are amplitude, propagation velocity and LOS relaxation.

Anatomical factors at the cardia

In addition to sphincter tone, position and length, other mechanical factors present at the gastro-oesophageal junction will influence overall LOS competence.

Angle of His

The 'flap valve' mechanism formed at the cardia (angle of His) has been shown to be an effective barrier to reflux.[12] In hiatus hernia, this angle is absent and may therefore explain one cause of GOR in this condition. Steiner[13] found that the cardioesophageal angle in infants with hiatus hernia was virtually absent and the oesophagus and stomach formed a straight tube.

Diaphragmatic crus

The 'pinchcock' action of the right crus of the diaphragm has also been shown to be a contributory factor in the overall valve-like action of the LOS. Indeed, the radial asymmetry of the LOS may be a direct result of the pinchcock action of the crus.[14] Anatomically, other extraluminal factors associated with the ARM may be contributions from the oblique gastric sling fibres and the phreno-oesophageal ligament.

Mucosal rosette

The convoluted folds of the oesophageal mucosa, held in apposition by the surface tension of mucosal secretions, form a mucosal 'rosette' or 'choke', which acts as a reflux barrier.[15] In oesophagitis, where the integrity of the distal oesophageal mucosa is compromised, it is likely that this factor will be absent, thus increasing the likelihood of GOR.

LOS vagal reflex

The oesophagus is extrinsically innervated by the vagus nerve although the majority of neural activity is controlled by the intramural myenteric plexus. Even so, a vagovagal reflux has been described[16] which plays an important role in reflux prevention. A reflex rise in LOS pressure has been shown to exist in response to an increase in intra-abdominal pressure. This is thought to be a physiological mechanism to protect the oesophageal mucosa from acid when gastric pressure exceeds LOS pressure. This reflex can be abolished by atropine and vagotomy and has been shown to be impaired in chronic reflux patients with oesophagitis.[17] This is an important finding and may help to explain why some patients with apparently good LOS tone and oesophageal body peristalsis, have severe reflux.

Saliva secretion

In humans, saliva is produced by glands in the mouth to lubricate food and contains a number of substances including bicarbonate, mucous and salivary enzymes which initiate the first stages of digestion. Salivary output varies widely from a minimal basal state to a maximum secretion when stimulated by mastication. Swallowed saliva is thought to be important in GORD as the volume and composition of saliva plays an important role in the neutralisation of refluxed acid. Many papers have been produced which show the importance of saliva in GORD.[18,19]

Gastric factors

Gastric motility and emptying

Any impairment of contractility or coordination of fundic or antral motor function may lead to gastric stasis and delayed gastric emptying of chyme. Conditions that induce gastric stasis (truncal vagotomy, visceral autonomic neuropathy) may therefore give rise to secondary GOR. So almost any disease that causes impaired gastric outflow and delayed gastric emptying (GE) may cause a rise in intragastric pressure and possible GOR. However, the evidence for this remains controversial, with some studies showing delayed gastric emptying[20] and others showing normal emptying in patients with GORD.[21]

Gastric acid secretion

The importance of hypersecretion of gastric acid as a major cause of GORD is an attractive hypothesis, after all, by far the most effective medical treatments are with acid-suppressing drugs. Even the 'non-systemic drugs' such as antacids, incorporate some form of antacid action in the way of neutralisation with alkaline substances. In spite of this, the role of acid secretion in the pathogenesis of reflux remains unclear. It was Castell[22] who coined the phrase, 'acid in the wrong place', with reference to GORD and this statement may well describe the underlying principle of reflux disease. A large number of studies have been performed to examine acid secretion in GORD and although a few have shown significant differences in basal and peak acid outputs in GORD patients, the majority show little difference in overall acid secretory levels compared with controls.[23]

Duodenogastric reflux

Duodenogastric refluxate may contain bile acids and pancreatic and duodenal enzymes which could cause oesophageal mucosal damage. There is evidence that pepsinergic activity and the presence of bile in the oesophagus is implicated in the pathogenesis of GORD and its complications.[24-26] The columnar lines oesophageal mucosa, named after one of the first to describe it in the 1950s, Norman Barrett, has led to the development of the disease entity 'Barrett's oesophagus'. The disorder, which is thought to be the end stage of chronic GORD, presents when the normal, squamous cell-lined distal oesophagus is replaced by gastric-like columnar epithelium. The condition has been shown to be associated with progression to carcinoma through the dysplasia, metaplasia sequence, although irrefutable evidence has not yet been shown. The addition of alkaline duodenogastric reflux to the acid refluxate may also have a role in the pathogenesis of Barrett's oesophagus.

Failure of the ARM

Failure of the ARM may result in reflux of gastric juice into the oesophagus and GORD. The failure may by primary, that is where the reflux barrier at the GO junction fails, or, secondary, where reflux is caused by oesophageal, gastric or other factors albeit with apparently normal LOS function. Table 10.2 outlines the factors that may contribute to GORD.

Gastro-oesophageal reflux disease

Gastro-oesophageal reflux (GOR) is the retrograde movement of gastric content into the oesophagus. It is experienced by many species of mammal including humans and in small amounts is a physiological phenomenon, providing it does not give rise to symptoms. Gastro-oesophageal reflux disease (GORD) is also associated with reflux of gastric contents into the oesophagus but by definition the reflux gives rise to symptoms and may subsequently cause the complications associated with the disease. These are oesophagitis, ulceration, stricturing and Barrett's oesophagus which may lead to adenocarcinoma. GORD is caused by failure of the physiological antireflux barrier which allows exposure of the poorly protected oesophageal mucosa to the injurious substances of digestion.

Table 10.2 *Postulated mechanisms contributing to failure of the antireflux mechanism*

Primary	LOS hypotension
	LOS overall length < 2 cm
	LOS intra-abdominal length < 1.5 cm
	Hiatus hernia
	Loss of angle of His (hiatus hernia)
	Crural diaphragm failure
	Loss of mucosal rosette (inflammation)
Secondary	Salivation production impairment
	Impaired oesophageal peristalsis (loss of 'pump' function)
	Gastric acid hypersecretion
	Gastric outlet impairment – gastroparesis
	Small intestinal outlet dysfunction
	Mechanical obstruction
	Motor dysfunction (visceral enteropathy)

Prevalence of GORD

GOR is very common, it has been estimated that up to 60% of the population will have symptoms of GOR at some time in their lives.[27] GORD represents up to 80% of benign oesophageal pathology and is a major drain on healthcare resources in terms of consultation, treatment and time off work. As physiological GOR is regarded as a normal phenomenon, the dividing line between what is regarded by clinicians as significant for pathological GOR is a difficult management problem. For example up to 40% of GORD patients have no oesophagitis at endoscopy[28] but may have severe symptoms. On the other hand some patients first present with dysphagia and a peptic stricture, but with only mild symptoms. The spectrum of GORD is therefore very broad and this leads to difficulties in management. In terms of treatment, some patients' symptoms are self-limiting and do not require initial medical intervention, although as symptoms frequently recur at irregular intervals, ultimately a medical consultation is often sought. Most patients, however, require therapy and this usually takes the form of antacids and alginates, H_2-receptor antagonists and proton pump inhibitors, depending on the severity of the disease. The problem is that symptoms are not a good guide to disease severity and relapse after healing courses of drugs is common. GORD is therefore a chronic and relapsing disease that may require lifetime therapy in some patients. It is not surprising therefore that in some cases, surgical intervention is sought in the form of an antireflux procedure (see Chapter 11).

Aetiology

Symptomatic GOR can appear at any period of life. It is common in the newborn, usually seen as post-feed vomiting and possetting. GOR in this group is probably due to incomplete maturation of the lower oesophageal sphincter (LOS) and development of oesophageal peristaltic function.[29] The predominant supine posture of Western babies and the frequency and volume of feeds may also be relevant to the GOR seen in the early months of life and subsequent GORD in later life.

The poor association between GORD and age suggests a multifactorial cause. It is postulated that an underlying anatomical or physiological defect may be activated by external factors such as obesity, life style, diet, stress or even another illness which can trigger the onset and perpetuation of reflux symptoms.

No association has been found between GORD and geographical location or ethnic groups, although there are some areas in the world where GORD is rare. Orientals have little in the way of reflux disease and one study has shown the Chinese to have supercompetent LOS tone when compared with control European values.[30] There is, however, a paucity of objective data on this subject and for the most part, we have to rely on prevalence figures from epidemiological studies for information regarding GORD world-wide. As data are scarce from all but the most developed countries (Europe, USA, Japan, Australia), an accurate estimate of prevalence is currently impossible.

Pathophysiology

Inappropriate, transient lower oesophageal relaxations (TLSOR) are the major cause of GORD accounting for 95% of reflux episodes in controls and 70% in patients with GORD. In patients, more of the TLSORs are accompanied by acid GOR than in controls although it is unclear whether the actual number of TLSORs is increased in patients.[31] TLSORs are increased after meals or with gastric distension but suppressed in the supine position. The actual mechanism of TLSORs is unclear but vagal stimulation is likely to be important.[15,16] Other mechanisms involved with GOR are:

1. Free GOR across the GO junction with no detectable basal LOS pressure.
2. GOR accompanying a transient increase in intra-abdominal pressure.
3. GOR at the moment of a deep inspiration.

Low basal LOS pressure is responsible for some GOR but there is likely to be a contribution from the putative vagovagal reflex rise in LOSP in response to intra-abdominal pressure increase as postulated by Olgivie and others.[15,16]

The major injurious agent in GORD is hydrochloric acid from gastric juice but pepsin or, in rare cases, alkaline secretions from the duodenum such as bile, pancreatic juice or other proteolytic substances may be important in the pathophysiology of the disease. Although GORD is caused predominantly by acid reflux it is unlikely that acid secretion *per se* is the primary cause of the disorder. The underlying problem is almost certainly caused by failure of the antireflux mechanism, although in terms of treatment, the most effective drugs given for symptom relief and mucosal healing are currently drugs that suppress or neutralise gastric acid. Drugs which augment the antireflux barrier in some way (prokinetic agents) are also advocated but at present may not be potent enough to act as efficiently as the acid inhibitors. It is noteworthy that the only other treatment for GORD when medical therapy fails is antireflux surgery. The primary aim of surgery is to restore the antireflux mechanism and not to suppress acid. Acid-reducing operations such as vagotomy or antrectomy are rarely advocated as effective surgical treatment for reflux unless complications or repeat surgery warrant the abolition of gastric acid secretion.

Clinical presentation

Typical

Patients usually present with heartburn, epigastric and retrosternal pain, regurgitation of acid-tasting fluid, dysphagia, odynophagia, globus and occasionally waterbrash.

Atypical

Some patients present with atypical symptoms such as cardiac like chest pain, respiratory symptoms of asthma or chronic wheezing, orolaryngeal symptoms including unexplained sore throat or hoarseness and palatal dental erosion. All these being associated with chronic intermittent exposure of the oral cavity, pharynx and airways to refluxed gastric juice.

Table 10.3 outlines the major symptoms associated with GORD. The list includes infants and children, GOR also being common in this group. Progression of symptoms is often associated with complications of GORD including oesophagitis, peptic stricture and Barrett's oesophagus.[32]

Because symptoms are such an unreliable guide to the presence or severity of GORD, objective investigation is essential to diagnose and treat the disease. Some clinicians advocate a trial of acid suppression as a diagnostic screening test. Although this is effective in some patients, this is a dangerous management route to advocate due to the possibility that other acid-related pathology may be responsible for the symptoms (duodenal ulcer, gastric ulcer, *Helicobacter pylori* antritis, gastric cancer). Acid suppression with proton pump inhibitors at normal doses may also not be effective in up to 15% of patients.[33,34]

Table 10.3 *Symptoms of gastro-oesophageal reflux*

	Adult	**Paediatric**
Typical	Heartburn Regurgitation Epigastric pain Retrosternal pain	Vomiting Haematemesis Perceived pain related to feeding (crying, back arching, irritability, poor feeding)
Atypical	Angina-like chest pain Dysphagia Nocturnal wheeze/asthma Laryngeal symptoms Rumination Toothwear Halitosis	Chronic wheeze Chest infection Bronchodysplasia Pneumonia Stridor Failure to thrive Near sudden infant death

Investigations

Radiology

Contrast studies yield information regarding structure and function although in recent years other methods such as endoscopy, manometry and pH have largely replaced radiology in the diagnosis of GORD.

Barium swallow/meal

Oesophageal body luminal changes such as diverticula, rings and webs can be identified. Luminal obstruction, benign strictures, carcinoma and LOS abnormalities (tight, lax) can also be identified. Two functional abnormalities of the oesophagus, achalasia and diffuse oesophageal spasm are usually diagnosed using barium swallows. In early cases the structural changes may be intermittent or more subtle and videofluoroscopy or manometry may be required to confirm the diagnosis. Generally, abnormalities of oesophageal motility are best assessed using dynamic techniques.

Videofluoroscopy

Videofluoroscopy allows repeated dynamic review and slow motion playback to examine motor function and coordination of swallowing. Barium-based liquids, or coated solids (marshmallow or bread)[35] are swallowed while the radiologist follows the passage of the medium along the oesophageal length. This type of radiology remains the best means of examination of the upper sphincter and is also useful in detection of motility abnormalities of the oesophageal body and lower sphincter.

Endoscopy and biopsy

Examination of the oesophagus

At gastroscopy, the endoscope is passed into the mouth (over a suitable guard) and visual examination of the oropharynx, oesophageal mucosa, sphincters and gastro-oesophageal junction are undertaken. Measurements of LOS position, the Z line and the presence of a hiatus hernia should be documented, the presence of any oesophageal pathology is identified and noted.

Mucosal abnormalities including oesophagitis, columnar lined oesophageal epithelium (Barrett's oesophagus), the presence of peptic strictures and mucosal infection or other damage should also be noted. Oesophagitis is graded according to severity of mucosal damage. A widely used grading system for oesophagitis was first described by Savary and Miller and adapted by others.[36]

Biopsies of the mucosa or deeper layers can be obtained to support visual or macroscopic findings by histopathology. Needle aspiration, punch or biopsy forceps and brush cytology are used to collect tissue. Vital stains are occasionally used in diagnostic endoscopy to aid recognition of mucosal abnormalities. Intravital stains such as methylene blue, Lugol's iodine[37] and Congo red have also been used to demonstrate preferential uptake by diseased tissue.

Manometry

The major role for oesophageal manometry in clinical use is the investigation of dysphagia and chest pain and other symptoms undiagnosed by radiology, endoscopy or pH monitoring. Recently, the development of ambulatory manometry is also proving useful in patients with intermittent or infrequent symptoms suggestive of oesophageal spasm.

Techniques

Static

Perfused tube   The mainstay technique for measurement of oesophageal motility is the water perfused tube technique. A soft, plastic, multilumen tube with side holes placed along its length is positioned at the desired site by intubation per oral or nasally. Each port is perfused with water by a pneumohydraulic pump at a flow rate determined by the desired frequency response of the system. Occlusion of the side hole by wall contractions of the oesophagus cause a rise in pressure. The pressure rise is detected by an in-line transducer connected to a recording device (analogue pen recorder or computer-driven system supported by an analogue to digital conversion unit).

Strain gauge microtransducers   Miniature strain gauges mounted on small, flexible catheters are becoming increasingly popular in the measurement of oesophageal motility. Although expensive (£500–£1000 per channel), they obviate the need for water perfusion and can be used more easily in ambulatory measurements.

Sleeve sensors   Because there is a tendency for the position of the LOS to alter in relation to a fixed point this makes accurate siting of a pressure sensor in the LOS difficult, especially for prolonged measurements. To overcome this problem, Dent *et al.*[10] devised a thin, 6 cm, open-ended, silastic sleeve which surrounded the most distal perfused port of a multilumen catheter, specifically to facilitate LOS measurements. The sleeve operates by straddling the high pressure zone of the LOS and records the average circumferential and axial pressure as a result of all forces acting on the sleeve.

For prolonged ambulatory studies of LOS pressure, a device called a 'sphinctometer' has been developed[38] and subsequently commercially manufactured (Gaeltec Ltd, Isle of Skye, UK). This device is sited at the most distal port of a multichannel microtransducer catheter and consists of a side-mounted strain gauge surrounded by a silicone oil-filled silastic tube of 6 cm in length of the same diameter as the catheter.

Motility measurement techniques

Pull-through

These techniques are most useful for sphincter assessment. This is achieved with either radially mounted sensors at the same level (minimum three (120°), maximum eight (45°)), or staggered along the length of the catheter where the radial LOS measurement is achieved during station pull-through. These catheters are essential to accurately map LOS pressure as it is known that sphincters including the LOS are radially asymmetric.

Station pull-through The recording ports are passed beyond the LOS and withdrawn in small increments (usually 0.5–1 cm), recordings being made at each station for a sufficient period to give a stable reading. Figure. 10.3 illustrates a pull-through in the oesophagus using

Figure 10.3
Station pull-through manometry across the LOS (ch3) with progressive pull through body with wet swallows ('wet') to demonstrate normal function.

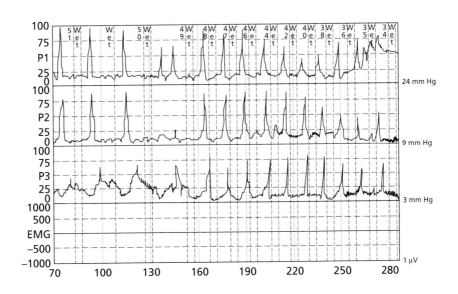

a three-channel catheter with radially mounted ports at 5, 10 and 15 cm from the tip (stations are identified at the top of the trace). The LOS, body and UOS are identified and the response of the sphincters and body are examined by 5 ml water boluses ('wet'). A normal peristaltic response is preceded and followed by UOS and LOS relaxation.

Rapid pull-through This technique, using similar equipment to that above, requires a steady, continuous withdrawal of the recording ports through the sphincter (0.5–1 cm/s) while the patient holds their breath. This is best achieved by a mechanical puller. This allows LOS pressures to be measured without interference of respiration.

Sphincter measurements

LOS LOS pressure measurements are used to document pressure, length and relaxation. Pressure measurements from radial ports at the same level has facilitated the production of three-dimensional images of LOS morphology in addition to the other data and is called 'vector volume'.[39] The technique, first developed in the anorectum, can be used to produce three-dimensional visual images of LOS pressure profiles which may be useful where sphincter defects are to be corrected, for example where reconstruction of the LOS is planned for hiatus hernia repair and fundoplication.

Upper oesophageal sphincter (UOS) This striated muscle sphincter has a tonal pressure substantially higher than the LOS and a dynamic response in keeping with striated muscle with a rapid velocity of opening and closure in response to swallowing. In consequence, the measurement of UOS function requires higher fidelity measuring equipment in comparison to the other parts of the oesophagus.

Manometric assessment of the UOS comprises measurements of position, intrinsic tone with due attention paid to radial asymmetry, relaxation and the relationship of relaxation to pharyngeal and oesophageal contractions. The perfused tube catheter does not have a frequency response fast enough to follow UOS dynamics so micro strain-gauge transducers are recommended for the accurate assessment of this sphincter. Static and station pull-through protocols are the most widely used methods to examine the function of the UOS and detailed information regarding the equipment and methodology have been well described.[40]

Prolonged ambulatory recordings

It has been recognised that the symptoms of GORD are often intermittent and that representative measurements may be better obtained by prolonged recordings. Furthermore, circadian changes in gut biorhythms require that measurements are made to span a normal daily cycle, i.e. in most cases for a minimum of 24 h. This requirement, together with the rapid development in computer technology has seen the introduction of digital recording systems. These have sufficient memory capacity and on-board computing processing power to allow high fidelity recordings from multichannel sensors for long periods, in some cases over many days. Equipment is battery powered, lightweight, portable and allows for almost total ambulation during measurement. This means that recordings can be made in near physiological conditions and patients can undergo studies in their homes and workplace. Event markers also allow for correlation between symptoms and abnormalities in the measured parameter. pH and pressure are the most widely measured parameters in the oesophagus using this technique. The addition of such technology has also added the ability to analyse recordings with sophisticated computer software programs. This has clinical benefits in the diagnosis of patients with intermittant oesophageal motor disorders.

Oesophageal pH measurements

As GORD and reflux oesophagitis are the two most common acid-related disorders of the oesophagus, an accurate diagnosis of GORD is highly desirable to discriminate physiological from pathological reflux and also to positively identify oesophageal acidification from other causes of dyspepsia and acid-related symptoms. As GORD diagnosis can be complicated by the absence of visible oesophagitis in up to 40% of patients and in a poor correlation with symptoms, a specific test to measure the presence of gastric juice in the oesophagus has been developed. Intraoesophageal pH was first described in the late 1960s,[41,42] refined by DeMeester *et al.*[43] and subsequently developed as an ambulatory technique.[44] Ambulatory pH measurement, is now held to be the best discriminator between physiological and pathological reflux and is regarded as the gold standard in the diagnosis of reflux disease. pH monitoring is simple and inexpensive to perform, with little discomfort to the patient and requires a minimum of specialised skills.[45]

pH measurement

Methodology

Sensors Miniature (< 2 mm), glass or antimony electrodes are available with either combined or external reference electrodes. Most antimony electrodes have a limited useful life of around 5 days continuous measurement due to oxidation of the sensor. Glass electrodes have a longer life and are reusable many times but are more fragile and also more expensive. A glass, cable-free radiotelemetry capsule is also available but is mainly used for research purposes.[46]

Recorders Ambulatory, outpatient oesophageal pH recordings are desirable in order to express GOR in as near a physiological setting as possible. Consequently recording devices are required to be suitable for domiciliary investigations. Recorders have seen much development since the initial introduction of prolonged, ambulatory pH monitoring in the 1980s. Most are digital, portable and solid-state[47] and incorporate event markers to document symptoms, meals and upright and supine periods, all important for the accurate diagnosis of pathological GOR. There are many companies internationally who produce pH recorders and all are capable of producing high quality measurements of oesophageal pH over a minimum of 24 h.

Procedure

The pH sensor is introduced transnasally or orally and positioned 5 cm proximal to the lower oesophageal sphincter, this being determined ideally by manometry. For investigators without manometry facilities there are commercially available LOS finders which consist of portable pressure indicators which detect the LOS high pressure zone. Other techniques using X-rays, endoscopy or pH withdrawal across the GOJ should be avoided as they do not accurately localise the LOS. For pH sensors with an external reference, the electrode is sited high on the chest over a bony area and secured with adhesive tape. The pH sensor lead is usually brought out nasally, affixed to the cheek with waterproof adhesive tape and connected to the recorder by routing the cable underneath the clothing. This enables the patient to undress without disconnection and is also more cosmetically acceptable.

pH measurements should be performed, ideally for a full 24 h. Practically, shorter periods are acceptable but the recording should be at least 20 h. It is essential to include at least one or two meals and the nocturnal period so the minimum period is probably around 18 h. This is to ensure that postprandial and nocturnal GOR is assessed. Studies should be performed under near physiological conditions and patients should be encouraged to perform normal daily activities where possible. During diagnostic tests, free access to normal meals, smoking and alcohol should be allowed, but these events should be documented. Antireflux medication should be withdrawn prior to study (5 days for proton pump inhibitors, 2 days for H_2 receptor antagonists and prokinetics and 24 h antacids and alginates). Where drug efficacy is questioned, pH monitoring may be performed while patients continue to take medication. This is particularly helpful when medication appears to be failing to control symptoms. Dual oesophageal and gastric pH recordings are particularly useful to detect failure of acid inhibitors and to document alkaline reflux, although the latter is rare (see below).

Figure 10.4 illustrates a 24 h oesophageal pH profile in a patient under consideration for antireflux surgery for long-term intractable reflux symptoms. It can be seen that the pH profile has numerous acidic episodes during both the day and the night time period and that symptom correlation is highly coincident with oesophageal acid-

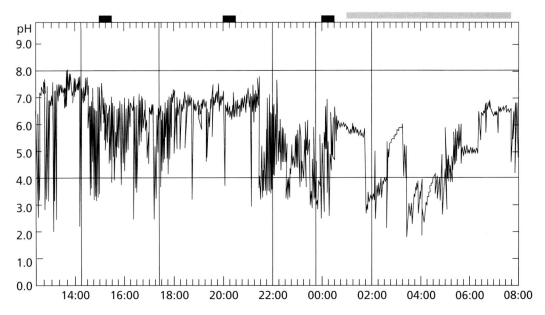

Figure 10.4 *24 h pH trace showing GOR. Meals(■) and sleep(▨) are marked and symptoms are indicated with the vertical lines.*

ification. Analysis of the recording revealed that acid exposure time < pH 4 was over 3 h of the 24 h recording (14.7%) in this patient which is important objective evidence when surgery is being considered.

Multichannel

Many recorders now have the capability of recording two or more channels of pH. With two or more sensors, the reference sensor is always positioned in the distal 5 cm above the LOS and the other sensors may then be positioned above or below at intervals set by the fixed inter-electrode distance (usually 5, 10, 15 or 20 cm). These studies are particularly useful in more detailed examinations of acid levels around the gastro-oesophageal junction or high in the oesophageal body.

Figure. 10.5 illustrates a two-channel 24 h recording in a patient with regurgitation and possible aspiration, causing night time choking and hoarseness. The proximal sensor is placed high in the pharyngeal oesophagus, 20 cm above the LOS. It can be seen that much of the GOR migrates to the upper electrode and this is highly suggestive of an association of GOR with the respiratory symptoms.

Combined with simultaneous oesophageal pH, gastric acid measurements can yield additional information regarding alkaline reflux[48] and the efficacy of acid suppression therapy.[33,34] Fig. 10.6 shows two two-channel pH recordings from a patient with reflux symptoms not controlled by high-dose proton pump inhibitor therapy. Sensors placed in the distal oesophagus (GOJ – 5 cm, ch1) and in the gastric body

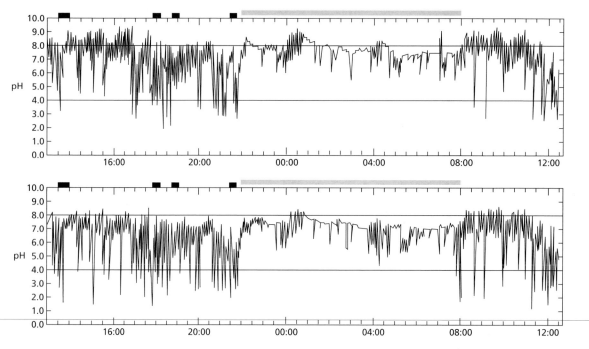

Figure 10.5 *Two channel 24 h pH recording. pH sensors are sited: ch1, 5 cm above LOS and ch2, 10 cm above LOS. Traces demonstrate distal oesophageal GOR and pharyngeal acidification in a patient with respiratory symptoms.*

(GOJ + 10 cm, ch2) detect GOR and gastric pH. The upper traces are with no therapy and the lower while the patient continued to take 40 mg omeprazole. GOR is present to a lower degree in the lower trace but the patient continues to be symptomatic as acid suppression is suboptimal even at the high dose (percentage of gastric pH < 4: without therapy > 90%, with therapy > 70%). At this dose of acid inhibition, gastric pH should be expected to be less than pH 4 only 20–30% of the 24 h period.

pH measurement with pressure

Multichannel digital data loggers are best used to investigate patients with unexplained, non-cardiac type and other atypical chest pain (NCCP) associated with GORD. The objective of such recordings is the simultaneous monitoring of oesophageal motility, LOS function and pH. This enables a comparison of abnormalities of motility and GOR and any correlation with symptoms. Technically, the recordings can be achieved easily, using solid-state multichannel microtransducers, combined with either one or two pH channels. The investigation is more demanding for the patient due to the presence of a larger catheter assembly, or two catheters (when pH and pressure are on separate catheters) and for the investigator because

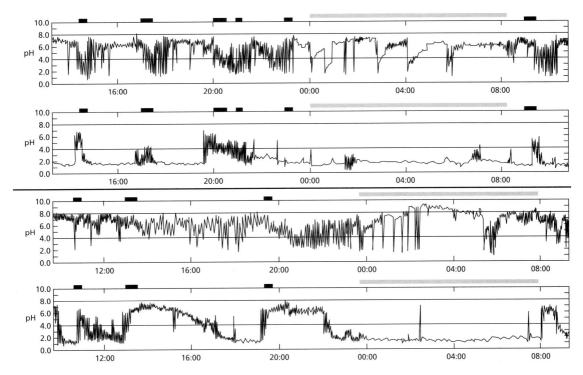

Figure 10.6 *Two channel 24 h pH recordings in a patient being considered for antireflux surgery. Upper recording off therapy. Lower recording on 20 mg omeprazole bd. pH sensors are sited: ch1, 5 cm above LOS and ch2, 10 cm below LOS. The 2nd recording demonstrates reduction of symptoms but continued suboptimal acid suppression with high doses of proton pump inhibition.*

of the demands of more complex analysis and interpretation of the recordings.

One publication[38] has suggested that the major use of combined recordings is the investigation of NCCP caused by diffuse oesophageal spasm or similar motility disorder. The test is also useful for exclusion of oesophageal pain as a cause of NCCP as, sometimes, patients with microvascular angina can be missed on initial cardiological investigations. At present, in our practice, combined recordings are limited to patients who have no oesophagitis, normal pH and stationary manometry but who remain symptomatic.

Figure. 10.7 illustrates a patient with high pressure contractions in the oesophageal body and LOS with and without simultaneous GOR and associated symptoms indicating chest pain. The abnormal motility was caused by a tight fundoplication and resulted in revision surgery. The infrequency of this type of abnormal motility is unlikely to be detected by conventional manometry and in this case prolonged manometry combined with pH was essential to determine the cause of symptoms in relation to the surgery.

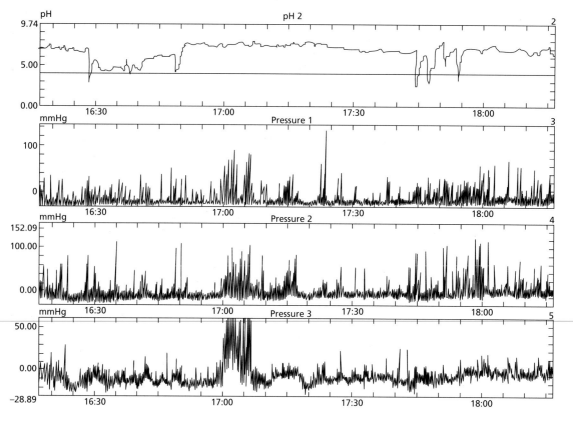

Figure 10.7 *Combined manometry with ambulatory pH. Ch1, distal oesophageal pH; ch2 and 3 oesophageal body motility; ch4, LOS pressure. The recording demonstrates that chest pain (vertical lines) can be attributed but not distinguishable from GOR (pH trace) or LOS spasm (ch4) in a patient with postfundoplication complications.*

Provocation tests

Provocation tests have been devised to simulate symptoms in a controlled setting. Acid-related symptoms may be provoked with instillation of hydrochloric acid into the oesophagus to mimic the pain induced by acid reflux[49] or by inducing reflux by structured activities such as raising intra-abdominal pressure or inversion of the patient (Standard Acid Reflux Test (SART), Acid Reflux Provocation Test (ARPT)). However, these tests have all but been abandoned except in special circumstances with the introduction of 24 h pH monitoring.

Provocation of pain by spasm

Atypical chest pain of non-cardiac origin thought to be caused by oesophageal spasm can be provoked artificially in the laboratory in an attempt to make a diagnosis, especially where symptoms are intermittent. The following procedures have been advocated as useful.

Balloon distension

This test involves inflating a latex balloon in the oesophageal body to elicit pain. The volume which initiates pain has been shown to be significantly lower in patients with various motility disorders than in controls.[50]

Pharmacological provocation

There are a number of pharmacological methods that have been developed in an attempt to elicit oesophageal pain in order to differentiate the symptoms of spasm. Parasympathomimetic substances including ergometrine and bethanecol were initially advocated, being injected intravenously (randomised with saline to avoid false positives) and recording any symptoms produced. If the patient complains of symptoms similar to those normally experienced, a diagnosis of pain of oesophageal origin can be made. The side effects of parasympathomimetics (bradycardia and hypotension) led to alternatives being sought. Edrophonium (tensilon), an anticholinesterase, is now advocated as a safer stimulant with fewer side effects and currently is the only drug used in pharmacological provocation of oesophageal symptoms.[51]

Pharmacological provocation is not widely used today and has largely been superseded by balloon distension and prolonged pH and manometry recording. It remains useful in the investigation of the difficult patient.

Oesophageal scintigraphy

Oesophageal scintigraphy has been adapted to investigate the oesophagus as an alternative to radiological investigation. Although scintigraphy lacks the fidelity of radiology as an imaging technique, it has the advantage of yielding dynamic data with objective measurements of oesophageal transit. Two techniques have been developed.

The basic technique involves labelling a liquid or solid meal with a short half-life gamma isotope, the most commonly used isotope being technetium-99m. A gamma camera with a large diameter head is required such that the whole of the oesophagus can be imaged simultaneously. Aqueous liquids (water, orange juice) or solids (egg) are mixed with a standard dose of isotope and swallowed by the patient during rapid acquisition of images (200–500 ms over the first 2 min, longer after this if stasis or GOR is being investigated). Data are stored by computer and replayed in sequence to measure the transit characteristics of the swallow. Condensed images can be simultaneously displayed and graphs generated to examine the bolus transit of the test meal and identify areas of hold-up or reflux. Gamma scintigraphy is useful in the examination of achalasia and other disorders of oesophageal motility and GORD, especially where complications may be suspected (Barrett's or stricture).[52]

Prolonged, ambulatory scintigraphy has been described[53] which utilises a portable selenium detector strapped to the chest over the epigastrium connected to a portable recorder. The technique is currently mainly a research tool but can examine the differential reflux of food against acid by simultaneous isotope detection and pH monitoring.

Motility disorders

These are disorders of oesophageal function usually causing dysphagia and chest pain or otherwise interfering with normal swallowing without any organic obstruction. The symptoms are caused by paralysis, spasm or incoordination of the oesophageal musculature. This may be due to interruption of the extrinsic nerve supply, destruction of the myenteric plexus or to disorders of the extrinsic nerve itself. This group of conditions represents a broad spectrum of poorly understood oesophageal abnormalities of unknown aetiology which can only be classified by their motility patterns. They may be classified as primary or secondary (Table 10.4).

Classification

The most frequent symptoms are dysphagia, chest pain and regurgitation of oesophageal contents. In disease of skeletal muscle the pharynx and upper third of the oesophagus will be disturbed whereas if smooth muscle is primarily affected, the dysmotility will be distal. Symptomatically, pharyngeal disorders are characterised by difficulty in initiating swallowing and by regurgitation into the nasopharynx and trachea, whereas disorders of the oesophagus and LOS result in dysphagia and chest pain. In addition, if food is retained in a dilated, atonic oesophagus, regurgitation can also occur.

Table 10.4 *Motility disorders of the oesophagus*

Primary (Oesophagus only involved)	Achalasia – vigorous achalasia Diffuse and segmental oesophageal spasm Symptomatic oesophageal peristalsis – 'nutcracker' Non-specific motility disorder (NSMD)
Secondary (Oesophagus involved in systemic condition)	Collagen vascular disease e.g. systemic sclerosis (scleroderma) Neuromuscular disorders (myasthaenia gravis) Diabetes mellitus Chagas' disease (*Trypanosoma cruzi*) Metastatic cancer Presbyoesophagus

Dysphagia due to motility disorders may be intermittent, is usually only slowly progressive and may be as severe for liquids as solids.

Chest pain due to oesophageal dysmotility may be spontaneous but is often triggered by eating or anxiety. It can be severe and may be indistinguishable from ischaemic cardiac pain.

Regurgitation of oesophageal contents typically occurs at night from an atonic dilated oesophagus with hold up at the cardia. The oesophageal residue can flow back due to gravity when the patient is supine and the patient wakes to find food soiling the pillow. This is typical in advanced achalasia.

Respiratory complications are due to overspill of retained oesophageal contents into the respiratory tract leading to nocturnal cough and wheeze or aspiration pneumonia.

Investigations

Barium swallow

This gives some indication of motility in the oesophagus and in certain well developed or advanced disorders with gross structural changes can be totally diagnostic. However, early and subtle abnormalities may be missed. The addition of a solid component to the examination, usually bread or marshmallow soaked in barium can increase the diagnostic yield (Table 10.5).

Upper gastrointestinal endoscopy

The main role of endoscopy is to exclude an organic narrowing or other mucosal abnormality in the oesophagus or GOJ. In particular, the endoscope should pass into the stomach with no resistance as a submucosal lesion of the cardia can masquerade as achalasia, leading to a false diagnosis: this has been labelled 'pseudoachalasia'.

Manometry

This is the most important investigation in evaluation of oesophageal motor dysfunction of the upper and lower sphincters and oesophageal body. Static studies are most useful in the detection of continuous abnormalities such as early achalasia, scleroderma and some cases of nutcracker oesophagus (Table 10.5). Prolonged, ambulatory studies are best used in cases where symptoms are intermittent or atypical, e.g. non-cardiac chest pain mimicking angina, diffuse oesophageal spasm and other non-specific disorders. In this case, the 'snapshot' view seen at static manometry may miss pathology which may only be present infrequently. It is also in this situation where provocation tests may have a role, i.e. edrophonium or balloon distension studies. The most important objective in these studies is to correlate symptoms with motor abnormalities.

Table 10.5 *Investigation findings of primary oesophageal motility disorders*

	Sx Dysphagia	Sx Chest pain	Sx Regurgitation	Barium swallow	Gastroscopy	Manometric findings Body motility	Manometric findings LOS
Achalasia	+++	+	++	Dilated oesophagus with food residue Hold-up at cardia	Dilated oesophagus with food residue Scope into stomach without resistance	No peristalsis Sometimes +ve baseline pressure Low amplitude contractions when oesophagus dilated 'Common cavity'	Absent or incomplete relaxation with normal or high pressure
DOS	++	+++	+	Tertiary contractions 'corkscrew'	Normal+/- Tertiary contractions	High amplitude Prolonged duration Repetitive waves Mixed peristaltic and simultaneous	Normal or high pressure Normal relaxation
Nutcracker	−	++	−	Normal	Normal	High amplitude Prolonged duration Normal peristalsis	Normal Occasionally high pressure
NSMD	+	+	+	Normal	Normal	Mixed peristaltic, simultaneous and incomplete propagation	Normal
Presbyoesophagus	+	+	+	Normal	Normal	As above Low amplitude	Normal or low pressure

Figure 10.8
Station manometry – achalasis. LOS pressure is very high with no relaxation on swallowing. Body motility is repetitive and aperistalic (simultaneous waves).

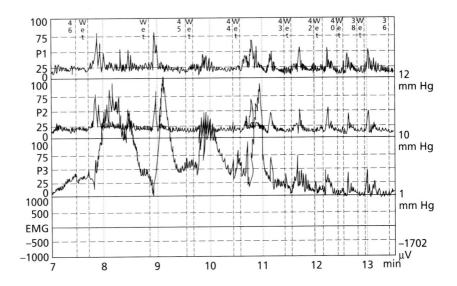

Primary motility disorders

Achalasia (failure of relaxation (Greek))

This is a disease of unknown aetiology characterised by the absence of peristalsis in the oesophageal body and failure of relaxation in the LOS in response to swallowing. Fig. 10.8 is a manometric record from a patient with a well-developed achalasia. The LOS pressure is high, the sphincter does not relax and contractions in the body are repetitive and 100% simultaneous with no residual peristalsis. Accumulation of food in the oesophageal body and subsequent dilation of the muscle wall lead to elongation and a sigmoid mega-oesophagus in long-standing cases. The food stagnation in the oesophagus is probably one factor in the increased incidence of squamous cell cancer in approximately 5% of patients with achalasia.

Achalasia is the most common primary motility disorder with an incidence of one case per 100 000 of the population per year in the UK. It occurs in all races and affects both sexes equally. Achalasia may occur at any age but it is most common from 30–70 years. The major symptoms are dysphagia and regurgitation and much less commonly, chest pain. Most patients give a long history prior to diagnosis.

Pathophysiology

Histological studies There are large amounts of histopathological data in achalasia but these have often been variable and contradictory. Abnormalities have been demonstrated in human tissues from the CNS in the dorsal motor nucleus of the vagus, in the vagal nerve trunks and in oesophageal smooth muscle. However, the most

Figure 10.9
Station manometry – diffuse oesophageal spasm. Trace demonstrates hypertensive (< 350 mmHg), mixed peristaltic and simultaneous waves with associated chest pain.

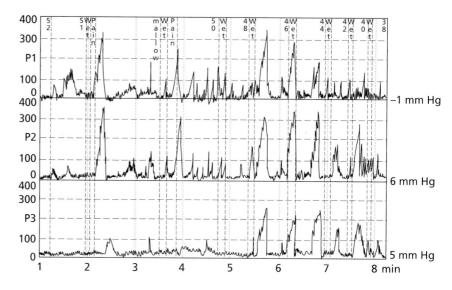

consistent changes are found in the oesophageal myenteric plexus with a reduction of ganglion cells.

Pharmacological studies These suggest denervation of the oesophagus but the site is unclear. Excitatory cholinergic innervation of the LOS appears intact but inhibitory innervation of the circular smooth muscle is impaired although the neurotransmitter is not known. The cause of the neuronal damage is not known but it has been suggested that it may be due to a neurotropic infection or an autoimmune process as both mechanisms could explain nerve damage being specific to the oesophagus.

Diffuse oesophageal spasm

This condition is characterised by simultaneous, sometimes high amplitude contractions in the oesophageal body, which are of prolonged duration and often repetitive in nature. Disordered waves are often more marked in the distal oesophageal body but may be restricted to a very localised segment. The contractions are often intermittent with patients retaining some peristaltic activity. The diagnosis is accepted in the presence of greater than 20% of simultaneous contractions after wet swallows. Fig. 10.9 is a manometric example showing high pressure waves (> 350 mmHg) of long duration associated with pain.

The major symptom is chest pain due to bolus impaction or the high amplitude contractions (sometimes greater than 3–400 mmHg). Dysphagia is as a result of the failure of peristalsis during the spasm. The disorder is commoner in middle age and affects both sexes equally. There appears to be a relationship to patients of an anxious personality. The high pressures generated during periods of spasm may lead to pulsion diverticula of the oesophageal mucosa and submucosa through the muscle layer, usually in the lower oesophagus: the so-called epiphrenic diverticulum.

Symptomatic oesophageal peristalsis ('nutcracker')

As the name suggests, this disorder is where the patient complains of chest pain and the manometry reveals prolonged high amplitude (> 180 mmHg) peristaltic contraction in the oesophageal body. LOS pressure may also be high but this is not necessary to make the diagnosis (Table 10.5). No other abnormality is detectable.

Non-specific motility disorder (NSMD)

Some patients with non-cardiac chest pain or dysphagia demonstrate abnormalities on manometry that are not specific for any named motor disorder (Table 10.5). The abnormality may be a single aberration (i.e. hypertensive LOS, abnormal wave pattern) or a combination of disordered wave activity. Progression of NSMD to other disorders (i.e. DOS or achalasia) have been demonstrated but there is no clear association.

References

1. Meyer GW, Auston RM, Brady CE, Castell DO. Muscle anatomy of the human oesophagus. J Clin Gastroenterol 1986; 8: 131.
2. Arey LB, Tremaine MJ. The muscle content of the lower oesophagus of man. Anat Rec 1933; 56: 315–20.
3. Cannon WB. Oesophageal peristalsis after bilateral vagotomy. Am J Physiol 1907; 19: 436–44.
4. Roman C, Gonelli J. Extrinsic control of digestive tract motility. In: Johnson LR (ed.) Physiology of the gastrointestinal tract (2nd edn) New York: Raven Press, 1987, pp. 507–53.
5. Mukhopadyhyay AK, Weisbrodt NW. Neural organisation of esophageal peristalsis: role of the vagus nerve. Gastroenterolgy 1975; 68: 444–7.
6. Meltzer SJ. On the causes of the orderly progress of the peristaltic movements in the esophagus. Am J Physiol 1899; 2: 266–72.
7. Christensen J. The innervation and motility of the esophagus. Front Gastrointest Res 1978; 3: 18–32.
8. Diamant NE, Sharkawy TY. Neural control of oesophageal peristalsis. A conceptual analysis. Gastroenterology 1977; 72: 546–56.
9. Furness JB, Costa M. Arrangement of the enteric plexus. In: Furness JB, Costa M (eds). The enteric nervous system, London: Churchill Livingstone, 1987, pp. 6–25.
10. Dent J, Hollaway RH, Toouli J, Dodds WJ. Mechanism of lower oesophageal sphincter incompetence in patients with symptomatic gastro-oesophageal reflux. Gut 1988; 29: 1020–8.
11. Kahrilas P, Dodds W, Hogan WJ. Effect of peristaltic dysfunction on esophageal volume clearance. Gastroenterology 1988; 94: 73–80.
12. Atkinson M, Summerling MD. The competence of the cardia after cardiomyotomy. Gastroenterology 1954; 92: 23–134.
13. Steiner GM. Gastro-oesophageal reflux. Hiatus hernia and the radiologist with special reference to children. Br J Radiol 1977; 50: 164–74.
14. Kaye MD, Showalter JP. Manometric configuration of the lower oesophageal sphincter in normal human subjects. Gastroenterology 1971; 61: 213–23.
15. Petterson GB, Bombech CT, Nyhus LM. The lower oesophageal sphincter mechanism of

opening and closure. Surgery 1980; 88: 307–14.

16. Ogilivie A, Atkinson M. Influence of the vagus nerve on reflux control of the lower oesophageal sphincter. Gut 1984; 25: 253–8.

17. Ogilvie A, James PD, Atkinson M. Impairment of vagal function in reflex oesophagitis. Q J Med 1985; 54: 61–74.

18. Helm JF, Dodds WJ, Pele L, Palmer DW, Hogan WJ, Teeter BC. Effect of esophageal emptying and saliva on acid clearance. N Engl J Med 1984; 310: 284–8.

19. Helm JF, Dodds WJ, Hogan WJ. Salivary response to esophageal acid in normal subjects and patients with reflux esophagitis. Gastroenterology 1987; 93: 1393–7.

20. McCallum RW, Berkowitz DM, Lerner E. Gastric emptying in patients with gastro-oesophageal reflux. Gastroenterology 1988; 80: 285–91.

21. Coleman SL, Rees WDW, Malagelada JR. Normal gastric function in reflux oesophagitis. Gastroenterology 1979; 76: A1115.

22. Castell DO (ed) The oesophagus. Boston: Little Brown, 1992.

23. Cadiot G, Sekera E, Mignon M. Gastric secretion in GORD. Front Gastrointest Res 1994; 22: 209–22.

24. Gillen P, Keeling P, Byrne PJ, Hennessy TPJ. Implications of duodenogastric reflux in the pathogenesis of Barrett's oesophagus. Br J Surg 1988; 75: 540–3.

25. Gotley DC, Morgan AP, Ball D, Owen RW, Cooper MJ. Composition of gastro-oesophageal reflux. Gut 1991; 32: 1093–9.

26. Iftikhar YF, Ledingham Sally J, Evans DF et al. Bile reflux in columnar lines Barrett's oesophagus. Ann R Coll Surg Engl 1993; 75: 411–16.

27. Jones R, Lydeard S. Prevalence of dyspepsia in the community. Br J Med 1989; 298: 30–2.

28. Richter JE, Castell DO. Gastroesophageal reflux. Pathogenesis, diagnosis and therapy. Ann Intern Med 1982; 97: 93–103.

29. Boix-Ochoa J, Canals J. Maturation of the lower oesophageal sphincter. J Pediatr Surg 1976; 11: 749–56.

30. Branicki FJ, Lam DKH, Tse CW et al. Why is symptomatic gastro-oesophageal reflux a rarity in the Chinese? Surg Res Commun 1990; 7: 119–26.

31. Holloway RH, Panagini R, Ireland AC. Criteria for objective definition of transient lower oesophageal relaxation of the lower oesophageal sphincter. Am J Physiol 1995; 268: G128–33.

32. Gillen P, Hennessy TPJ. Barrett's oesophagus. In: Hennessy TPJ, Bennett J, Cuchieri A (eds) Reflux oesophagitis. London: Butterworths, pp. 87–111.

33. Klinkenborg-Knoll E, Meuwissen SG. Combined gastric and oesophageal 24 hr pH monitoring and oesophageal manometry in patients with reflux disease resistant to omeprazole therapy. Aliment Pharmacol Ther 1990; 4: 485–95.

34. Kadirkamanathan SS, Evans DF, Wingate DL. Investigation of gastro-oesophageal reflux and acid secretion in patients unresponsive to therapeutic doses of omeprazole. Gut 1994; 35: S12.

35. Morris DL, Jones JA, Evans DF et al. An objective evaluation of the Angelchik anti-reflux prosthesis in the treatment of gastro-oesophageal reflux. Br J Surg 1985; 72: 1017–20.

36. Little AG, DeMeester TR, Kircner PT, O'Sullivan GC, Skinner DB. Pathogenesis of oesophagitis in patients with GERD. Surgery 1980; 88: 101–7.

37. Sugimachi K, Kitamura K, Baba K, Ikebe M, Kuwano H. Endoscopic diagnosis of early cancer of the oesophagus with Lugol's iodine. Gastrointest Endosc 1992; 38: 657–61.

38. Barham CP, Gotley DC, Miller R, Mills A, Alderson D. Ambulatory measurement of oesophageal function: clinical use of a new pH and motility recording system. Br J Surg 1992; 79: 1056–60.

39. Bombeck CT, Vaz O, De Salvo J, Donahue PE, Nyhus LM. Computerised axial manometry of the oesophagus. A new method for assessment of anti-reflux operations. Ann Surg 1987; 206: 465–72.

40. Wilson J, Heading RC. The proximal sphincters. In: Kumar D, Wingate DL (eds), Illustrated guide to gastrointestinal motility, 2nd edn. Edinburgh: Churchill Livingstone, 1993, pp. 357–72.

41. Spencer J. Prolonged pH study in the study of gastro-oesophageal reflux. Br J Surg 1969; 56: 912–15.

42. Pattrick FG. Investigation of GOR in various positions with a two-line pH electrode. Gut 1970; 11: 659–67.

43. DeMeester TR, Johnson LR, Joseph GJ, Toscano MS, Hall AW, Skinner DB. Patterns of gastroesophageal reflux in health and disease. Ann Surg 1976; 184: 459–69.

44. Branicki FJ, Evans DF, Hardcastle JD, Ogilvie AL, Atkinson M. Ambulatory monitoring of oesophageal pH in reflux oesophagitis using a portable radiotelemetry system. Gut 1982; 23: 992–9.

45. Richter JE (ed). Ambulatory oesophageal pH monitoring. New York: Igaku-Shoin, 1991.

46. Evans DF, Pye G, Bramley R, Clark AG, Dyson TJ, Hardcastle JD. Measurement of gastrointestinal pH in normal ambulant human subjects. Gut 1988; 29: 1035.

47. Evans DF. Twenty-four hour ambulatory oesophageal pH monitoring: an update. Br J Surg 1987; 74: 157–61.

48. Mattioli S, Felice V, Pilotti V, Bacchi ML, Pastina M, Gozzetti G. Indications for 24 hr gastric pH monitoring by single or multiple pH probe in clinical research and practice. Dig Dis Sci 1992; 37: 1793–801.

49. Bernstein LM, Baker LA. A clinical test for the oesophagitis. Gastroenterology 1958; 34: 760–81.

50. Barish CF, Castell DO, Richter JE. Graded esophageal balloon distension: a new provocative test for non-cardiac chest pain. Dig Dis Sci 1986; 31: 1292–8.

51. de Caestecker JS, Pryde A, Heading RC. Comparison of intravenous edrophonium and oesophageal acid perfusion during oesophageal manometry in patients with non-cardiac chest pain. Gut 1989; 29: 1029–1034.

52. Tolin RD, Malmud LS, Reilley J, Fisher RS. Oesophageal scintigraphy to quantitate oesophageal transit. Gastroenterology 1979; 76: 1402–9.

53. Washington N, Greaves JL, Iftikhar SY. A comparison of gastro-oesophageal reflux in volunteers assessed by ambulatory pH and gamma monitoring after treatment with either Liquid Gaviscon or Algicon Suspension. Aliment Pharmacol Ther 1992; 6: 579–88.

11 Treatment and complications of GORD

Stephen E. A. Attwood
John Bancewicz

General advice Therapy for gastro-oesophageal reflux disease (GORD) has usually been started a long time before the patient reaches the surgical gastroenterologist. Indeed the patient has usually tried a variety of remedies before he or she seeks medical attention at all. These may include simple medications and avoidance of precipitating factors such as hot or spicy foods and hot or alcoholic liquids. The list of possible foods that might be avoided is extensive and includes coffee, chocolate, fats and specific preparations of alcohol such as red wine, spirits and beers. Although these are often advised against there is little evidence that avoiding them has any long-term benefit. Although it is traditional for a physician to advise changes in life style they have usually been tried already without success. The role of obesity in GORD is significant and in motivated patients a strict diet associated with appropriate exercise can improve symptoms and the quality of life dramatically. Unfortunately, in clinical practice this is rarely achieved.

Minor modification of the type and timing of meals, volume of each meal, and elevation of the head of the bed (using 10–15 cm blocks under the legs of the bed at the head end, and not just pillows) are common conservative measures resorted to but in most patients who reach a surgeon these measures have only temporising effects. However it is worthwhile to advise the patient to stop smoking. One of the great difficulties about stopping smoking is the habit of previous nicotine addicts to eat excessively. This seems to be a way for the ex-smoker to relieve stress and excess weight gain is a very common result of advising a patient to give up smoking. In the context of gastro-oesophageal reflux disease this can have the disastrous effect of worsening the symptoms and making the patient even less ideal for subsequent surgical intervention.

Medical therapy

Simple antacids

In patients with pathological acid gastro-oesophageal reflux simple antacids only relieve symptoms temporarily and have no effect on oesophagitis or other complications.

Alginates (e.g. Gaviscon)

The same can be said about alginates but they are popular with many patients as they are fairly effective in producing immediate symptom relief from severe heartburn during episodes of acid reflux.

Acid suppression (H2-receptor antagonists, proton pump inhibition)

The first effective treatment for GORD came with drugs that suppress the production of acid by the stomach. The H2-receptor antagonists (cimetidine, ranitidine, famotidine and nizatidine) all have symptomatic efficacy when given in adequate dosage.[1] When they were first used in the 1970s they revolutionised the medical approach to reflux symptoms as they significantly improved quality of life in patients with GORD[2] and in some patients (25%) produced resolution of endoscopic oesophagitis.[3] The proton pump inhibitors, introduced in the late 1980s with omeprazole, and more recently lanzoprazole and pantoprazole have much greater efficacy in both symptom reduction and healing of oesophagitis. Published healing rates depend on the proportion of patients in the series with higher grades of oesophagitis. The severity of disease in patients in a family practice will be much less than that in a hospital specialist practice and whereas 90% of patients in general practice will have endoscopic healing after 4 weeks proton pump inhibition this may drop to 60–70% in a typical hospital practice.[4,5] Certainly, patients with established grade 2 or 3 oesophagitis using the Savary Miller grading system[6] will have healing rates at the lower end of this range. Whether failure is due to inadequate acid suppression or due to other agents in the refluxed material such as bile or duodenal juice is not yet understood.

In those patients who have responded well to proton pump inhibitors symptoms will recur in more than 50% within a few months of cessation of the drug. Since persistent symptoms and rapid relapse of symptoms are a common problem, long-term (maintenance) acid suppression is now commonly prescribed. This is with half standard doses of the proton pump inhibitors (omeprazole 10 mg daily or lanzoprazole 15 mg daily). As these drugs are expensive the decision on long-term use must take into account cost-effectiveness. Using powerful acid suppression in the long term has not been shown to have any significant deleterious effect, although concerns have been expressed about potential gastric epithelial proliferation from the resulting hypergastrinaemia. However, to date, there has been no direct evidence of any carcinogenic effects of long-term proton pump inhibition. Recent studies have shown a higher incidence of gastrointestinal infections such as *Campylobacter* gastroenteritis in patients taking proton pump inhibitors, due to the failure of the stomach to kill ingested bacteria.[7]

Prokinetic agents (cisapride, metoclopramide, domperidone)

Cisapride has therapeutic benefit on its own which is roughly equivalent to that of the H2 antagonists. It is also synergistic when in combination with H2 antagonist acid suppression. Studies have not shown an objective benefit of combining the proton pump inhibitors with cisapride. In GORD there is often a significant reduction in the ability of the oesophagus to clear refluxed acid. As well as improving peristalsis prokinetics may enhance gastric emptying and so reduce the potential volume of refluxed gastric juices. However, neither metoclopramide nor domperidone have been shown to have an independent beneficial effect on the classic symptoms of gastro-oesophageal reflux. Cisapride has a measurable effect on the lower oesophageal sphincter function but it is probably not clinically significant.

Mucosal protection (sucralfate)

The recent investigations of bile content in the refluxed juices in the oesophagus and stomach has raised awareness of the non-acid injurious agents. Mucosal protectants such as sucralfate are effective in the stomach but their value in the lower oesophagus is not well studied. Compliance with sucralfate is sometimes poor as it is not pleasant to take.

Helicobacter pylori eradication

There is no documentation of any benefit of *Helicobacter* eradication treatment in GORD but, since other peptic disorders are commonly coincidental, the abdominal symptoms may be improved by the eradication of ulceration with *H. pylori* infection. *H. pylori* has been found in the stomach and in columnar epithelium of the lower oesophagus but the relationship of *Helicobacter* to Barrett's oesophagus or to lesser degrees of intestinal metaplasia around the gastric cardia has not been clarified.[8,9] Recent work has also shown that the presence of pathological duodenogastric reflux may be secondary to the *H. pylori* infection in the antroduodenal mucosa, rather than the cause of the infection. The relevance of this in clinical practice has yet to be determined. If this hypothesis is proven to be true then *H. pylori* eradication would take on a new dimension in GORD.

Surgical therapy

The principle underlying the surgical management of gastro-oesophageal reflux disease is the creation or augmentation of the barrier

Table 11.1 *Indications for antireflux surgery*

Failure of medical therapy to control symptoms of heartburn or volume regurgitation
Recurrent stricture while on medical therapy
Barrett's oesophagus
Aspiration pneumonia or nocturnal choking
Malnutrition due to reflux, especially in children or mental handicap.
Patient preference over life-long medical therapy
With cholecystectomy when GORD co-exists with symptomatic gallstones
With Heller's myotomy for achalasia

between the oesophagus and stomach. The mechanical prevention of reflux does not distinguish between the varying nature of the content of refluxed material, nor is it affected significantly by the precise underlying cause of the reflux.[10–12]

Indications for surgical management (Table 11.1)

Failure of medical treatment

The primary indication for surgery is the failure of medical treatment and general advice measures. The definition of failure of medical treatment in our unit is the failure to control symptoms while on an adequate dose of acid suppression, which usually is a standard dose of proton pump inhibitor for many months. Indeed many of our patients have been on double doses of proton pump inhibition for some months and still have symptoms of heartburn and voluminous regurgitation.

The definition of failure can be based on persistent symptoms either while on medication or soon after stopping. In this, as with many indications, the decision is balanced between the reliance on medication and the patient's wish to be free of recurrent symptoms and free of medication, considered in the light of their operative fitness, age and expectations from life. In patients with persistent symptoms while on proton pump acid inhibition and who are fit for anaesthesia (ASA 1 or 2) there is a clear indication for antireflux surgery. In young patients (i.e. < 60 years) whose symptoms are controlled with a proton pump inhibitor but wish to be free of their drugs for reasons of convenience or economy the decision on a surgical option is more debatable. Much of this debate rests not on the efficacy of surgery but the associated mortality. This issue has been raised recently because of the transient rise in perioperative mortality after laparoscopic antireflux surgery. The cost-effective argument does not hold any strength if the mortality rates are significant. Certainly there is a group of severe refluxers who require higher than standard doses (e.g. omeprazole 40 mg bd) and in these patients the cost effectiveness of surgical options becomes an important question.

Recurrent stricture was seen by some as an indication for surgery[13] although the majority of patients are now successfully managed by endoscopic dilatation and long-term acid suppression.

Respiratory complications

The development of respiratory complications of reflux including aspiration pneumonia and nocturnal choking are clear indications for surgical intervention. The relationship of asthma and reflux is less clear cut and although the two conditions may co-exist the expectations of improvement in asthma should be guarded and in asthmatic patients antireflux surgery should be performed on the basis of the reflux symptoms and not as a treatment of the asthma.

In children aspiration and malnutrition are serious complications of GORD and they often occur in conditions of mental handicap. In these situations antireflux surgery is highly effective.

Barrett's oesophagus

The development of Barrett's columnar lined lower oesophagus is often not associated with particularly severe initial symptoms but the very high incidence of strictures, ulceration, the risk of perforation and haemorrhage and the risk of dysplasia and subsequent cancer has raised the issue of surgery for prevention of complications and encouraged a more frequent use of the surgical option. The only studies that have prospectively compared medical and surgical treatment of Barrett's oesophagus[14-16] have shown clear benefit for surgery in relation to both the symptoms and quality of life as well as a reduction in complications.

At present there is little evidence that treatment (medical or surgical) reduces the incidence of carcinoma in Barrett's oesophagus. Ortiz *et al.*[16] have documented a reduction in malignant degeneration after antireflux surgery compared to a medically treated control group of patients with Barrett's oesophagus. However, none of these studies included long-term proton pump inhibition and as this is now the standard form of acid suppression for patients with Barrett's oesophagus firm conclusions cannot be drawn. Theoretically if duodenal juice has a role in the pathogenesis of carcinoma of the lower oesophagus and cardia then antireflux surgery would be preferable to acid suppression alone in patients with Barrett's oesophagus. This hypothesis has yet to be adequately tested.

Patient preferences

Patients' perceptions and preferences vary and they require a responsive and adaptable professional approach. In the context of a safe and competent surgical service some patients will choose surgery whereas others will opt for long-term medical therapy. In the absence of complications it is probably wisest to present the alternatives without expressing an opinion and await the patient's own decision. In the presence of some of the more serious complications of aspiration and malnutrition then a more definite recommendation for surgery is justified. It is essential that the patient make an informed decision and it is useful for the surgical department to have its own audit for the purposes of describing the frequency of success and the risks of complications in the hands of the surgeons involved. For instance in our unit 90% of patients are Visick 1 or 2 after operation and these patients are very satisfied with the result. (See complications of antireflux surgery, below.) The final decision must rest with the patient.

Quality of life values are the most objective final outcome measures but have not been measured. When they have been measured, surgical treatments have been preferred. However, the only studies to date with representative prospective comparison used the less effective acid suppression of H2 antagonists and compared them to open surgery.[14] Cost-benefit analyses have been published by a small number of authors and give some advantage in favour of surgery but it must be remembered that centres publishing results probably have above average surgical results and as such bias the costs in favour of the surgical series. A broad-based estimate of the costs of the average surgical service versus the more standardised drug treatment costs needs to be assessed.

Combination of cholecystectomy with antireflux surgery
Many patients with gallstones and symptoms of abdominal discomfort have pathological acid gastro-oesophageal reflux and this is known to get worse after cholecystectomy.[17] Since up to 30% of gallstone patients will have residual abdominal symptoms after cholecystectomy it is reasonable to consider the extent of reflux disease in patients listed for cholecystectomy. This consideration should include an upper gastrointestinal (GI) endoscopy and if oesophagitis is present an oesophageal manometry and pH study. With the knowledge of the degree of reflux and perhaps some identification of its relationship to symptoms it will be possible to make a decision on the need for combined cholecystectomy and antireflux surgery or the need for postoperative medication.

Preoperative investigations

The investigation of gastro-oesophageal reflux disease has already been discussed (Chapter 10) but it must be emphasised that some specific investigations are a prerequisite to establishing a high standard in antireflux surgery technique. An assessment of surgical suitability includes identifying the patient's comorbidity, obesity and concomitant medication.

Endoscopy
Endoscopy is a prerequisite because oesophageal tumour must be excluded, strictures dilated and the degree of oesophagitis documented. The position of the squamocolumnar junction and the relationship

and size of any hiatus hernia should be assessed. Although the presence of a large hiatus hernia is no contraindication to surgery it might influence the approach (thoracic rather than abdominal) or it might influence the decision on the use of minimal invasive techniques.

Manometry

Manometry is essential to exclude primary motility disorders and document the presence of propagating peristalsis. The presence of a weak amplitude is not a contraindication to antireflux surgery as the oesophageal motility often improves after effective antireflux surgery, but the knowledge of peristaltic strength may influence the type of wrap chosen. Manometry is also essential to precisely place a pH probe for subsequent monitoring.

Oesophageal pH and bile monitoring

Documentation of pathologic reflux is absolutely essential before undertaking antireflux surgery.[18] The majority will have acid detected on pH monitoring but a few (especially after previous vagotomy and pyloroplasty) will have abnormal bile monitoring. The technique of bile reflux monitoring, using a portable spectrophotometer, applied in a manner similar to a 24-hour pH probe, has allowed quantitation of the exposure time of the oesophagus or stomach to bilirubin, and by implication, duodenal juice.[19] Although the role of bile reflux monitoring has yet to be defined in gastro-oesophageal reflux disease the measurement of bile reflux is helpful in patients who fail to respond to acid suppression and may help to plan operative intervention. This is especially so when concomitant gastric pathology may indicate the need for bile diversion such as the creation of a Roux-en-Y gastro-enterostomy instead of, or in addition to, a Nissen fundoplication.

Patient information and consent

The surgical therapy for gastro-oesophageal reflux disease modifies a patient's quality of life but in many cases it does not affect survival and its effects must be balanced against the effects of not operating. It is essential that the patient participates in the decision and understands what the specific indications are in his or her case. They must also be aware of all the potential problems that might occur as a result of surgery. It is our practice to discuss the list of complications emphasising the important potential but rare problems. These include the short-term probability of some dysphagia for the first month or two after antireflux surgery. The patient must be aware of the risks of recurrent symptoms, the risks of difficulties with belching and vomiting and the possibility of gas bloat discomfort. The patient should be aware that they might lose some weight after surgery (of course in the obese this may be a beneficial side effect of surgery) and this weight loss may be associated with an alteration in satiety level, or with a postoperative dysphagia.

For all of these problems it is useful to have a well audited practice so that as well as taking active steps to minimise the frequency of such outcomes, it is also possible to give a patient a realistic estimate of the likelihood of these problems in the hands of the surgeon in question. Conversely it is useful to indicate to the patient the likelihood of symptom resolution and the chance of being free from acid suppression or prokinetic mediation for the future. Since the advent of laparoscopic surgery it has become important to discuss the approach to the surgical field and the possibility of needing to convert to an open operation should be clearly stated. It is our view that this counselling of the patient is essential and should be recorded in writing at the time of the discussion and form the major part of the interactive process of providing informed consent.

Mechanism of action of antireflux operations

Antireflux surgery seems to work equally well when reflux occurs in the presence of a normal lower oesophageal sphincter pressure as it does when the sphincter is mechanically defective. Exactly how the procedures work is debated and the following list of possible mechanisms of action indicate the lack of consensus on the exact mechanics of a successful fundoplication.

1. The floppy valve principle of the abdominal oesophagus means that when the gastric luminal pressure rises the lower oesophagus is compressed by the fundus of the stomach surrounding it.
2. There may be a reduction in the triggering of 'transient lower oesophageal relaxations'.
3. Exaggeration of the flap valve at the angle of His where the oesophagus joins the stomach.
4. Increase in the residual or resting pressure in the lower oesophageal sphincter as measured during swallowing in postoperative manometric studies.
5. A reduction in the volume of the gastric fundus aiding gastric emptying.
6. Prevention of the shortening of the abdominal oesophagus during gastric distension (balloon neck principle).

The absolute increase in lower oesophageal sphincter pressure is not important.[20] Indeed no change in resting pressure is required to produce an effective antireflux fundoplication. Over the past 20 years there has been a gradual reduction in the length of the Nissen wrap together with an understanding of the need to use a floppy wrap. This has resulted in procedures which are as effective but better tolerated with fewer side effects of dysphagia and gas bloat.

Techniques of antireflux surgery

There are many types of antireflux operation. Although this may indicate that none is perfect, most have excellent results in expert hands. It should be clearly understood that the experience of the individual surgeon is at least as important as the technical merits of the various operations. Variation can be reduced, but not eliminated, by good technical descriptions and good surgical training. The most successful protagonists of the various methods have usually performed many hundreds of their favoured operations by the time they teach them or write about them and are well aware of the potential pitfalls. Few surgeons have extensive experience of a wide variety of different types of operation and performing many different types of operation inevitably dilutes experience and is probably undesirable.

All the major antireflux procedures may be performed using minimal access techniques. This has added a new dimension to old controversies, but does seem to be making surgery more acceptable to patients.

Nissen 360° fundoplication

This is probably the most popular antireflux operation world-wide.[21] To perform a classic Nissen fundoplication the oesophagus is mobilised and separated from the diaphragmatic hiatus. Any hiatus hernia is reduced into the abdominal cavity and the upper part of the fundus of the stomach is mobilised by dividing some or all of the short gastric vessels. The vagus nerves are preserved. The mobilised gastric fundus is brought around behind the oesophagus and sutured anteriorly to the remainder of the fundus using non-absorbable sutures. The wrap is kept loose, the so-called floppy Nissen. This may be judged by eye, but a convenient guide is a 50 French gauge Maloney mercury dilator in the oesophagus and a finger or 38 gauge Hegar dilator between the plication and the oesophagus. The length of the wrap is also kept short, i.e. 1–2 cm. Many types of suture may be used. DeMeester uses a single horizontal mattress suture of prolene, placed over Teflon pledgets to create a wrap that is 1 cm long. One of the authors (JB) uses Goretex sutures placed over multiple small Teflon pledgets, again with a 1 cm wrap (Fig. 11.1). No method has a 100% success rate, but there is a very low incidence of wrap disruption with suitable sutures. The lowermost suture includes the anterior wall of the oesophagus at the cardia to help anchor the wrap in the correct position and stop slippage. Removal of the fat pad at the cardia is helpful to allow accurate placement of the sutures. Crural repair should be performed to avoid herniation of the fundoplication into the chest.

Rosetti–Nissen fundoplication

Rosetti modified the classic Nissen so that the part of the stomach used to create the wrap around the oesophagus is the anterior wall of the fundus.[22] It is brought behind the oesophagus as in the classic Nissen and sutured to the remainder of the fundus anteriorly

Figure 11.1 *Floppy Nissen fundoplication.*

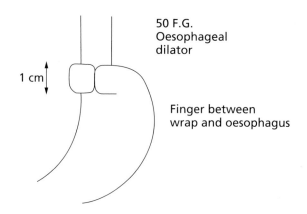

50 F.G. Oesophageal dilator

1 cm

Finger between wrap and oesophagus

(Fig. 11.2). With both the Rosetti and the classic Nissen operations the hepatic branch of the vagus nerve is preserved, if at all possible, as this makes a useful natural limit to the lowermost part of the fundoplication and reduces the postoperative complication of 'slipped Nissen'.

The logic behind the Rosetti modification is to allow adequate fundus to be involved in the wrap without the need for mobilisation of the greater curve and separation of the short gastric vessels from the spleen.

The two major variations of the Nissen operation have their protagonists and there are still strong opinions as to whether the short gastric vessels should be divided or not.[23] The controversy has recently been heightened by the introduction of laparoscopic fundoplication. Laparoscopic division of the short gastric vessels can be tedious, especially in obese subjects and the Rosetti approach has therefore become favoured by laparoscopists. It is likely that the controversy will continue for some time.

Luostarinen *et al.*[24] have compared the results of mobilisation of the greater curvature in a randomised prospective study. This showed no difference in postoperative symptoms, but there was a significant increase in operating times with the classic Nissen. Hunter *et al.*[25] have reported their clinical results with the different types of plication and have found a higher incidence of postoperative dysphagia if the short gastric vessels are not divided.

Partial fundoplication

A number of surgeons have described fundoplication operations in which the fundus is wrapped partially round the oesophagus rather than the full 360° of the Nissen. The rationale is to reduce the potential side effects of full fundoplication which can produce overcompetence of the cardia.

Toupet

Toupet[26] described a partial posterior wrap where the gastric fundus is laid behind the oesophagus and sutured to the left lateral and right lateral

Figure 11.2
*Rossetti–Nissen
fundoplication*

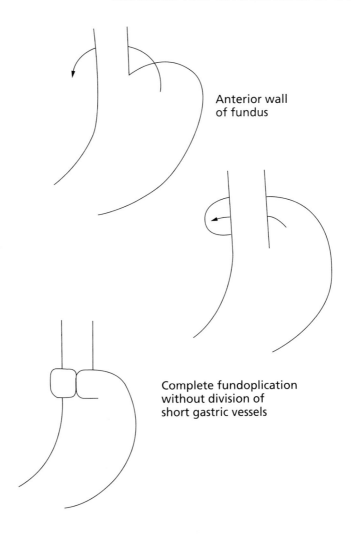

Anterior wall
of fundus

Complete fundoplication
without division of
short gastric vessels

walls of the oesophagus, creating a 180° posterior wrap. The wrap is also sutured to the diaphragmatic crura on each side to prevent herniation. This ensures strong suture lines and eliminates tension (Fig. 11.3).

Lind

Lind[27] described a procedure very similar to the Toupet operation with a 300° posterior fundoplication. The fundoplication is fashioned and two rows of sutures are placed between the oesophagus and the cuff of fundus in the left and right lateral positions. A third row is placed anteriorly leaving a 60° bare area anteriorly. The hiatus is repaired if necessary (Fig. 11.4).

Belsey 'Mark IV'

The Besley 'Mark IV' is a 240° partial fundoplication which requires a thoracic approach. In this procedure the oesophagus is mobilised up

Figure 11.3 *Toupet posterior hemi-fundoplication.*

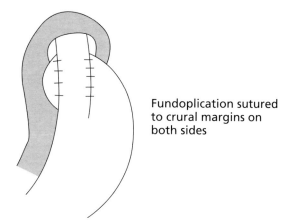

Fundoplication sutured to crural margins on both sides

Figure 11.4 *Lind 300° fundoplication.*

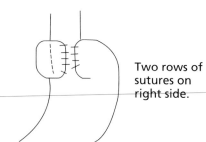

Two rows of sutures on right side.

to the aortic arch and then sutured to the gastric fundus and to the diaphragm to reduce any hernia and to wrap the fundus over the anterior two-thirds of the oesophagus.[28] It is a well established and successful operation, but is somewhat difficult to perform. A minimally invasive video-assisted thoracic approach has been described, but it has not so far been presented in the peer reviewed surgical literature.

Dor

The Dor procedure is an anterior hemifundoplication.[29] Good results have been reported from individual centres, but a small randomised prospective study showed results that were somewhat inferior to the Hill procedure.[30] The Dor fundoplication is particularly useful as an adjunct to Heller's myotomy for achalasia as it is non-obstructive and may reduce the risk of gastro-oesophageal reflux and oesophagitis after a myotomy.

Watson

The Watson[31] procedure involves reduction of any hiatus hernia, suture of the gastric fundus to the diaphragm accentuating the angle of His, creating an anterior hemifundoplication by suture of the fundus of stomach to the left lateral wall of the oesophagus and closure of the crura (Fig. 1.5).

Figure 11.5
Watson procedure. The completed procedure after accentuation of the angle of His and 120° anterolateral fundoplication. From Watson A et al. Br J Surg 1991; 78: 1090.

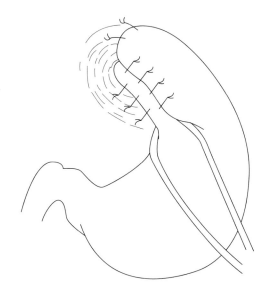

Hill

Hill[32] described a procedure which is usually regarded as a gastropexy rather than a fundoplication. However, it also tightens the cardia and, when complete, looks similar to a fundoplication. The essential aspect of the Hill procedure is suture of the anterior and posterior phreno-oesophageal bundles to the pre-aortic fascia and the median arcuate ligament. It was highly successful in the hands of Hill and his trainees and is still practised by a number of surgeons. It has not gained favour widely because of difficulties in understanding the anatomical principles. In addition Hill emphasised the use of peroperative manometry to achieve good results and the need for this may have been another disincentive.

Collis Nissen

The Collis Nissen procedure is useful in patients whose oesophago-gastric junction cannot be reduced below the diaphragm. It uses a tube of gastric lesser curve to recreate an abdominal length of oesophagus around which a Nissen wrap is created. This is a most useful procedure in patients with a short oesophagus and can avoid thoracotomy in all but the most extreme cases. It is conveniently created using a circular end to end stapler 9 cm from the angle of His and a linear anastomotic stapler from this hole up to the angle of His (Fig. 11.6).

Complete or partial fundoplication?

The relative merits of the full 360° Nissen fundoplication operation and the partial fundoplication operations have been hotly debated for many years. No one disputes that the Nissen is highly effective in controlling reflux, but it is easy to produce an overcompetent cardia that causes symptoms of dysphagia and gas bloat. Conversely there

Figure 11.6
*Collis–Nissen
procedure.*

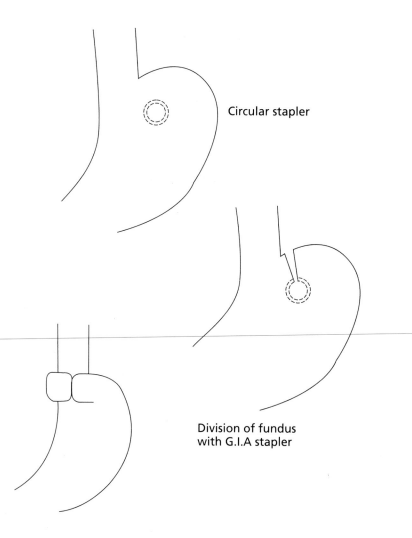

Circular stapler

Division of fundus
with G.I.A stapler

is fairly wide agreement that partial fundoplication reduces the chance of overcompetence, but there is the worry that it may be a less durable antireflux repair because of the nature of the tissues that are sutured.

With the passage of time the weaknesses of the different operations have been reduced. The advent of the floppy Nissen[33] was a significant advance and DeMeester[11] has emphasised the importance of keeping the length of the Nissen wrap as short as possible. Suture materials and suture techniques have also improved and although there has been no formal study this may have improved the durability of partial fundoplication.

Several prospective randomised studies of different antireflux operations have been done.[34,35] However, such studies are difficult to do, the numbers of patients entered has been small and the studies therefore lack the statistical power for firm conclusions to be drawn. Lundell *et al.*[36] have recently reported a comparative study of the Nissen and

Toupet operations; 137 patients were entered (72 Toupet, 65 Nissen) making this a study of moderate statistical power. Both operations gave comparable reflux control, but there was a higher incidence of flatulence following Nissen fundoplication. This is an important study that demonstrates that the Toupet operation is a good one. Enthusiasts of the Nissen procedure will no doubt counter by pointing out that the type of Nissen fundoplication that was done in the trial was 2–3 cm long as opposed to the 1 cm length that is now common. In addition there was a higher than expected incidence of symptomatic herniation of the Nissen fundoplication into the thorax. This was due to a policy of not routinely performing a crural repair.

A prosthetic collar of silicone[37] (the Angelchik prosthesis) was introduced to provide an easier and more standardised method than fundoplication and it fulfilled many of the requirements of a successful antireflux operation. Its introduction was associated with a number of complications relating to migration of the prosthesis but this was corrected by design improvements and is no longer a problem. Randomised comparison with a Nissen operation showed that it was equally effective[38] but in the author's opinion there is no advantage in using a prosthetic device rather than a fundoplication.

Antireflux surgery is sometimes performed as an adjunct to Heller's myotomy. It is an option which is used variably by experienced surgeons depending on the perceived risk of post-myotomy reflux. This depends on the degree of mobilisation of the cardia and the extent to which the myotomy is carried onto the stomach. After Heller's myotomy, some surgeons recommend suturing part of the fundus to the cut edges of the oesophageal muscle to keep them apart. This amounts to a Dor type of fundoplication.

Laparoscopic antireflux surgery

Many reflux operations have now been performed with laparoscopic techniques, or less commonly by thoracoscopy or video-assisted thoracic surgery (VATS). There is no doubt that fundoplication can be done safely and effectively with minimal access techniques.[39,40] There are no specific contraindications to the laparoscopic approach. Some surgeons prefer not to attempt mobilisation of a large hiatal hernia, and as with all laparoscopy care needs to be taken in patients who have had previous abdominal surgery. Although follow-up periods are inevitably still rather short the results in good hands seem indistinguishable from those of open surgery.

The disadvantage of laparoscopic antireflux surgery, as with laparoscopic cholecystectomy has been the problem in intraoperative injury, particularly during the 'learning curve' period. Unrecognised oesophageal perforation has caused several deaths, but it is likely that this problem will greatly reduce with experience of the technique.[25,41]

Training in laparoscopic surgery is now well organised in many countries so that the trainee surgeon can participate in simulator training followed by formal operative training in the operating theatre.

Such structured training is essential because of the limitations of movement imposed by laparoscopy and the difficulties this creates for such ostensibly simple tasks as suturing. Laparoscopic instrumentation is also improving steadily and is likely to improve further the safety of this type of surgery.

Postoperative care

Little in the way of specific aftercare is required following antireflux surgery. Nasogastric intubation is widely used. Some say that intubation may reduce the risk of early disruption of the fundoplication, but its value has not been tested. Indeed there is much good evidence that nasogastric tubes often cause more harm than good and we do not use them routinely, even after open surgery. Following laparoscopic surgery gastrointestinal function returns to normal so quickly that intubation is completely unnecessary. We allow fluids ad lib on the first postoperative day and a soft diet on the second day. Drains are also unnecessary. Dietary restrictions after fundoplications relate more to the presence or absence of dysphagia than anything else.

Prophylaxis for deep vein thrombosis (DVT) is essential. It should be remembered that laparoscopic surgery increases the risk of thromboembolic complications because of the reduction of venous return that is caused by the pneumoperitoneum and by the use of the modified lithotomy position for operative access.

Postoperative assessment

Any surgeon performing antireflux surgery needs to have some form of ongoing audit of the results with symptom review and objective testing. Ideally, clinical evaluation should be methodical and objective. For this purpose standard questionnaires are useful together with evaluation of the patient by someone who is not a member of the surgical team.

Endoscopy should be performed at some stage after surgery to document improvement in oesophagitis and to establish the presence of an intact fundoplication. Our own studies have shown that assessment at 6–9 months after operation will detect most recurrences.[42]

pH monitoring should also be encouraged, but it is somewhat uncomfortable and not always popular with patients. Nevertheless it is the only truly objective measure of reflux. As with endoscopy it is prudent to wait 6–9 months after surgery to detect most recurrences.

Routine and methodological audit is one of the most effective stimuli for consistent surgical performance and needs to be encouraged.

Complications of antireflux surgery

Mortality

In most series of antireflux operations a certain morbidity rate is inevitable. Many series have been reported without mortality and it would be hoped that the overall incidence of postoperative mortality is less than 0.1%. Such events are usually related to patient factors such as respiratory complications in children or more recently to laparoscopic misadventures. It is hoped that training standards will prevent the learning curve of minimally invasive techniques resulting in excess mortality.

Visick grade

Although it can be expected that 85–90% of patients will be happy with their results with a Visick grade of 1 or 2 there will be a 10–15% rate of postoperative symptoms. In many of these patients the symptoms are less severe than the preoperative state because of the fairly tight indications for operation. However, they might become a more serious issue if the indication for surgery includes those patients well controlled on proton pump inhibitors.

Persistent symptoms

Persistent heartburn may occur in 5–8% of patients and is due to either a disruption of a fundoplication or to unsuspected distal pathology such as delayed gastric emptying (secondary to duodenal ulceration in most cases). To minimise the risk of wrap disruption DeMeester devised a horizontal mattress suture buttressed with a Teflon pledglet. Another additional measure is the use of a second layer of sutures to approximate the two gastric walls in the fundoplication. In patients with persistent or recurrent heartburn the use of a proton pump inhibitor may be more effective than preoperatively and should be tried before considering revision surgery.

Recurrence of the hiatus hernia can occur and is more likely in patients who have not had a crural closure.

Wrap too long or too tight

Problems relating to a wrap that is too tight or too long include persistent dysphagia, gas bloat, difficulty with belching and inability to vomit. Gas bloat was once a common complication when long and tight Nissen wraps were employed and this complication gave the whole arena of antireflux surgery a bad reputation in the 1970s. Modifications of technique, particularly the emphasis of short and floppy fundoplications have corrected this and gas bloat is now extremely rare. Although initial dysphagia is common (up to 3 months after surgery) persistent dysphagia is rare occurring in 3–5%. After 3 months it is an indication for re-operation, as endoscopic dilatation is usually unhelpful. This is due to the underlying muscle tension in the fundoplication rather than fibrosis in the oesophageal wall. Dysphagia was a common reason for removing the Angelchik prosthesis. It has been described that after removal of such a prosthesis the residual fibrous tissue limits the expansion of the oesophagogastric junction and is sufficient to maintain reflux control.

Slipped Nissen

A 'slipped Nissen' is a characteristic but rare complication. Dysphagia and abdominal discomfort occur when the fundoplication slips down the lesser curve of the stomach creating an hour glass deformity seen on contrast radiology. It should be prevented by fixing the wrap to the oesophagus and by preserving the hepatic branch of the vagus nerve in the lesser omentum, and ensuring that the wrap is above this. The diagnosis of a slipped Nissen is a definitive indication for revision surgery.

Peroperative complications

Complications which can occur peroperatively include perforation of the oesophagus and pneumothorax. Both of these have become more common since the introduction of laparoscopic techniques. It should be a cardinal rule that if a good view of the operating field cannot be achieved at laparoscopy then conversion to an open laparotomy be undertaken without delay. The time at which both of these complications can occur is during the posterior dissection of the oesophagus and a dry field, appropriate retraction of the oesophagus, proper mobilisation under direct vision and avoiding the use of curved dissectors where the tip of the instrument may be out of view should prevent these serious complications.

Splenectomy

Splenectomy can be required for bleeding during the mobilisation of the gastric fundus and seems equally common with the open or laparoscopic approach (1%). Patients do need to be warned of the risk of splenectomy and the consequences in terms of infection prophylaxis.

Incisional hernia was possibly the commonest complication after open antireflux surgery and should now be rarely seen.

Chest complications

Atelectasis, chest infection and pulmonary embolus are possible respiratory and circulatory disturbances that occur with either open or minimally invasive approaches and routine DVT prophylaxis and respiratory exercises and appropriate use of antibiotics should be standard.

Complications of GORD

Barrett's oesophagus

Columnar epithelial lining of the lower oesophagus is the most prevalent complication of GORD. It affects 10% of patients with symptomatic reflux who present to a hospital and it is important because of its frequent association with stricture, ulceration and other benign complications and because of its association with malignant degeneration.

Barrett's oesophagus is an acquired condition which is almost invariably associated with chronic excess gastro-oesophageal reflux.[43,44] Precisely why Barrett's mucosa grows in some patients with reflux but not in others is poorly understood. Gray et al.[45] suggested that a reduction in the swallowed salivary epidermal growth factor may have some bearing, but what causes such a reduction is not understood. The mechanism of epithelial replacement is also not understood. Acid/peptic damage may denude the squamous mucosal lining of the oesophagus[46] and be replaced by a creeping substitution up from the gastric mucosa[47], by regeneration of the epithelium from residual glands in the base of the oesophagus[48] or by a transformation of the maturation of normal cells toward a glandular rather than a squamous differentiation. Such transformation has been well documented in the dog model and in humans after oesophagogastrostomy.[49]

The precise frequency of Barrett's oesophagus in the community is hard to establish although the post mortem results of Cameron et al.[50] at the Mayo Clinic indicate that many people have Barrett's oesophagus (3.7 per 1000 population) but are not diagnosed in life. A large multicentre study of 14 898 upper gastrointestinal endoscopies in Italy has shown a prevalence of 3.2 per 1000 cases in persons without symptoms rising to 80 per 1000 in those who complain of heartburn.

The reason for clinical interest in Barrett's oesophagus is the high frequency of complications. The benign problems include stricture (usually in the squamocolumnar junction) and ulceration which is prone to bleeding and perforation.[51]

Clinical investigations show that patients with Barrett's oesophagus consistently have a severe degree of gastro-oesophageal reflux.[52] This is associated with a general foregut dysmotility with very weak oesophageal peristalsis, incompetent lower oesophageal sphincter and often delayed gastric emptying or duodenogastric reflux. The end result is manifested by a very high exposure of the lower oesophagus to acid. More recent studies have shown a raised exposure to bile. Whether the bile or duodenal content of the refluxed material is important in the pathophysiology of Barrett's oesophagus or its complications has yet to be determined.[53–55]

A major concern about Barrett's oesophagus is its propensity to develop into adenocarcinoma of the oesophagus. The precise frequency of malignant degeneration is still in some doubt with European series showing incidences of 1:50–60 patient years[15,56,57] and in American series 1:200–250.[58,59] The size of the problem is difficult to put into perspective and some have compared it to the risk of getting lung cancer after 30 years of heavy smoking. Whether there is any relationship of Barrett's oesophagus with the recent dramatic rise in adenocarcinoma of the lower oesophagus and cardia is not known.[60] It could be that all such tumours begin in areas of intestinal metaplasia in the lower oesophagus and cardia. The conventional restriction of the term

Barrett's oesophagus to a circumferential lining of 3 cm of columnar mucosa in the lower oesophagus limits the application of this terminology in this situation.

Assessing the risk of cancer developing in an individual patient with Barrett's oesophagus has focused on the measurement of markers of malignant potential from biopsy specimens. The intestinal type of metaplasia is thought to be the epithelial type which undergoes malignant degeneration and it is thought to progress through stages of dysplasia from low grade through high grade and then to invasive carcinoma. Unfortunately there are usually no macroscopic signs and the identification of these changes rests on the chance of sampling the right area during random biopsy. The cost effectiveness of surveillance programmes for Barrett's oesophagus has not been established and many units have looked for other markers of potential malignancy such as *P53*, proliferating cell nuclear antigen (PCNA), silver staining nucleolar organiser regions (AgNOR), carcino-embrionic antigen (CEA), ornithine decarboxylase, gene allelic deletions (17p), E-cadherin, transforming growth factor, flow cytometric assessment of aneuploidy or indices of epithelial cell turnover. Although alterations of these markers are detectable in series of patients with Barrett's oesophagus their predictive value in an individual case is not clinically useful.[61-66]

Surveillance endoscopy has in the past been recommended for all those patients with a Barrett's oesophagus in whom an oesophagectomy might be considered if a tumour were to develop, but it is now realised that this is an overwhelming task to undertake and not justified by the frequency of the carcinoma.[67-72] It may be that only those patients with persistent dysplasia after acid suppression therapy should be considered and work on genetic markers or evidence of DNA damage and repair may in the future allow fine tuning of surveillance to those at especially high risk.[68-71]

The treatment of established malignancy in Barrett's is along standard lines described in Chapter 5. However, the treatment of a patient with high-grade dysplasia is controversial because of the documentation by Altorki *et al.*[72] and others that when the oesophagus is resected in such patients 50% of them can be found to have invasive carcinoma in the resected specimen. Their argument is that in surgical centres with low operative mortality figures (< 10%) the right time to consider oesophagectomy is before the carcinoma has become obvious endoscopically or clinically as at this stage the overall survival is less than 25%, compared to the expected 90% 5-year survival rate of a cancer confined to the mucosa. In a fit patient with high-grade dysplasia we would advise getting a second pathologist to review the specimen and then if there is no dispute about the grade of dysplasia an oesophagectomy should be recommended.

Treatment of Barrett's oesophagus

Despite the measured severity of reflux being at the severe end of the spectrum, the severity of symptoms is often less severe than would be expected.[73,74] In clinical practice this has an important effect on management decisions. In the absence of significant symptoms many gastroenterologists choose to allow patients to remain untreated until symptoms demand action. Some physicians treat all patients with a Barrett's oesophagus with long-term proton pump inhibition.[75] An alternative viewpoint is the value of early antireflux surgery to prevent complications developing[14–16] although the comparisons in these series were predominantly with H$_2$ receptor antangonists.

Regression of Barrett's mucosa is not an end point in treatment that has any established value. The associated reflux must be stopped and the best way to do this is with the creation of a reflux barrier. Discussion about regression of Barrett's raises the possibility of removing the risk of malignant degeneration. However, although some reports of regression have been published there are insufficient numbers in the literature to make any assessment about malignant potential. Regression only occurs in about 10% of patients on treatment, either by proton pump inhibition or surgery.[15,76,77]

Active removal of the mucosa has been proposed over the past few years as an option and there are now a number of ways of doing this. It must be emphasised that the value of such manoeuvres has yet to be determined and any such treatment should be subject to proper scrutiny. Ablation of mucosa in the hope that normal squamous mucosa will grow should only be undertaken where there is adequate control of the refluxate. This may be by high dose proton pump inhibition or by antireflux surgery. The methods of mucosal destruction include laser (Nd-YAG), argon beam-directed plasma coagulation or by photodynamic therapy with infrared light after protoporphyrin administration.

Stricture

Stricture in the absence of a Barrett's oesophagus usually occurs in the elderly (> 75 years) many of whom are not suitable for antireflux surgery. At all ages, patients require an endoscopy to confirm the diagnosis and exclude malignancy. Endoscopic dilatation followed by powerful acid suppression is effective in the majority of patients. Preparation of the patient for endoscopic dilatation is the same as for a diagnostic endoscopy, although more patients would prefer sedation for this intervention. Once the stricture has been observed and biopsied a guide wire is passed through the stricture. It is important that the guide wire passes easily through the narrowing. If not and there is doubt about placement of the wire then radiological guidance should be sought. Some would recommend that all dilatations should be performed under X-ray control. The endoscope is then removed and a dilator passed over the wire. There are numerous types of dilator – tapered soft bougies (such as the Savary Guillard and the Key-Med advanced dilators), semi-rigid shouldered dilators (Celstin) and metallic olives (Eder-Puestow). Another alternative is a balloon passed through or alongside the endoscope and direct visualisation of the dilatation as it proceeds.

After dilatation of a stricture it is important to pass the scope through the area to assess the quality of the dilated stricture, to ensure no perforation and to check the stomach and duodenum distally. Minor bleeding may have occurred but stops without intervention. Patients can be dilated as day cases and may swallow fluids after 2 h and eat a solid diet when comfortable – within 24 h.

Repeated dilatation is required in some patients. In fit young patients the need for repeated dilatation (> 3) while on proton pump inhibitors is an indication for antireflux surgery. The application of antireflux surgery is still needed for stricture but special precautions need to be taken to avoid dysphagia as patients with peptic stricture often have a very weak peristaltic amplitude, and persistent dysphagia may be a problem.[78,79] Very rarely a resistant benign stricture in an elderly patient requires further action such as the insertion of an expanding metallic stent.

Areas of research interest and therapeutic potential

The introduction of minimal invasive surgery to gastro-oesophageal reflux disease has reawakened interest in surgical therapy for GORD. At the same time the expense of medical treatments has raised concerns about the cost effectiveness of treatment. Indeed the world's largest pharmaceutical profits now come from acid suppression and the commonest indication for their prescription is GORD. The potential for savings is enormous. There is now a need for a proper randomised comparative assessment of medical and surgical therapy to establish the place of antireflux surgery in the armamentarium of GORD therapy. Such a trial should be multicentre and applied to patients who are well controlled symptomatically on proton pump inhibition. For those patients not well controlled on medication there is a definitive indication for antireflux surgery.

There is the real possibility that in the future intraluminal endoscopic suturing at the angle of His or cardia may allow the creation of an anti-reflux barrier without the need for transcutaneous instruments. Of course such a procedure, if successful, would be applicable across a much wider age range and disease spectrum compared to current practice as many older or infirm patients would become potential candidates. This work is in its infancy but is ongoing in a number of centres.

The value of antireflux therapy in prevention of adenocarcinoma in Barrett's oesophagus has been raised in recent papers and further work must examine the relationship between the risk of malignancy and the continued damage due to refluxed gastric juice. The study of bile reflux is in its infancy as until recently the normal values for oesophageal and gastric exposure to bile were not known and comparisons of the disease states with normal were hampered. However, it is clear that bile (and therefore duodenal juice) does reach the oesophagus in patients with GORD and Barrett's oesophagus and it remains to be determined whether this is important in the development of the condition or its complications.

In this context the removal of the abnormal epithelium as well as the cessation of reflux in Barrett's oesophagus may be required to normalise the life expectancy of these patients. The methods of restoring the normal squamous lining to the lower oesophagus mentioned above need further evaluation and long-term study.

References

1. Barlow A, Watson A, Attwood SEA, Dixon JS, Johnson NJ. A double blind cross-over comparison of the effects of ranitidine 300 mgs qds, 150 mgs bd and placebo on intragastric acidity and intraoesophageal pH. Gullet 1992; 2: 63–9.

2. Colin-Jones DG. Histamine-2-receptor antagonists in gastro-oesophageal reflux. Gut 1989; 30: 1305–8.

3. Armstrong D, Blum AI and the Rezitic Study Group. Full dose H2 receptor antagonist prophylaxis does not prevent relapse of reflux oesophagitis. Gut 1990; 31: 134–6.

4. Bate CM, Keeling PWN, O'Morain CA *et al*. A comparison of omeprazole and cimetidine in reflux oesophagitis; symptomatic, endoscopic and histological evaluations. Gut 1990; 31: 968–70.

5. Hetzel DJ, Dent J, Reed W *et al*. Healing and relapse of severe peptic esophagitis after treatment with omeprazole. Gastroenterology 1988; 95: 903–12.

6. Savary M, Miller G. Der Oesophagus-Lehabuch und edoskopischer Atlas. Solothurn: Gassmann, 1977.

7. Neal K, Scott HM, Slack RCB, Logan RFA. Omeprazole as a risk factor for campylobacter gastroenteritis: case controlled study. BMJ 1996; 312: 414–15.

8. Paull G, Yardley JH. Gastric and esophageal *Campylobacter pylori* in patients with Barrett's esophagus. Gastroenterology 1988; 95: 216–18.

9. Trakai E, Ortiz GA, Butti AL, Sambuelli R, Armando R. Organisms of the *Campylobacter* type in Barrett's esophagus. Acta Gastroenterol Laninoam 1987; 17: 85–96.

10. Jamieson GG. Anti reflux operations: how do they work? Br J Surg 1987; 74: 155–6.

11. DeMeester TR, Bonavina L, Albertucci M. Nissen fundoplication for gastroesophageal reflux disease. Evaluation of primary repair in 100 consecutive patients. Ann Surg 1986; 204: 9–20.

12. Kauer WKH, Peters JH, DeMeester TR, Ireland AP, Bremner CG, Hagan JA. Mixed reflux of gastric and duodenal juices is more harmful to the esophagus than gastric juice alone. The need for surgical therapy re-emphasized. Ann Surg 1995; 222: 525–33.

13. Naef AP, Savary M. Conservative operations for peptic esophagitis with stenosis in columnar-lined lower esophagus. Ann Thorac Surg 1972; 13: 543–51.

14. Spechler SJ. VA Study Group. Comparison of medical and surgical therapy for complicated gastroesophageal reflux disease in veterans. N Engl J Med 1992; 326: 786–91.

15. Attwood SEA, Barlow AP, Norris TL, Watson A. Barrett's oesophagus: the effect of anti-reflux surgery on symptom control and the development of complications. Br J Surg 1992; 79: 1021–4.

16. Ortiz A, Martinez de Haro LF, Parilla P *et al*. Conservative treatment versus antireflux surgery in Barrett's oesophagus: long term results of a prospective study. Br J Surg 1996; 83: 274–8.

17. Jazrawi S, Walsh TN, Byrne PJ *et al*. Cholecystectomy and oesophageal reflux: a prospective evaluation. Br J Surg 1993; 80: 50–3.

18. DeMeester TR, Johnson GJ, Joseph GL *et al*. Patterns of gastroesophageal reflux in health and disease. Ann Surg 1976; 184: 459–69.

19. Bechi P, Balzi M, Becciolini A *et al*. Gastric cell proliferation kinetics and bile reflux after partial gastrectomy. Am J Gastroenterol 1991; 86: 1424–32.

20. Bancewicz J, Mughal M, Marples M. The lower oesophageal sphincter after floppy Nissen Fundoplication. Br J Surg 1987; 74: 162–4.

21. Nissen R. Gastropexy and fundoplication in surgical treatment of hiatus hernia. Am J Dig Dis 1961; 6: 954–9.

22. Rosetti M, Hell K. Fundoplication for the treatment of gastroesophageal reflux in hiatal hernia. World J Surg 1977; 1: 439–44.

23. Jamieson GG, Duranceau A. What is a Nissen fundoplication? Surg Gynecol Obstet 1984; 159: 591–3.

24. Luostarinen M, Koskinen M, Reinikainen P, Karvonen J, Isolauri J. Two antireflux operations: floppy versus standard Nissen fundoplication. Ann Med 1995; 27: 199–205.

25. Hunter JG, Swanstrom L, Waring JP. Dysphagia after laparoscopic antireflux surgery. The impact of operative technique. Ann Surg 1996; 224: 51–7.

26. Toupet A. Technique d'oesophago-gastroplastie avec phrenogastropexie appliquee dans la cure radicale des heries hiatales et comme complement de l'operation d'Heller dans les cardiospasmes. Mem Academ Chir 1963; 89: 384–9.

27. Lind JF, Burns CM, MacDougall JT. 'Physiological' repair for hiatus hernia – manometric study. Arch Surg 1965; 91: 233–7.

28. Baue AE, Belsey RHR. The treatment of sliding hiatus hernia and reflux oesophagitis by the Mark IV technique. Surgery 1967; 62: 396–495.

29. Dor J, Humbert P, Paoli JM *et al.* Traitmen396–495.

29. Dor J, Humbert P, Paoli JM *et*Nissen modifiee. Press Med 1967; 75: 2563–9.

30. Civello IM, Castrucci G, Cotogni P, Fichera A, Amato A, DeGiovanni L. L'intervento di Hill modificato nel trattamento chirurgico dell'ernia jatale. Minerva Chir 1989; 44: 2129–35.

31. Watson A. A clinical and pathophysiological study of a simple effective operation for the correction of gastrooesophageal reflux. Br J Surg 1984; 71: 991–5.

32. Hill LD, Tobias JA. An effective operation for hiatal hernia: an eight year appraisal. Ann Surg 1967; 166: 681–8.

33. Donahue PE, Bombeck CT. The modified Nissen fundoplication – reflux prevention without gas bloat. Chir Gastroenterol 1977; 11: 15–27.

34. Thor KBA, Silander T. Long term randomised prospective trial of the Nissen procedure versus a modified Toupet technique. Ann Surg 1989; 210: 719–24.

35. Walker SJ, Holt S, Sanderson CJ, Stoddard CJ. Comparison of Nissen total and Lind partial transabdominal fundoplication in the treatment of gastrooesophageal reflux. Br J Surg 1992; 79: 410–14.

36. Lundell L, Abrahamson H, Ruth M, Rydberg H, Lonroth H, Olbe L. Long term results of a prospective randomized comparison of total fundic wrap (Nissen–Rosetti) or semifundoplication (Toupet) for gastro-oeso-phageal reflux. Br J Surg 1996; 83: 830–5.

37. Angelchik JP, Cohen R. A new surgical procedure for the treatment of gastroesophageal reflux and hiatal hernia. Surg Gynecol Obstet 1979; 148: 246–8.

38. Stuart RC, Dawson K, Keeling P, Byrne PJ, Hennessy TPJ. A prospective randomised trial of Angelchik prosthesis versus Nissen fundoplication. Br J Surg 1989; 76: 86–9.

39. Hinder RA, Philippi CJ. The technique of laparoscopic Nissen fundoplication. Surg Laparosc Endosc 1991; 2: 265–9.

40. Hinder RA, Philippi CJ, Wetscher G *et al.* Laparoscopic Nissen fundoplication is an effective treatment for gastrooesophageal reflux disease. Ann Surg 1994; 220: 472–83.

41 Callard JM, deGheldere CA, DeKock M *et al.* Laparoscopic anti-reflux surgery: what is real progress. Ann Surg 1994; 220: 146–54.

42. O'Hanrahan T, Marples M, Bancewicz J. Recurrent reflux and wrap disruption after Nissen fundoplication: detection, incidence and timing. Br J Surg 1990; 77: 545–7.

43. Dahms BB, Rothstein FC. Barrett's esophagus in children: a consequence of chronic gastroesophageal reflux. Gastroenterology 1984; 86: 318–23.

44. DeMeester TR, Attwood SEA, Smyrk TC, Therkildsen DH, Hinder RA. Surgical therapy in Barrett's esophagus. Ann Surg 1990; 212: 528–42.

45. Gray MR, Donnelly RJ, Kingsnorth A. Role of salivary epidermal growth factor in the pathogenesis of Barrett's columnar lined oesophagus. Br J Surg 1991; 78: 1461–6.

46. Hennessy TPJ, Edlich RF, Buchin RJ, Tsung MS, Prevost M, Wangensteen OH. Influence of gastro-oesophageal incompetence on regeneration of oesophageal mucosa. Arch Surg 1968; 97: 105–7.

47. Bremner CG, Lynch VP, Ellis FH. Barrett's esophagus: congenital or acquired? An experi-

mental study of esophageal mucosal regeneration in the dog. Surgery 1970; 68: 209–16.

48. Gillen P, Keeling P, Byrne PJ, West AB, Hennessy TPJ. Experimental columnar metaplasia in the canine oesophagus. Br J Surg 1988; 75: 113–15.

49. Hamilton RH, Yardley JH. Regeneration of cardiac type mucosa and acquisition of Barrett's musoca after esophagogastrostomy. Gastroenterology 1977; 72: 669–75.

50. Cameron AJ, Zinsmeister AR, Ballard DJ, Carney JA. Prevalence of columnar-lined (Barrett's) esophagus. Comparison of population-based clinical and autopsy findings. Gastroenterology 1990; 99: 918–22.

51. Limburg AJ, Hesselink EJ, Kleibeuker JH. Barrett's ulcer: cause of spontaneous oesophageal perforation. Gut 1989; 30: 404–5.

52. Iascone C, DeMeester TR, Little AG, Skinner DB. Barrett's oesophagus: functional assessment, proposed pathogenesis, and surgical therapy. Arch Surg 1983; 118: 543–9.

53. Gillen P, Keeling P, Byrne PJ, Healy M, O'Moore RR, Hennessy TPJ. Implication of duodenogastric reflux in the pathogenesis of Barrett's oesophagus. Br J Surg 1988; 75: 540–3.

54. Champion G, Richter JE, Vaezi MF et al. Duodeno-gastroesophageal reflux: relationship to pH and importance in Barrett's esophagus. Gastroenterology 1994; 107: 747–54.

55. Attwood SEA, DeMeester TR, Bremner CG, Barlow AP, Hinder RA. Alkaline gastroesophageal reflux: implications in the development of complications in Barrett's columnar-lined lower esophagus. Surgery 1989; 106: 764–70.

56. Robertson CS, Mayberry JF, Nicholson DA, James PD, Atkinson M. Value of endoscopic surveillance in the detection of neoplastic change in Barrett's oesophagus. Br J Surg 1988; 75: 760–3.

57. Hameeteman W, Tytgat GNJ, Houthoff HJ, van den Tweel JG. Barrett's esophagus: development of dysplasia and adenocarcinoma. Gastroenterology 1989; 96: 1249–56.

58. Cameron AJ, Ott BJ, Payne WS. The incidence of adenocarcinoma in columnar-lined (Barrett's) esophagus. N Engl J Med 1985; 313: 857–9.

59. Spechler RW, Robbins AH, Rubins CE et al. Adenocarcinoma and Barrett's oesophagus:

an overrated risk. Gastroenterology 1984; 87: 927–33.

60. Blot WJ, Devesa SS, Kneller RW, Fraumeni JF. Rising incidence of adenocarcinoma of the esophagus and gastric cardia. JAMA 1991; 265: 1287–9.

61. Belladonna JA, Hajdu SI, Bains MS, Winawer SJ. Adenocarcinoma in situ of Barrett's esophagus diagnosed by endoscopic cytology. N Engl J Med 1974; 291: 895–6.

62. Hamilton SR, Hutcheon DF, Ravich WJ, Cameron JL, Paulson M. Adenocarcinoma in Barrett's esophagus after elimination of gastroesophageal reflux. Gastroenterology 1984; 86: 356–60.

63. Garewal HS, Sampliner R, Alberts D, Steinbronn K. Increase in ornithine decarboxylase activity associated with development of dysplasia in Barrett's esophagus. Dig Dis Sci 1989; 34: 312–14.

64. Hamilton SR, Smith RRL. The relationship between columnar epithelial dysplasia and invasive adenocarcinoma arising in Barrett's esophagus. Am J Clin Pathol 1987; 87: 301–12.

65. Rabinovitch PS, Reid BJ, Haggitt RC, Norwood TH, Rubin CR. Progression to cancer in Barrett's esophagus is associated with genomic instability. Lab Invest 1988; 60: 65–71.

66. Sampliner RE, Steinbronn K, Garewal HS, Riddell RH. Squamous mucosa overlying columnar epithelium in Barrett's esophagus in the absence of antireflux surgery. Am J Gastroenterol 1988; 83: 510–12.

67. Achkar E, Carey W. The cost of surveillance for adenocarcinoma of the esophagus. Am J Gastroenterol 1988; 83: 291–4.

68. Spechler SJ, Goyal RK. Barrett's esophagus. N Engl J Med 1986; 315: 362—71.

69. Reid BJ, Weinstein WM, Lewin KJ et al. Endoscopic biopsy can detect high-grade dysplasia or early adenocarcinoma in Barrett's esophagus without grossly recognizable neoplastic lesions. Gastroenterology 1988; 94: 81–90.

70. Reid BR, Haggitt RC, Rubin CE, Rabinovitch PS. Barrett's esophagus: correlation between flow cytometry and histology in detection of patients at risk for adenocarcinoma. Gastroenterology 1987; 93: 1–11.

71. Hamilton SR, Smith RRL, Cameron JL. Prevalence and characteristics of Barrett

esophagus in patients with adenocarcinoma of the esophagus or esophagogastric junction. Hum Pathol 1988; 19: 942–48.

72. Altorki NK, Sunagawa M, Little AG, Skinner DB. High grade dysplasia in the columnar lined oesophagus. Am J Surg 1991; 161: 97–100.

73. Johnson DA, Winters C, Spurling TJ, Chobanian SJ, Cattau EL Jr. Esophageal acid sensitivity in Barrett's oesophagus. J Clin Gastroenterol 1987; 9: 23–7.

74. Ball CS, Norris T, Watson A. Acid sensitivity in reflux oesophagitis with and without complications. Gut 1988; 29: 799–801.

75. Hameeteman W, Tytgat GN. Healing of chronic Barrett ulcers with omeprazole. Am J Gastroenterol 1986; 81: 764–6.

76. Brand DL, Ylvisaker JT, Gelfand M, Pope CE. Regression of columnar esophageal (Barrett's) epithelium after anti-reflux surgery. N Engl J Med 1980; 302: 844–8.

77. Sampliner RE, Kogan FJ, Morgan TR, Tripp M. Progression-regression of Barrett's esophagus. Gastroenterology 1985; 88: 1567.

78. Zaninotto G, DeMeester TR et al. Esophageal function in patients with reflux-induced strictures and its relevance to surgical treatment. Ann Thorac Surg 1989; 47: 362–8.

79. Watson A. The role of anti-reflux surgery combined with fibreoptic dilatation in peptic oesophageal stricture. Am J Surg 1984; 148: 346–9.

12 Benign ulceration of the stomach and duodenum

John Wayman
Simon A. Raimes

Introduction

Few areas of surgery can have seen such dramatic changes in practice in the last few years as surgery for peptic ulcer disease. With the advent of modern medical treatments the need for elective surgery in cases of peptic ulcer disease has become extremely rare. Operations that were once the 'bread and butter' of both general surgeons and their trainees have virtually disappeared from all but specialist practice. Current treatment strategies for both the elective and more importantly, emergency treatment of peptic ulcers have to take account of modern medical treatment and also decreasing surgical experience.

The need for hospital admission of patients with peptic ulceration has fallen markedly in the last 50 years together with the need for elective surgery. This is due to a decrease in incidence that is quite separate from the advances in treatment. Nevertheless, the incidence of complications of peptic ulceration such as perforation and haemorrhage have remained constant and the mortality has risen in the last decade. The role of surgery in peptic ulceration has become the surgery of resistant ulcers, of ulcer complications and surgery for the sequelae of previous ulcer operations.

Epidemiology

Study of the epidemiology of peptic ulceration is frequently flawed. Since the introduction of H_2 antagonists (H2RA), proton pump inhibitors (PPI), and eradication therapy for *Helicobacter pylori* (HP), most cases of peptic ulcer disease are treated in the community.[1] A decline in incidence of peptic ulcer disease based on hospital admission statistics owes more to these changes in treatment approaches than to true change in the incidence of disease. Hospital admission data are more accurately applied in situations where hospital admission has remained mandatory; the incidence of perforation has shown little change with time.[2] This still does not take account of changes in iatrogenic aetiological factors, such as the increasing use of non-steroidal inflammatory drugs (NSAIDs).

Mortality from peptic ulcer disease accounted for less than 1% of deaths in England and Wales in 1990.[3] Mortality statistics suggest that death from the complications of peptic ulcer disease is much more common in the elderly and especially females. In the UK, there has been a small increase in the rate of peptic ulcer perforation in elderly women since 1960.[4] In contrast the incidence of perforation in males and younger female patients has fallen.[5] It is postulated that this difference is largely due to the increased prescription of NSAIDs.

Factors that affect the incidence of peptic ulcers

Temporal

The incidence and prevalence of peptic ulcer disease varies with time, sex, geography and socioeconomic development. Both duodenal and gastric ulceration appear to be diseases of the twentieth century although their incidence has fluctuated. It has been suggested that this is due to a cohort phenomenon secondary to antecedent fluctuating economic prosperity and recession.[6] Since 1960, a period of relative prosperity in the West, the incidence of peptic ulcer disease has fallen in keeping with this hypothesis, whereas it has remained high in the underdeveloped world.

Geographic

Study of geographic variation is confounded by inconsistency of data collection and diagnostic criteria. Such studies have illustrated regional variation in the relative frequencies of duodenal and gastric ulceration and their complications.[7] Even within the UK, regional variation has been observed with an increasing incidence of perforated duodenal ulcer South to North.[5]

Socioeconomic variation

Closely allied to temporal and geographical variation is socioeconomic variation. Contrary to the 'traditional' portrayal of the patient with duodenal ulceration as affluent and the patient with gastric ulceration as poor, this characterisation is not valid; both are more common in the poorer classes.[8] The observation that incidence varies according to occupation and educational attainment is similarly closely related to socioeconomic disparity.[9]

Aetiology *Helicobacter pylori* overshadows all other factors implicated in the pathogenesis of peptic ulcer disease. Most peptic ulcers treated in modern practice are caused by *Helicobacter* infection or NSAID ingestion. Other factors, particularly smoking, may facilitate ulcerogenesis in the presence of one or other of the former causative factors. There remains a small group of patients with idiopathic ulceration in whom there are several possible aetiological factors.

Diet

There is no strong evidence for the role of diet in the aetiology of either duodenal or gastric ulceration. Cohort studies in the US have shown an association between caffeine consumption at a young age and a propensity to peptic ulceration later in life.[10] In the same study milk was shown to be protective, whereas alcohol had no effect.

Acid/pepsin

Reports conflict with respect to the relative roles of acid and pepsin in the aetiology of duodenal and gastric ulcers.

Duodenal ulcers

Patients with duodenal ulceration have been shown in several studies to have increased gastric acid production at night and during the day and have greater peak secretion levels. This may be due to a larger parietal cell mass, increased sensitivity of parietal cells to gastrin or an increased production of gastrin from the gastric antrum. It is postulated that increased acid production together with the increased gastric emptying recognised in some patients with duodenal ulceration leads to an increased exposure of the duodenum to gastric acid and pepsin.[11]

Gastric ulcers

There appear to be several different types of gastric ulcer each with having a different pathogenesis:

Type 1 – Lesser curve ulcers which are preceded by chronic atrophic gastritis. These ulcers are generally associated with low basal and peak acid output. Interestingly they appear to develop at the junction between the antral gastrin-secreting mucosa and the parietal cells of the body.

Type 2 – Associated with duodenal ulcer disease. They are usually HP-positive and produce normal or increased amounts of gastric acid.

Type 3 – Prepyloric ulcers within 2 cm of the pyloric ring. They are associated with a diffuse antral gastritis and increased acid production.

Type 4 – Proximal gastric ulcers in the parietal cell mucosa of the body or fundus. They are usually close to the oesophagogastric junction and associated with chronic atrophic gastritis.

Smoking

Patients who smoke are more prone to peptic ulceration and are more likely to die from the complications of ulceration than non-smokers.[12] The precise mechanism by which smoking contributes to ulceration is not proven, but may lie partly in decreasing epithelium haemoperfusion while enhancing the acid-secreting capacity of parietal cells.[13] It is known that those who smoke are more likely to fail both medical and surgical ulcer treatment.

Associated disease

Diseases associated with peptic ulceration are chronic liver disease, hyperparathyroidism and chronic renal failure, particularly during dialysis and after successful transplantation. Other disease associations have been observed, but are probably biased by the fact that patients under close medical supervision and regular attenders are more likely to have investigations performed and the diagnosis made than infrequent attenders of medical care.

Non-steroidal anti-inflammatory drugs and aspirin

The association between NSAIDs, gastritis and gastroduodenal ulceration has been known for some time. Use of NSAIDs is associated with an increase in the prevalence of gastric and duodenal ulceration, particularly complicated cases and especially in the elderly where the risk of bleeding is increased between two- and fourfold compared with non-NSAID users.[14] It should be appreciated that perhaps one-third of patients who develop ulcers while on NSAIDs would have had underlying ulcer disease.[15] A useful source of information for the role of aspirin in peptic ulceration comes from controlled trials of therapy for thromboembolic disease. These consistently indicate a twofold increase in risk of upper gastrointestinal bleed for patients given aspirin-containing regimens compared with controls.[16]

Helicobacter pylori

This is a spiral-shaped Gram negative microaerophilic bacterium that colonises gastric epithelium and mucus. Humans are its only known host. The discovery of HP, formerly *Campylobacter*, has revolutionised our understanding of the pathogenesis of peptic ulceration.[17] *Helicobacter* organisms have been isolated from areas of antral gastritis seen in association with duodenal ulceration, areas of gastric metaplasia adjacent to areas of duodenal ulceration and also areas of chronic active gastritis, the precursor of gastric ulceration.[18]

Transmission of infection

There is considerable evidence to support the theory of person to person transmission of infection. Areas where people live in close proximity, such as the Third World and institutionalised patients in the West, show a high prevalence of infection.[19] The clustering of infection within families with identical strains of organisms also supports this argument.[20] Accidental and experimental ingestion of the organism leads to infection.[21,22] Whether transmission is by oral–oral or faecal–oral contact is not clear since organisms have been isolated from both the faeces and saliva of infected patients.

Epidemiology of infection

Many of the previously observed socioeconomic, geographical and temporal trends in the prevalence of peptic ulcer are more likely to be a reflection of prevalence of HP infection. Hence the prevalence of infection is higher in developing countries (70% by the age of 20) compared with Western countries (60% by the age of 65).[23,24] HP is present with a presumed causative role in 95–99% of cases of non-NSAID-induced duodenal ulceration.[25,26] However, it has been estimated that only 10% of patients infected with HP will in fact go on to develop an ulcer. The clinical outcome of infection appears to be related to an interplay of organism and host factors.

Bacterial factors that predict clinical outcome

Genetic studies of HP suggest that there are strains which share similarities and are each associated with a particular disease; one subgroup associated with gastritis alone, one with gastritis and ulceration, and another with complicated ulcer disease.[27] Analysis of strains of bacteria isolated from ulcer and non-ulcer patients reveals that certain factors, particularly the bacteria's ability to adhere to epithelial cells and release toxins, may facilitate infection and ulcerogenesis.[28,29] Studies *in vitro* show that certain strains of HP exert a characteristic cytopathic effect on mammalian cells in culture with the formation of intracytoplasmic vacuoles.[30] About 50–60% of strains can be induced to release this vacuolation cytotoxin *in vitro*, although all strains possess the *vacA* gene that encodes it. Another marker of virulence is the protein product of the cytotoxin-associated gene A (*cagA*). The function of the high molecular weight (128 kDa) cagA gene product is unknown, but expression strongly correlates with severity of gastritis and development of peptic ulceration. The cagA-linked gene *picB* (Permits Induction of Cytokines) has recently been identified.[31] This has been shown to be necessary for enhanced interleukin 8 release from cultured cells which may be one factor responsible for the increased mucosal inflammation seen in association with cagA-positive strains.

Patient factors which predict clinical outcome

The host epithelium not only provides a protective barrier, but also initiates immune inflammatory responses to infections which may be deleterious to the host. HP binds preferentially to Lewis antigens on the surface of gastric epithelial cells.[32] Lewis antigens form part of the complex which determines blood group, particularly blood group O. This may be the explanation for the long-observed tendency for duodenal ulceration to occur in patients of blood group O. The age at which infection was acquired may have some bearing on the clinical outcome. Childhood infection is associated with a pan-gastritis similar to that found in gastric ulceration and gastric cancer, but different from that observed in cases of duodenal ulceration.[33]

Proposed mechanism of mucosal injury

Direct injury

The precise mechanism by which HP exerts its ulcerogenic effects is not established. The observation that ulceration occurs in the duodenum only in areas of gastric metaplasia colonised by HP suggests that direct local damage to the epithelium plays at least some part. It is probable that release of cytokines from the organism itself, or by the patient's cellular response to infection, is relevant to this process.[34] Cytotoxic substances released from the bacterium itself include membrane lipopolysaccharide, urease (which acts as a chemotoxin for monocytes and neutrophils *in vitro*), the vacuolating cytotoxin and heat shock proteins. These have a deleterious effect on the mucus layer and mucosal protection allowing acid to permeate directly to the epithelial cells thereby causing cellular injury. This in turn excites chemotaxis of leucocytes to the scene, with release of further cytokines and production of damaging oxygen free radicals which exacerbate and perpetuate this mucosal insult.[35]

Increased gastric acid production

HP causes antral gastritis and increased gastrin and pepsinogen release (hyperpepsinogenaemia I). Acid production in the more proximal stomach inhibits the colonisation by bacteria and inhibition of gastric acid secretion by antisecretory drugs facilitates the proximal migration of organisms. This relative sparing of the body of the stomach facilitates normal and in many cases increased gastrin-induced acid production. Gastrin release may be exaggerated due to the local action of cytokines from the inflammatory cells on the albeit reduced G cell mass.[36] The function of the G cells is further augmented by the reduced capacity of adjacent D cells to secrete the acid inhibitory peptide somatostatin.[37] Eradication of HP lowers gastrin levels and hence acid secretion by approximately two-thirds.[38]

Management strategies for peptic ulceration (Figs 12.1 and 12.2)

Endoscopic confirmation

Patients with dyspeptic symptoms should undergo endoscopic examination to confirm the presence of an ulcer and exclude other potentially serious pathology. Gastric ulcers must be carefully biopsied as there is a risk that an apparently benign gastric ulcer is in fact an early malignancy.[39] Direct endoscopic inspection, adequate tissue biopsy and expert histological interpretation are essential to identify dysplasia and neoplasia. Repeat endoscopy to confirm healing and re-biopsy are essential for all gastric ulcers.

Figure 12.1
Proposed management protocol for cases of duodenal ulceration

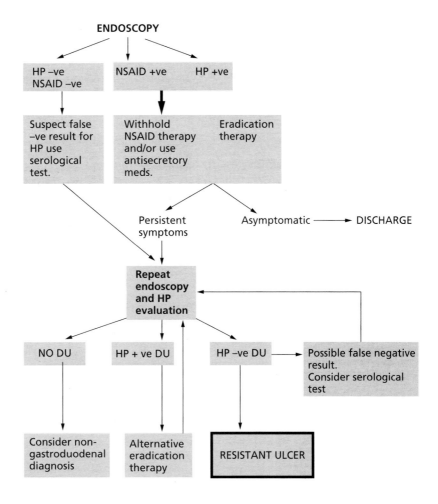

Diagnosis of *Helicobacter* infection

HP infection can be determined non-invasively by carbon isotope (^{13}C or ^{14}C)–urea breath test, serologically by ELISA, or using endoscopic biopsy material by functional assay of urease activity (*Campylobacter*-like organisms (CLO) test), and histological analysis with and without immunohistochemical stains. False negative diagnosis occurs in about 5–15% of cases depending on the laboratory experience. Several drugs including proton pump inhibitors, bismuth and antibiotics temporarily suppress HP and render functional assays falsely negative. In the absence of NSAID ingestion HP infection is so likely in cases of duodenal ulceration that a negative test result should be viewed with some scepticism. In view of the poor predictive value of a negative result, further testing by an alternative method, particularly serologically, or even empirical treatment with subsequent re-evaluation may be justified.[40]

Figure 12.2
Proposed management protocol for cases of gastric ulceration

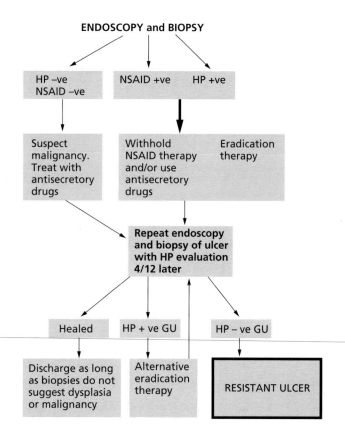

Determination of NSAID or aspirin ingestion

Careful inquiry is needed to elucidate whether NSAIDs or aspirin are being taken regularly. Ingestion is especially common among the elderly, but patients may fail to declare such information unless specific inquiry is made.

Treatment of peptic ulcers

NSAID-induced ulceration

HP should be tested for and eradicated even in patients taking NSAIDs. Half of patients on NSAIDs with peptic ulceration have HP infection contributing to ulceration.[41] There is some suggestion that the ulcerogenic effects are synergistic.[42] NSAIDs should be stopped or their dose reduced if cessation is absolutely contraindicated. If continued NSAID use is deemed necessary, most ulcers will heal with H_2 receptor antagonist therapy or, more quickly, with proton pump inhibitors. Maintenance therapy is likely to be required in some form.

Eradication of *Helicobacter pylori*

Eradication of HP leads to a cure of peptic ulcer disease.[43] Once eradication has been achieved, re-infection rates are less than 0.5% in developed countries.[44] Ulcer recurrence in the absence of HP infection is rare according to studies with up to 7-year follow-up.[45] Patients presenting with haematemesis do not re-bleed if HP is successfully eradicated.[46]

There is no consensus on the optimum treatment for HP. Although underlying infection must be eradicated by antibiotic therapy, conventional anti-ulcer therapy is also necessary to facilitate mucosal healing and symptom relief.

Antimicrobial drugs

Successful eradication of HP is inhibited by the inaccessibility of the habitat (between the adherent mucus gel and the epithelial cell surface) in which it exists and by antimicrobial resistance (especially to metronidazole) of some strains.[49] In order to overcome these factors prolonged therapy with complex multiple drug regimens has been suggested and proven nearly completely (98–100%) effective.[50] However, poor compliance and cost suggests that such aggressive therapy should be reserved for resistant infection.

The choice of antibiotic regimen should take account of previous antibiotic exposure and local prevalence of antibiotic resistance. Classical triple therapy consists of colloidal bismuth, metronidazole and tetracycline or amoxycillin. The most recent evidence suggests that a one week 'triple therapy' course of a proton pump inhibitor, with clarithromycin and either metronidazole or amoxycillin will cure HP infection in 90% of cases.[51,52] Currently UK and European guidelines suggest a one week, twice daily dose of a proton pump inhibitor and two of clarithromycin, metronidazole or amoxycillin. This regimen has an acceptable balance of efficacy in association with good compliance, effectiveness against metronidazole-resistant strains of HP and acceptable cost.[53] Failure to eradicate HP by one regimen should prompt the prescription of a second course of treatment after consideration of previous antibiotic exposure and sensitivities. A quadruple regimen (a proton pump inhibitor with 'classical' triple therapy) is justified in these circumstances. Inevitably more studies are being carried out to devise better strategies and further guidelines will be issued. As with other infectious diseases, consultation with microbiologists and development of local antibiotic policies should be considered with resistant *Helicobacter* infection.

Antisecretory drugs

H2 antagonists selectively and competitively block the class 2 histamine receptors of parietal cells to reduce secretion of gastric acid and pepsin.

Misoprostol, an analogue of prostaglandin E_1, inhibits the secretion of acid and proteolytic enzymes at the same time as increasing bicarbonate and mucus secretion.

Pirenzepine is a specific antagonist for muscarinic M_2 receptors which reduce gastric acid secretion by a pharmacological interruption of the vagus.

Proton pump inhibitors inhibit the Na^+/K^+-ATPase which is the final common pathway through which histamine, vagal acetylcholine and gastrin stimulate gastric acid production. This class of drugs induces virtual achlorhydria. The long-term effects and risks of this remain unknown. The choice of therapy is largely an economic one. H2RAs and proton pump inhibitors are both effective ulcer healing agents. Proton pump inhibitors are more effective in cases of gastric ulcer, whereas the differences between the two in cases of duodenal ulceration is less marked.[47,48]

Investigation of ulcers which fail to heal (Fig. 12.3)

The natural history of peptic ulceration has been transformed by pharmacological and bacteriological developments. The stage at which one defines failure of medical treatment is open to conjecture. Duodenal ulcers are generally considered refractory if healing is not evident by eight weeks and gastric ulcers if healing is not at least progressing by twelve weeks.[40]

Persistent symptoms without refractory ulcer

Endoscopic re-evaluation of duodenal ulcers should differentiate between a refractory ulcer and persistent symptoms despite ulcer healing. If satisfactory ulcer healing and HP eradication are demonstrated, alternative diagnoses should be considered.

Persistent *Helicobacter* infection

The first step in the evaluation of refractory ulcers should be to confirm successful eradication of HP. Biopsies should be repeated at the same time as the endoscopy when failure of healing is confirmed. A higher than usual rate of false negative results should be anticipated with carbon isotope breath tests within the first three weeks after eradication therapy due to suppression of bacterial function, but not necessarily eradication. Serum antibody titres can be expected to fall after successful eradication but this is slow (up to six months) and variable.

Possible causes of failure of HP eradication are antibiotic resistance (most commonly to metronidazole) or if the patient has failed to comply with the prescribed regimen. The former may be overcome by appropriate modification of the eradication regimen.

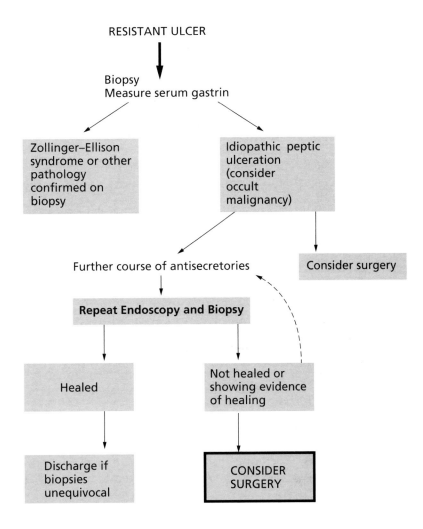

Figure 12.3
Proposed management protocol for resistant ulcers

Failure of ulcer healing if HP negative

Ingestion of NSAIDs should be re-evaluated. Surreptitious aspirin ingestion has been observed and if suspected can be established by assay of plasma salicylate levels. Any other factor which may be facilitating ulceration such as smoking or intercurrent disease should be sought and eliminated where possible. Smoking in particular is associated with failure of medical treatment of peptic ulcer disease.

The truly resistant ulcer

Resistant ulcers are of two types.

1. **Refractory resistant ulcer** is an ulcer which fails to heal despite the exclusion of *Helicobacter pylori* infection and ingestion of ulcerogenic drugs.
2. **Relapsing resistant ulcer** is an ulcer which heals initially but recurs

in the absence of *Helicobacter pylori* or ingestion of ulcerogenic drugs.

Refractory or relapsing ulceration should prompt multiple biopsies of the ulcer margin and base to identify the several neoplastic, infectious and inflammatory conditions that can mimic peptic ulcer. Gastric ulceration should be viewed with caution and biopsied from the outset. A diagnosis of Zollinger–Ellison should be suspected in cases of *Helicobacter* negative, non-NSAID-induced refractory ulceration and especially where there is ulceration of the second part of the duodenum or large confluent ulcers in the duodenum.

Treatment of idiopathic refractory ulceration

Where no cause for persistent ulceration can be found it may be necessary for the patient to take long-term antisecretory drugs. Alternatively, elective surgery may be considered in this highly selected group of patients. Inherent in this decision is a careful calculation of the relative risks and benefits of surgery (see below) against the potential risks and costs of continued medical treatment. The risks of complications of persistent ulcer disease, the degree of disability experienced by patients and their fitness for surgery should all be considered in the decision of whether or not to operate. In the case of refractory gastric ulcers there is the concern of unidentified malignancy. Hypergastrinaemia should be excluded prior to a decision to treat a refractory ulcer surgically.

Zollinger–Ellison syndrome

In 1955 Zollinger and Ellison[54] described a condition of a non-insulin secreting tumour of the pancreas associated with gastric hypersecretion and fulminant peptic ulcer disease.[54]

Clinical features

The syndrome typically presents with epigastric pain, although 40% of patients complain of diarrhoea and weight loss and a third present with oesophagitis only.[55] The disease may present with perforation, haemorrhage, oesophageal stricture, jejunal ulceration or anastomotic breakdown. The condition should also be suspected when a duodenal ulcer coexists with primary hyperparathyroidism or metastatic adenocarcinoma of unknown origin.

Historically Zollinger–Ellison (ZE) syndrome was only recognised after a protracted course of ulcer disease leading to a delay in diagnosis of 3–9 years.[56] Diagnosis should be now considered early in the small group of patients who fail to respond to medical treatment.

Pathology

Although originally described as a pancreatic endocrine tumour, the definition has also come to include extrapancreatic gastrin-secreting tumours. Where the condition is due to a pancreatic tumour, in two-thirds of cases the tumour will be multifocal within the pancreas,[57] at least two-thirds will be histologically malignant[58] and one-third will already have demonstrable metastases by the time of diagnosis.[59] The most common extra-pancreatic site is in the wall of the duodenum. These extrapancreatic tumours rarely metastasise to the liver and, even though they do metastasise just as frequently to regional lymph nodes, they tend to have a better prognosis than primary pancreatic tumours.[60]

Multiple endocrine neoplasia

A quarter of patients with ZE syndrome have other endocrine tumours as part of a familial multiple endocrine neoplasia (MENI) syndrome. This group of patients have a much worse prognosis than sporadic ZE syndrome, in part due to the multifocal nature of the tumour within the pancreas. Cure is rarely possible in this group and treatment is conservative with attempted surgical resection being contra-indicated.

Sporadic gastrinomas

The majority of cases of ZE syndrome arise sporadically. Such tumours are more likely to occur in extrapancreatic sites than familial types. Prognosis is better in this group of patients.

Diagnosis

The diagnosis of ZE syndrome can be established by radioimmuno-assay of serum gastrin levels and measurement of gastric acid hypersecretion. Diagnosis may be confirmed by the finding of fasting hypergastrinaemia. False-positive results may occur in cases of achlorhydria such as ingestion of antisecretory drugs, postvagotomy, pernicious anaemia and atrophic gastritis. Hypergastrinaemia may also be detected in conditions which increase antral G cell gastrin production, such as gastric outlet obstruction and antral G cell hyper-plasia, and conditions which impair the elimination of gastrin from the body, such as renal failure. If there is diagnostic uncertainty or the basal serum gastrin level is marginal, dynamic assay of serum gastrin following secretin (or alternatively calcium or glucagon) provocation may be required. Gastrin response to a standard meal helps to differ-entiate hypergastrinaemia due to antral G-cell hyperplasia, which will result in an increase in serum gastrin levels, whereas no response would be expected in cases of gastrinoma.

Treatment

There are two main aims of treatment in patients with ZE syndrome; treatment for the effects of the excessive hormone production and treatment directed at the tumour itself with resection if possible.

Treatment of gastric hypersecretion

Before the introduction of H_2 receptor antagonists in the mid-1970s a total gastrectomy was often necessary to control the gastric hypersecretion and prevent recurrent and life-threatening complications. Lesser acid-reducing operations were associated with a very high recurrence rate. Complete resolution of symptoms follows adequate acid suppression, although very large doses of H2RAs were often needed. Since parietal cell vagotomy reduces the need for H_2 antagonists by 75%, parietal cell vagotomy at the time of exploratory laparotomy has been advocated.[61] The introduction of the more potent proton pump inhibitors has led to a more acceptable twice daily dosing. The consensus has moved to a general acceptance of omeprazole as the preferred therapy with parietal cell vagotomy becoming infrequently used.[62] A recently published study with 16 years follow-up of cases of proximal gastric vagotomy in Zollinger–Ellison syndrome has once more fuelled debate over the long-term antisecretory treatment of this condition.[60] This report illustrates that only 30–40% cure rates can be expected in patients undergoing exploratory laparotomy and that 30–60% of patients cured by surgery will be able to discontinue antisecretory medications. Hence the argument has swung back in favour of parietal cell vagotomy at the time of exploratory laparotomy. This is appropriate especially for women of child-bearing age for whom the teratogenic risks of proton pump inhibitors remain unknown. Patients in whom exploratory laparotomy is not indicated due to obvious dissemination should not be considered for surgery and are treated with a dose of PPI 'titrated' against endoscopic and symptomatic response. Patients in whom metastases are only discovered at the time of laparotomy should also be treated with PPIs.

Treatment of tumour

Preoperative localisation

A tumour of the pancreas should be sought and localised by computed tomography (CT). Percutaneous ultrasonography is of little benefit but endoluminal and intraoperative ultrasonography have proved useful in identifying tumours as small as 4 mm in diameter especially when situated in the duodenal wall. More elaborate diagnostic tools including selective angiography and splenic venous catheter sampling of blood gastrin levels improve the detection of both solitary gastrinomas and metastases. These techniques are more sensitive than CT or even intraoperative ultrasonography by 16 and 28% respectively.[63] Liver metastases can frequently be detected by conventional imaging but somatostatin receptor scintigraphy with [^{111}In]DTPA-DPhe1 octreotide has proved a more sensitive investigation which may prevent unnecessary surgical exploration.

Surgical excision of primary gastrinoma

How aggressively surgery should be pursued in cases of gastrinoma is controversial. Surgical exploration and resection is generally recommended in all cases without MEN1 where there is no evidence of metastases. Others advocate a more aggressive Whipples procedure for cases with local lymph node metastasis and multiple duodenal gastrinomas. On balance, if a resectable solitary or multiple gastrinomas can be identified, surgical management should be considered in view of the high risk of malignancy. Patients with MEN1 and those with diffuse liver metastases should not be treated surgically.

Surgical strategy

Exploration of the pancreas despite failure of preoperative investigations to localise a tumour is controversial. If surgical exploration is performed then the pancreas must be mobilised along its entire length, inspected, palpated and if the facilities are available re-scanned intra-operatively. If a tumour cannot be localised by these means, the next step in the search should be directed toward the duodenum. Transillumination may reveal tumours within the duodenal wall and palpation via a duodenotomy may identity tumours within the medial wall of the duodenum. If no tumour is identified then at most an acid-reducing operation should be performed; there is no place for blind pancreatic resection. Further non-operative localisation tests should be repeated 6–12 months later, but further surgery only contemplated if a tumour is definitely detected.

Elective surgery for peptic ulceration

In developed Western countries very few patients will now even be considered for an elective ulcer procedure. There will still be rare patients with ulcers resistant to treatment in whom all the common aetiological factors have been excluded. Throughout the second half of this century elective surgical treatment has been reserved for those with non-healing or rapidly recurring symptomatic ulcers and for those who do not comply with their treatment. On the basis of the concept that peptic ulcer disease is a spectrum of a disease rather than a single entity, those undergoing surgery were generally at the worst end of this spectrum. With the development of increasingly strong antisecretory drugs the indications have narrowed even further and by the late 1980s very few elective ulcer operations were required. The discovery of the importance of eradication of *Helicobacter pylori* in the healing and maintenance of ulcer healing has narrowed the indications even further.

Duodenal ulcer surgery

Definitive surgery for duodenal ulcer evolved around the concept of acid reduction either by resection of most of the parietal cell mass, vagal denervation of the parietal cells or resection of the antral gastrin-producing cells. The balance lay in minimising the chance of ulcer recurrence while at the same time trying to avoid the symptomatic side-effects and metabolic sequelae of the procedure that would effect the patient for the rest of their life.

The trend by the mid-1970s was towards highly selective or proximal gastric vagotomy (HSV or PGV) which denervated the parietal cell mass, but left the antrum and pylorus innervated. This allowed a gastric emptying pattern, that although not completely normal, did not require a drainage procedure.[64] This was the first ulcer procedure that did not involve bypass, destruction or removal of the pylorus and as a result has significantly fewer side effects than other ulcer operations.

HSV in most series has a mortality of well under 1%.[65] The incidence of side effects such as early dumping, diarrhoea and bile reflux is also very low.[66] The main concern with their operation, whether for duodenal or gastric ulcer, has been the recurrence rate. In the best hands recurrence rates of 5–10% have been achieved.[67,68] Many others had not been able to produce this level of excellence and even at the time of the introduction of H_2 antagonists the truncal versus highly selective vagotomy debate continued. Once cimetidine was available, recurrent ulceration became a less significant problem as patients who had undergone an unsuccessful vagotomy could be treated with H_2 receptor antagonists and actually appeared to be more sensitive than patients who had not had their parietal cells denervated.[69] Improvement in the intraoperative testing of completeness of vagotomy and particularly the use of the endoscopic congo red test have also improved the performance of HSV and lessened the risk of ulcer recurrence.[70,71]

Anterior seromyotomy with posterior truncal vagotomy probably denervates the proximal stomach more consistently.[72] This operation has never been compared with HSV in a large trial and so its place in ulcer surgery remains uncertain. It has proved that the posterior vagal trunk can be divided and the patient not experience significant diarrhoea, provided the pylorus is intact and innervated. There is now no place for truncal vagotomy with either destruction, bypass or excision of the pylorus because of the life-long risk of diarrhoea, which in a significant proportion of patients is socially disabling.[73]

Some surgeons, particularly in the USA, advocated the use of truncal vagotomy and antrectomy suggesting that this operation is the most effective for reducing acid secretion and has a very low recurrence rate of about 1%. The procedure was subsequently modified to a selective vagotomy and antrectomy, leaving the hepatic and coeliac fibres of the vagi intact. This did reduce the incidence of side effects, especially diarrhoea, though dumping was still a problem. Bile gastritis and oesophagitis were also troublesome side effects unless a Roux-en-Y reconstruction was used, though recurrent stomal ulceration was then more frequent unless a more extensive gastric resection was performed (see below). The perfect ulcer operation has remained elusive and indeed there is none that has no side effects or risks.

By the early 1980s it was becoming apparent that the introduction of H_2 antagonists had significantly narrowed the indications for elective ulcer surgery and that recurrent ulceration rates after HSV were rising. There were several studies that attempted to address this concern by comparing HSV with selective vagotomy and antrectomy. Overall the balance of opinion considered that the higher rate of ulcer recurrence, but better side effect profile of HSV were preferable as it was easier to treat recurrent ulcers than other more debilitating side effects which the patient would suffer for the rest of their life.[67,74,75]

The last paper of importance about HSV was a report from Johnston's group in Leeds in 1988.[76] This confirmed that as the group of ulcer patients undergoing elective surgery became more selected the recurrence rate after HSV was increasing. Looking at the group of duodenal ulcer patients who were refractory to healing with a three month course of full-dose H_2 antagonists (1 g of cimetidine or 300 mg of ranitidine per day) they found an 18% recurrent ulcer rate at two years rising to 34% at five years. In comparison the respective figures for those who had healed on H_2 antagonists, but did not wish to take long-term maintenance therapy, were 1.5% and 3%. In the past the single most important factor in determining ulcer recurrence after HSV was the surgeon who had performed the operation.[69] However, in the H_2 antagonist-resistant group even the best surgeon had a 3-year recurrence rate of over 20%. There are presently no figures available for those patients who are *Helicobacter* negative and are refractory to healing with proton pump inhibitors, but the recurrence rate would be predicted to be very much higher. It has to be concluded that HSV will almost certainly not have a place in the treatment of refractory duodenal ulcers in the late 1990s. Since the operation is so operator-dependent few trainee surgeons will have the opportunity to learn the correct technique, and indeed those who have already done so will have scant opportunity to maintain their experience. Surgery for benign ulcers will have to be centralised to a few specialised units.

Recommended operations for refractory duodenal ulcers
At present no one knows what operation should be recommended for refractory duodenal ulcer. After eradication of *Helicobacter* and exclusion of other causes of persistent ulceration, there remains a very small number of patients with aggressive ulcer disease who are often female and smokers. If they are under 60 and otherwise healthy surgery should be considered. In view of the predicted poor results of HSV in this group of patients it is likely that resection of the antral gastrin-producing mucosa and either resection or vagal denervation of the parietal cell mass is necessary. The operations that could be considered include the following (Fig. 12.4).

Selective vagotomy and antrectomy
Selective denervation is preferred because of a lower incidence of side effects. It is not an easy procedure, in particular the dissection around

Figure 12.4
Surgical treatment of refractory duodenal ulcers

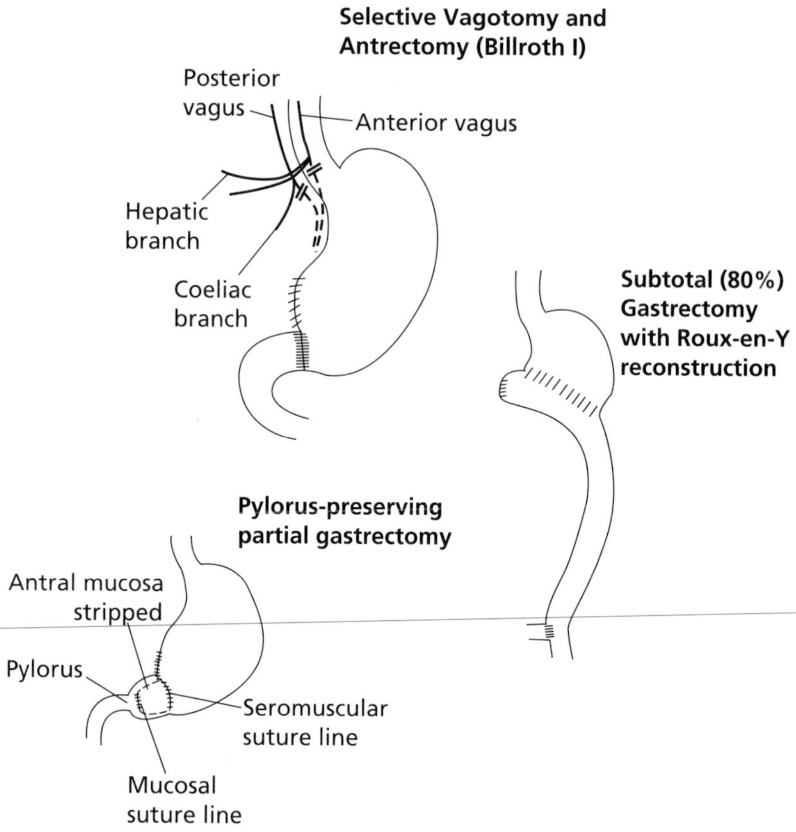

the lower oesophagus and cardia has to be done very carefully. The vagotomy should be performed before the resection and tested intra-operatively. The reconstruction should either be a gastroduodenal (Billroth I) anastomosis or a Roux-en-Y gastrojejunostomy. The latter is associated with less problems with bile reflux into the gastric remnant and oesophagus, but a higher risk of stomal ulceration and so at least a two-thirds gastrectomy is advised.

Subtotal gastrectomy

Removal of a large part of the parietal cell mass is sound in theory and indeed ulcer recurrence after this operation is unusual. However, there is a high incidence of postprandial symptoms and in particular epigastric discomfort and fullness that significantly limits calorie intake. Importantly there is a high incidence of long-term nutritional and metabolic sequelae that require life-long surveillance and can be difficult to prevent, particularly in women.

Pylorus-preserving gastrectomy

There is interesting work from China on a form of highly selective vagotomy with resection of about 50% of the parietal cell mass and the antral mucosa, but preserving the pyloric mechanism and the vagus nerves to the distal antrum and pylorus.[77] This operation is physiologically sound and may prove to be nearer to the ideal operation for refractory ulcers in the West. Further clinical experience is yet to be reported.

Surgery for gastric ulcer

Surgical treatment for benign gastric ulcer is now very rarely required as failure to heal after exclusion of aetiological factors and up to 6 months treatment with a PPI is extremely uncommon. Type 2 and 3 ulcers should be treated in the same way as duodenal ulcers – it is important to realise that HSV is not recommended for prepyloric ulcers. The choice of operation for a type 1 ulcer is between excision of the ulcer with HSV or Billroth 1 partial gastrectomy. The recurrence rate is higher after HSV/excision, but the operative mortality is lower and side effects fewer after this procedure. There are no reliable data on which to base a recommendation for surgical treatment of refractory gastric ulcers in the late 1990s.

Laparoscopic peptic ulcer surgery

Interest in minimally invasive procedures has led to many publications proving the feasibility of laparoscopic definitive ulcer operations. The simple fact is that the issue is not whether the operation can be done, but whether it needs to be done. The indications for laparoscopic surgery are exactly the same as for open procedures.

Surgery for the complications of peptic ulcers

Although the number of patients requiring elective surgery has declined, the number who require surgery for the complications of peptic ulcer disease has remained constant.[78,79]

Perforation

With the changing emphasis towards medical treatment of peptic ulcers, surgery is now mainly performed in the emergency situation. Those requiring emergency surgery are a selected group of high risk patients with higher mortality.[80] There is a spectrum of treatment options for peptic ulcer perforation. At one extreme is conservative non-surgical treatment and at the other is early operation involving definitive antiulcer procedures at the same time.

Conservative management
Study of the natural history of perforated peptic ulcers suggests that they frequently seal spontaneously by omentum or adjacent organs.[81] Since 1951 the argument for conservative management has been advocated, but never gained widespread acceptance. Taylor showed that

the mortality in his series of patients with peptic ulcer disease was half that of the contemporary reported mortality for perforation treated surgically.[82] More recently a small, randomised controlled trial comparing conservative treatment with surgical treatment showed no difference in morbidity or mortality.[83] Eleven of 40 patients treated conservatively, 11 ultimately required surgical treatment; these cases were more often over 70 years of age. Hence some authors advocate an initial, closely monitored trial of conservative therapy of parenteral broad spectrum antibiotics, intravenous fluid resuscitation and nasogastric aspiration in patients under the age of 70. Such a policy requires careful interval assessment by an experienced surgeon with a low threshold for performing laparotomy if clinical improvement is not apparent. One of the chief concerns with the conservative approach is the uncertainty of the diagnosis made on clinical grounds alone as upper abdominal peritonitis may be caused by other pathology that may not respond to conservative measures.

Open surgery

In most centres the treatment of choice for patients with perforation of the duodenum is still laparotomy, peritoneal lavage and simple closure of perforation usually by omental patch repair.[84] Additional biopsy of perforated gastric ulcers is mandatory. This simple treatment is safe and effective in the long-term, especially when combined with *Helicobacter* eradication and pharmacological acid suppression.[85,86] Traditionally there has been a school of thought that at the time of emergency laparotomy, definitive ulcer surgery should be performed. In particular HSV has been strongly advocated to reduce the risk of recurrent ulceration and its complications.[87] The advances in understanding of the treatment of ulcers together with the decrease in experience of elective antiulcer surgery have made this argument no longer tenable. The indications for emergency definitive surgery are exactly the same as the criteria for elective surgery and are now be extremely rare in the patient presenting with an acute perforation.

Laparoscopic surgery

Over recent years there has been a movement towards minimally invasive surgery in the acute situation.[88] Laparoscopic treatment of peptic ulcer perforation was first reported in 1990.[89] The limited series available suggest that laparoscopically performed omental patching is feasible, safe and has comparable results to open surgery and with less postoperative discomfort.[90] Recent developments of tissue adhesive glue and repair of perforation by falciform ligament patch repair have had some success.[91,92] Where the expertise and experience are available, a laparoscopic approach followed by appropriate ulcer treatment seems to be emerging as the therapeutic strategy of choice for peptic ulcer disease. Though technically feasible, laparoscopic definitive surgery has no place in the emergency treatment of peptic ulcer disease for the same reasons described above.

Pyloric stenosis

Gastric outlet obstruction can result from peptic ulcer disease of the duodenum or prepyloric region. It is a condition usually associated with chronic relapsing ulceration and is now fairly uncommon in the western world.

Resuscitation and medical therapy

Initial management should consist of aggressive parenteral fluid and biochemical restoration with nutritional and vitamin supplementation as necessary. Nasogastric intubation with a wide bore tube allows gastric wash out of undigested food and so reduces antral stimulation. Aggressive parenteral antisecretory therapy and *Helicobacter* eradication, if appropriate, are used.

In cases where the obstruction has been due to oedema and spasm, the situation can be expected to resolve once medical treatment has healed the ulcer. In cases where the obstruction is due to fibrosis and cicatrisation of a pyloric ulcer, some form of intervention will be necessary.

Endoscopic treatment

The group of patients who develop gastric outflow obstruction are generally elderly, often with intercurrent disease who tolerate major surgery poorly. Minimally invasive approaches are often appropriate in the first instance. Initial reports of successful resolution of pyloric stenosis following endoscopic balloon dilatation were challenged due to the relatively high number of cases which ultimately required open surgery (50% within 2 years).[93,94] Nevertheless this remains a useful first-line endoscopic procedure which can be repeated on several occasions with good long-term results in up to 80% of patients.[95] The main risk of endoscopic dilatation is perforation and the procedure should only be performed on patients who have been appropriately worked-up for surgical intervention if needed. Only if a combination of intensive medical treatment and dilatation fails to re-open the gastric outlet is surgery indicated.

Surgery

The most appropriate operation to perform in cases of gastric outlet obstruction must take into account all those factors outlined for elective surgery of gastric and duodenal ulceration. The procedure must also restore drainage of the stomach. There are no published series that prove which procedure best achieves these aims. Initial fears about the capacity of a large atonic stomach to resume function have not been realised. The operation with least complications is simple pyloroplasty (or gastro-enterostomy where the inflammation around the pylorus is particularly intense), with highly selective vagotomy. Antrectomy and selective vagotomy or subtotal gastrectomy are more aggressive alternatives less likely to result in re-stenosis but with a higher mortality and incidence of both short- and long-term side effects.

Laparoscopic surgery for pyloric stenosis

In keeping with the trends for minimally invasive surgery, laparoscopic highly selective vagotomy with balloon dilation has been attempted with some success in cases of pyloric stenosis.[95] This has not been proven to be superior to dilatation and long-term acid suppression. More recently laparoscopic truncal vagotomy and gastroenterostomy has proven a technically feasible solution with good symptomatic response at six months follow-up.[96] This operation cannot be recommended as a definitive ulcer procedure. Laparoscopic techniques may have a role in the future for patients who have failed endoscopic balloon dilatation therapy, but are not a first-line intervention for pyloric stenosis.

Management of the complications of previous ulcer surgery

Although there are few patients now being considered for ulcer surgery, there are still a considerable number attending gastroenterology and surgical clinics with the side effects of previous ulcer operations. Recurrent ulceration has always been regarded as the marker of failure of an ulcer operation, but in fact is relatively easy to treat when compared with the other life-long sequelae of these procedures.

The specialist upper gastrointestinal surgeon should be aware of the intricacies of treating these problems if they are not to make the same mistakes as their predecessors. It is important to take a very careful history and confirm the subjective impression with objective evidence from appropriate investigations. The first line in treatment is medical and dietary – further surgery should only be contemplated after failure of conservative measures. It should be appreciated that among those with these sequelae is a group of chronically unhappy individuals who have probably persuaded a previous surgeon of their need for a surgical solution to their 'ulcer symptoms'. These same patients will, through perseverance and lack of response to other treatments, try and persuade the surgeon to embark on further surgical endeavours with an equally unsuccessful outcome. That is not to say that there are not patients who have a significant diminution in the quality of their life as a result of the side effects of previous surgery – these patients are also unhappy individuals and for a good reason. The art of managing these problems is to identify those who really will benefit from corrective surgery.

Recurrent ulceration

Most ulcer recurrences present clinically within 5 years of the initial operation and are rare after 10 years. Since there have been very few

Table 12.1 *Causes of abdominal pain after ulcer operations*

Recurrent ulcer
Early dumping syndrome
Non-specific pain
Alkaline enterogastric reflux
Small stomach syndrome
Roux-en-Y syndrome
Gallstones
Carcinoma

---

elective ulcer operations in the last 10 years, recurrence is now mainly seen after attempts at emergency definitive ulcer procedures for ulcer complications. Almost inevitably these recurrences are due to an incomplete vagotomy by an inexperienced trainee. There are rarer causes of recurrence that should be considered and so a logical step-wise approach to the investigation is suggested.

Endoscopic confirmation of recurrence

This is an essential first step unless the patient presents with a perforation. There are multiple causes for abdominal pain after ulcer surgery and so recurrence must be proven rather than assumed (Table 12.1). If the ulcer is gastric then multiple biopsies are mandatory; an early recurrence may represent a missed carcinoma whereas a late recurrence may be due to malignant change in the postoperative stomach.

Test for Helicobacter

The first step in the treatment of recurrent ulcers is to eradicate HP and then to repeat the endoscopy and confirm healing and eradication. If the ulcer is healed then no further investigation is required. If the patient is HP negative or the ulcer does not heal then the investigation pathway should be initiated.

Exclude other aetiological factors

Ingestion of aspirin or NSAIDs must be carefully sought and these drugs stopped irrespective of the HP status, at least until proven ulcer healing. They should only be reintroduced for strong clinical reasons and then under endoscopic surveillance. Smokers should cease their habit and further surgery should not even be contemplated until this has been achieved.

Gastrin level

ZE syndrome is a rare cause of recurrent ulceration and so gastrin estimation need only be considered in those who are HP negative and not taking aspirin/NSAIDs or who have an unhealed or multiple recurrent ulcers. Investigation is then along the lines previously described. Antral exclusion is a cause of recurrent ulceration after a Billroth II gastrectomy where a small cuff of antrum has been included in the 'duodenal' closure. In the alkaline environment of the duodenal stump the G cells produce excessive gastrin.

Test for incomplete vagotomy

If the other steps have been followed then this stage is rarely reached. In the past patients underwent acid secretion studies all of which are now becoming obsolete because of lack of ongoing experience. Tests involving acid secretion induced by hypoglycaemia by giving subcutaneous insulin are regarded as dangerous. Sham feeding tests are probably the safest for measuring the vagal phase of gastric acid secretion.

A far more acceptable and simpler test for incomplete vagotomy is the endoscopic congo red test. This can be performed in the endoscopy room and involves giving the patient 6 μg/kg of subcutaneous pentagastrin 15 min before testing. The empty stomach is then lavaged with about 200 ml of congo red solution (3 g/l) in 0.5% sodium bicarbonate solution. The excess fluid is aspirated through the gastroscope and the entire mucosa observed after 2 min. Parietal cells that still have a vagal innervation turn the dye black – in a complete vagotomy there should be no black areas within 2 min. The test not only confirms whether the vagotomy is incomplete, but also maps out the incomplete trunk or fibres.

Consider surgery

Before contemplating further surgery high dose PPIs should be prescribed until healing occurs. If healing does not occur with this treatment then the suspicion should arise that the ulcer is not peptic or the patient is ingesting undeclared drugs or not complying with the treatment. Further investigation is imperative. Once the ulcer has healed then a lower maintenance dose should be prescribed and a repeat gastroscopy performed 4 weeks later. If the patient is over about 60 years of age or poses any anaesthetic risk then long-term maintenance treatment is preferable if the ulcer remains healed. In the younger patient surgery is probably indicated, but with the realisation that the process followed has selected the patients with ulcer disease at the very worst end of the ulcer spectrum. In such cases the antrum has to be resected along with completion of an incomplete vagotomy. Attempted completion of an incomplete vagotomy is not recommended as the sole operative measure as there is still a high recurrence rate in this group of patients. If the previous vagotomy was complete then a 75% gastrectomy is recommended. It is important to involve the fully informed patient in the decision-making before undertaking this type of procedure.

Dumping syndrome

This is uncommon in patients who have an intact and innervated pylorus as it is due to rapid and uncontrolled gastric emptying. It is

Table 12.2 *Symptoms of the early dumping syndrome*

Cardiovascular and vasomotor	Gastrointestinal
Sensation of warmth	Nausea
Flushing	Vomiting
Sweating	Eructations
Palpitations	Epigastric fullness
Breathlessness	Borborygmi
Weakness	Diarrhoea
Feeling of faintness	
Loss of consciousness	

most common after gastrectomy, but does also occur after truncal and selective vagotomy. The dumping syndrome ('early dumping') occurs during or very soon after eating and comprises various cardiovascular and gastrointestinal symptoms (Table 12.2). Most patients experience more than one of these symptoms and in the very worst cases most or all may occur. Early dumping should not be confused with the poorly named 'late dumping' which is due to reactive hypoglycaemia and produces symptoms about 2–3 h after eating. Many patients experience dumping symptoms in the early weeks after surgery, but in most cases the symptoms are mild and improve considerably with simple dietary adjustments that patients often discover for themselves.

The diagnosis is usually made on the history. In less clear cases the patient should keep a diary card recording foods eaten and symptoms experienced. When there is still doubt then a 'Dumping Provocation Test' may give objective proof of the cause of postprandial symptoms.[97] This involves giving a hypertonic glucose drink which may cause severe symptoms and should be performed under medical supervision.

Medical treatment

The mainstay of treatment is dietary manipulation and this should involve a dietician with expertise in this type of problem. Meals with a high refined carbohydrate content and hypertonic liquids such as soups should be avoided. Meal size may have to be reduced and liquids taken separately. If these measures are not sufficient then various substances and drugs taken before meals can be tried. Pectin or guar gum delay gastric emptying, but exacerbate early satiety and pectin may precipitate diarrhoea attacks. The somatostatin analogue octreotide given subcutaneously before eating has been reported to be effective although experience with this agent is limited.[98,99]

Surgical treatment (Fig.12.5)

The main reason for dumping after truncal vagotomy is the drainage procedure and to a lesser extent the loss of receptive relaxation in the

Figure 12.5
Surgical treatment for dumping syndrome or enterogastric reflux

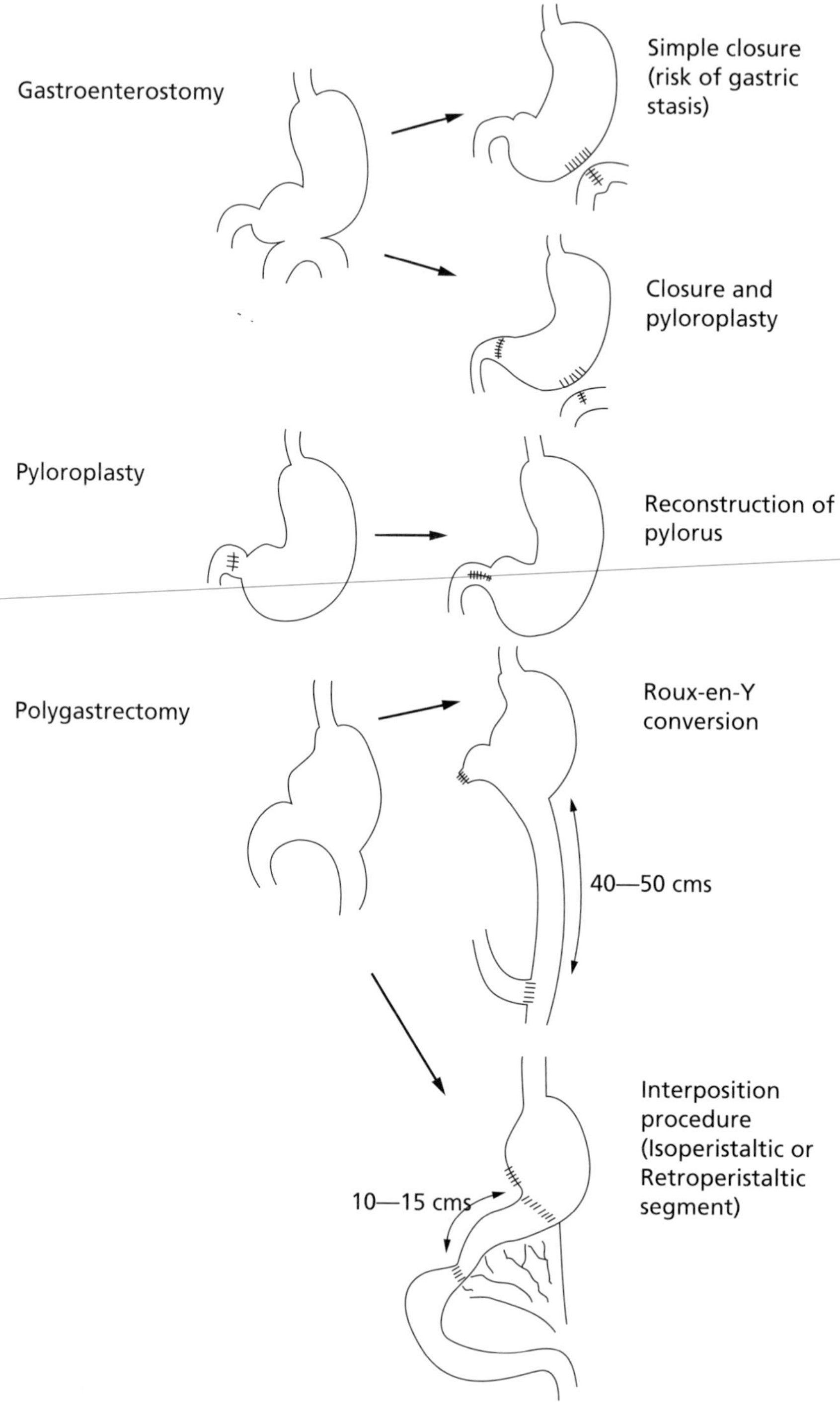

Gastroenterostomy

Simple closure (risk of gastric stasis)

Closure and pyloroplasty

Pyloroplasty

Reconstruction of pylorus

Polygastrectomy

Roux-en-Y conversion

40—50 cms

Interposition procedure (Isoperistaltic or Retroperistaltic segment)

10—15 cms

upper stomach. Reversal of the drainage procedure does stop dumping, but at the cost of delayed gastric emptying of solids and resulting gastric stasis. Reconstruction of the pylorus has produced variable results.[100,101] Simple closure of a gastroenterostomy also risks new symptoms resulting from gastric stasis, though it is claimed that conversion to a pyloroplasty avoids this and does improve dumping symptoms. Modern prokinetic agents are helpful in treating stasis, although strict dietary measures are also necessary.

There are several options for improving dumping after a gastrectomy. The simplest is conversion of the drainage to a Roux-en-Y reconstruction.[102] The benefial effect of this procedure is thought to be due to transection of the neural plexuses resulting in a decrease in the frequency of isoperistaltic contractions in the long jejunal limb together with retrograde contractions from ectopic pacemakers in the limb that effectively slow gastric emptying.[103] The only significant risk is the Roux-en-Y syndrome which produces a functional gastric outlet obstruction and left upper quadrant discomfort after eating.[104] There is also a risk of stomal ulceration if the vagotomy is incomplete. The other options are the insertion of either an isoperistaltic or antiperistaltic 10–15 cm jejunal segment in the proximal jejunum or between the gastric remnant and duodenum. These complex procedures have a significant serious complication rate and variable success for early dumping.

Diarrhoea

This may be part of a severe dumping attack, but more commonly is a complication of operations that include a truncal vagotomy. Postvagotomy diarrhoea is usually episodic with the patient complaining of discrete attacks of explosive watery diarrhoea associated with extreme urgency. Attacks may occur at any time of day, although are more common in the mornings. The frequency varies from a continuous form occurring every day to an episodic form every few days. Patients who have had a cholecystectomy are much more prone to postvagotomy diarrhoea and have a particularly severe form. This is the most troublesome side effect of truncal vagotomy and in the severe form may be socially disabling and does not improve with time.[73] Unlike early dumping the attacks are often precipitated by a relatively small osmotic load. Diarrhoea after gastric resection is usually due to dumping, but occasionally is due to bacterial overgrowth in the proximal small intestine. In such cases faecal fat levels are elevated, vitamin B_{12} levels low and the diarrhoea tends to be continuous. Diagnosis is made by aspiration of jejunal contents or the $[C^{14}]$glycocholate breath test.

Medical treatment

The first step in treatment is dietary and in particular the avoidance of refined carbohydrates. Patients are advised to substitute sugar in their hot drinks by a sweetener. Patients who have had a concomitant cholecystectomy benefit from cholestyramine taken morning and evening, although there are concerns about the long-term use of this drug. The key to successful treatment is prevention of attacks and loperamide taken in small doses on a prophylactic basis has proved to be very successful.[105] The treatment should be started with 2 mg first thing each morning and increased in 2 mg increments – it is very rare for a patient to need more than 4 mg a day when loperamide is taken in this way. This drug has a very long half-life and need only be taken once a day.

Surgical treatment

This is rarely, if ever, indicated for postvagotomy diarrhoea. The only operation that has proved effective is a distal ileal onlay graft.[106] There are concerns about the long-term effects of this type of operation. Small intestinal bacterial overgrowth after gastrectomy may be treated with courses of antibiotics, although if persistent and due to stasis may necessitate reconstruction.

Enterogastric reflux

Reflux of alkaline duodenal juices into the stomach occurs in any operation where the pylorus has been destroyed, bypassed or removed. Bile reflux is more common after gastrectomy and particularly more extensive resections with Billroth II reconstruction because of the long afferent limb and small gastric remnant. It may cause a symptomatic gastritis, reflux oesophagitis and bile vomiting. The patient complains of persistent epigastric discomfort sometimes made worse by eating and frequently associated with intermittent vomiting of small amounts of bile with or without food. The patients develop nutritional problems because of inadequate calorie intake. The diagnosis is not always easy and it is important to exclude recurrent ulceration as the cause of these symptoms. If objective evidence is required then the ^{99m}technetium HIDA scan is usually helpful.[107]

Medical treatment

This is often not very effective and should start with an intensive course of medication to allow recovery of the gastric and oesophageal mucosa. Aluminium hydroxide binds bile acids, but the effect is short-lived. Altacite plus is useful for bile gastritis as is sucralfate with both acting as a mucosal protective in addition to binding bile acids. Cholestyramine taken at night helps reduce the bile salt pool and decreases exposure of the stomach and oesophagus during the night. A combination of these drugs should be tried initially. Prokinetic agents may also be prescribed, but may worsen dumping and diarrhoea.

Surgical treatment

Surgical reconstruction is indicated in severe cases. As with dumping a gastroenterostomy should be closed or the pylorus reconstructed, but

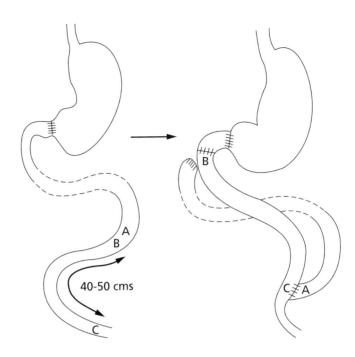

at the same time warning the patient that they may swap their bile reflux symptoms for problems with gastric emptying. A possible compromise operation is the 'duodenal switch' procedure in which a Roux limb is brought up to the divided duodenum (see Fig. 12.6).[108] Patients who have had a gastric resection should have a Roux-en-Y reconstruction with a long limb of at least 40 cm. As previously discussed this type of procedure is not itself free of side effects. The most troublesome side effect is a functional obstruction leading to delayed gastric emptying. If there has been no vagotomy or the vagotomy is incomplete then there is a high incidence of stomal ulceration when the initial operation was for duodenal or prepyloric ulceration. Both these problems are largely solved by resecting at least 75% of the stomach, but this does then lead to a risk of long-term nutritional problems (Fig 12.5). Other experts recommend a less radical resection, but with long-term maintenance H2RAs to prevent recurrent ulceration.

Small stomach syndrome

This presents as early satiety and early postprandial pain. It is thought to be due to a loss of reservoir function and is a common symptom after subtotal and total gastrectomy. In many patients it is multifactorial and can be due to early dumping, Roux syndrome, reduced gastric capacity and when there has been a vagotomy, loss of receptive relaxation in the proximal stomach. The importance of early satiety is that it can lead to significant nutritional problems with weight loss and specific deficiencies; this is discussed in more detail in Chapter 5. The dietary and medical treatments are also discussed in Chapter 5. Prokinetic agents are worth trying for postvagotomy emptying problems, though they may make diarrhoea worse. Surgical treatment with the construction of an intestinal pouch may be indicated after an extensive gastric resection, but is very much the territory of the super-specialist – the operations for this and other postgastric surgery problems are well described in Maingot's Abdominal Operations.[109]

Nutritional problems

These occur for three reasons:

1 The extent of gastric resection leading to restriction of meal size;
2 Severity of postprandial symptoms that also indirectly limit meal size.
3 Presence of bacterial overgrowth which particularly leads to fat malabsorption.

Nutritional sequelae are virtually unknown after HSV, uncommon after truncal vagotomy, but are a frequent long-term problem after gastrectomy. They are discussed in detail in Chapter 5.

Gastric cancer after previous ulcer surgery

There is evidence of an increased risk of gastric cancer after previous gastric resection. By convention the diagnosis of cancer within 5 years of the original operation is classed as a missed diagnosis. Stump cancer in the remnant stomach is usually seen 15–20 years after the first operation and is more common if the original operation was for a gastric ulcer. The aetiological factors include hypochlorhydria, allowing the growth of anaerobic bacteria that produce carcinogens from ingested nitrates and nitrosamines. Enterogastric reflux may also be important and it has been observed that most stump cancers develop close to the anastomosis. The role of *Helicobacter pylori* in stump cancer has not yet been established. If HP does have a role in the hypochlorhydric stomach then we may see an increased incidence in gastric cancer even after vagotomy procedures, although no significant evidence of this has emerged as yet. The important message clinically is to endoscope any patient who develops new upper abdominal symptoms at any time after previous ulcer surgery.

References

1. Kurata JH, Honda GD, Frankl H. Hospitalisation and mortality rates for peptic ulcers: a comparison of a large health maintenance organisation and US data. Gastroenterology 1982; 83: 1008–16.
2. Coggon D, Lambert P, Langman MJS. Twenty years of hospital admissions for peptic ulcer in England and Wales. Lancet 1981; i: 302–4.
3. Mortality statistics, cause. England and Wales 1990. Office of Population, Censuses and Surveys: HMSO, 1991.
4. Walt R, Katschinski B, Logan R, Ashley J, Langman M. Rising frequency of ulcer perforation in elderly people in the United Kingdom. Lancet 1986; i: 489–92.
5. Brown RC, Langman MJS, Lambert PM. Hospital admissions for peptic ulcer during 1968–1982. Br Med J 1976; 1: 35–7.
6. Susser S, Stein Z. Civilisation and peptic ulcer. Lancet 1962; i: 115–18.
7. Langman MJS. The epidemiology of chronic digestive disease. London: Arnold, 1979.
8. Mendelhoff AI. What has been happening to duodenal ulcer? Gastroenterology 1974; 67: 1020–2.
9. Friedman GD, Siegelaub AB, Seltzer CC. Cigarettes, alcohol, coffee and peptic ulcer. N Engl J Med 1974; 290; 469–73.
10. Paffenberger PS, Wing PL, Hyde RT. Chronic disease in former college students. XIII. Early precursors of peptic ulcer. Am J Epidemiol 1974; 100: 307–15.
11. Maddern GH, Horowitz M, Hetzel DJ, Jamieson GG. Altered solid and liquid gastric emptying in patients with duodenal ulcer disease. Gut 1985; 26: 689–93.
12. McCarthy DM. Smoking and ulcers – time to quit. N Engl J Med 1984; 311: 726.
13. Parente P, Lazzaroni MOS, Baroni S, Bianchi Porro G. Cigarette smoking, gastric acid secretion and serum pepsinogen 1 concentrations in duodenal ulcer patients. Gut 1985; 26: 1327–32.
14. Faulkner G, Prichard P, Sommerville K, Langman MJS. Aspirin and bleeding ulcers in the elderly. Br Med J 1988; 297: 1311–13.
15. Griffin MR, Piper JM, Daugherty JR, Snowden M, Ray WA. Non-steroidal anti-inflammatory drug use and increased risk for peptic ulcer disease in elderly persons. Ann Intern Med 1991; 114: 735–40.
16. Group AR. A randomised controlled trial of aspirin in persons recovered from myocardial infarction. JAMA 1980; 243: 661–9.
17. Warren RJ, Marshall BJ. Unidentified curved bacilli on gastric epithelium in active chronic gastritis. Lancet 1983; i: 1273–75.
18. Dixon MF. *Helicobacter pylori* and peptic ulceration: histopathological aspects. J Gastroenterol Hepatol 1991; 6: 125–30.
19. Berkowicz J, Lee A. Person to person transmission of *Campylobacter pylori* (letter). Lancet 1987; ii: 681–2.
20. Drumm B, Perez-Perez G, Blazer M, Sherman P. Intrafamilial clustering of *Campylobacter pylori* infection. N Engl J Med 1990; 312: 359–63.
21. Morris A, Nicholson G. Ingestion of *Campylobacter pyloridis* causes gastritis and raised fasting gastric acid. Am J Gastroenterol 1987; 82: 192–9.
22. Langenberg W, Rauws EAJ, Oudbier JH, Tygat GNJ. Patient to patient transmission of *Helicobacter pyloris* infection by fibreoptic gastroduodenoscopy and biopsy. J Infect Dis 1991; 61: 307–11.
23. Megraud F, Boussens J, Ruble MP *et al.* Seroepidemiology of *Campylobacter pylori* infection in various populations. J Clin Microbiol 1989; 27: 1870–3.
24. Pounder RE, Ng D. The prevalence of *Helicobacter pylori* infection in different countries. Aliment Pharmacol Ther 1995; 9 (Suppl 2): 33–9.
25. Rauws EAJ, Langenberg W, Houthoff HJ, Zanen HC, Tygat GNJ. *Campylobacter pyloridis*-associated chronic antral gastritis. Gastroenterology 1988; 94: 33–40.
26. NIH consensus conference. *Helicobacter pylori* in peptic ulcer disease. JAMA 1994; 272: 65–9.
27. Go MF, Tran L, Chan KY *et al.* REP-PCR finger print analysis reveals gastro-duodenal disease specific clusters of *Helicobacter pylori* strains. Am J Gastroenterol 1993; 88: 1591.
28. Hessey ST, Spenger J, Wyatt JI. Bacterial adhesion and disease activity in *Helicobacter*-associated chronic gastritis. Gut 1990; 31: 134–8.
29. Tee W, Lambert JR, Pegorer M, Dwyer B.

Cytotoxin production by *Helicobacter pylori* more common in peptic ulcer disease. Gastroenterology 1993; 104: A789.

30. Leunk RD. Production of a cytotoxin by *Helicobacter pylori*. Rev Infect Dis 1991; 13: S686–9.

31. Tummuru MKR, Sharma SA, Blaser MJ. *Helicobacter pylori* picB, a homolog of the *Bordatella pertussis* toxin secretion protein, is required for induction of IL-8 in gastric epithelial cells. Mol Microbiol 1995; 18: 867–76.

32. Boren T, Falk P, Roth KA, Larson G, Normak S. Attachment of *Helicobacter pylori* to human gastric epithelium mediated by blood group antigens. Science 1993; 262:1892–5.

33. The Eurogast Study Group. An international association between *Helicobacter pylori* infection and gastric cancer. Lancet 1993; 391: 1359–62.

34. Playford R. Cytokines and *Helicobacter pylori* – a growth area. Gut 1996; 39: 881–2.

35. Dunn B. Pathogenic mechanisms of *Helicobacter pylori*. Gastroenterol Clin North Am 1993; 22: 43–57.

36. Graham DY, Go MF, Lew GM, Genta RM, Rehfeld JF. *Helicobacter pylori* infection and exaggerated gastrin release. Effects of inflammation on progastrin processing. Scand J Gastroenterol 1993; 28: 690–4.

37. Graham DY. Lechago J. Antral G-cell and D-cell numbers in *Helicobacter pylori* infection; effect of *Helicobacter pylori* eradication. Gastroenterology 1993; 104: 1655–60.

38. El-Omar E, Panman I, Dorrain CA, Ardill JES, McColl KEL. Eradicating *Helicobacter pylori* infection lowers gastrin-mediated acid secretion by two thirds in patients with duodenal ulcer. Gut 1993; 34: 1060–5.

39. Podolsky I, Storms PR, Richardson CT, Peterson WL, Fordtran JS. Gastric adenocarcinoma masquerading endoscopically as benign gastric ulcer: a five-year experience. Dig Dis Sci 1988; 33: 1057–63.

40. Soll AH. Medical treatment of peptic ulcer disease – practice guidelines. JAMA 1996; 275: 622–9.

41. Laine L, Martin-Sorensen M, Weinstein WM. Non-steroidal antiinflammatory drug-associated gastric ulcers do not require *Helicobacter pylori* for their development. Am J Gastroenterol 1992; 87: 1398–402.

42. Heresbach D, Raoul JL, Bretagne JF *et al.* *Helicobacter pylori*: a risk and severity factor of non-steroidal anti-inflammatory drug induced gastropathy. Gut 1992; 33: 1608–11

43. Coghlan JG, Gilligan O, Humphries H *et al.* *Campylobacter pylori* and recurrence of duodenal ulcers: a 12 month follow up study. Lancet 1987; ii: 1109–11.

44. Graham DY, Lew GM, Klein PD *et al.* Effect of treatment of *Helicobacter pylori* infection on the long term recurrence of gastric or duodenal ulcer. Ann Intern med 1992; 116: 705–8.

45. Forbes GM, Glaser ME, Cullen DJE *et al.* Duodenal ulcer treatment with *Helicobacter pylori* eradication: seven year follow up. Lancet 1994; 343: 258–60.

46. Graham DY, Heaps KS, Ramirex FC *et al.* Treatment of *H. pylori* reduces the rate of rebleeding in complicated peptic ulcer disease. Scand J Gastroenterol 1993; 28: 939–42.

47. Banatvala N, Davies GR, Abdi Y, Clements L, Rampton DS, Hordie JM. High prevalence of *Helicobacter pylori* metronidazole resistance in migrants to East London: relation with previous nitroimidazole exposure and gastroduodenal disease. Gut 1994; 35: 1562–6.

48. de Boer W, Driessen W, Jansz A, Tytgat GNJ. Effect of acid suppression on efficacy of treatment for *Helicobacter pylori* infection. Lancet 1995; 345: 817–19.

49. Lind T, Velduyzen van Zanten SJO, Unge P *et al.* Eradication of *Helicobacter pylori* using one week triple therapies combining omeprazole with two antimicrobials. The MACH 1 study. Helicobacter 1996; 1: 138–44.

50. Misiewicz JJ, Harris AW, Bardham KD, Levi S, Longworthy H. One week low-dose triple therapy for eradication of *Helicobacter pylori*: a large multicentre, randomised trial. Gut 1996; 38 (suppl): A1.

51. Malfertheiner P, Megraud F, O'Morain C *et al.* Current European concepts in the management of *Helicobacter pylori* infection – the Maastricht consensus report. Eur J Gastroenterol Hepatol 1997; 9: 1–2.

52. Maton PN. Omeprazole (review) N Engl J Med 1991; 324: 965–75.

53. Howden CW, Jones DB, Peace KE, Burget DW, Hunt RH. The treatment of gastric ulcer with anti-secretory drugs: relationship of pharmacological effect to healing rates. Dig Dis Sc 1988; 33: 619–24.

54. Zollinger RM, Ellison EH. Primary peptic ulcerations of the jejunum associated with islet cell tumours of the pancreas. Ann Surg 1955; 142: 709–23.

55. Bondeson AG, Bondeson L, Thompson NW. Stricture and perforation of the oesophagus: overlooked threats in Zollinger–Ellison syndrome. World J Surg 1990; 14: 361–3.

56. Jaffe BN. Surgery for gut hormone-producing tumours. Am J Med 1987; 82 (Suppl 5B): 68–76.

57. Ellison EH, Wilson SD. The Zollinger–Ellison syndrome: re-appraisal and evaluation of 260 registered cases. Ann Surg 1964; 160: 512–20.

58. Stabile BE, Pessaro E. Benign and malignant gastrinoma. Am J Surg 1985; 149: 144–50.

59. Zollinger RM, Ellison EC, O'Darisio TM, Sparks J. Thirty years of experience with gastrinoma. World J Surg 1984; 8: 427–35.

60. McArthur KE, Richardson CT, Barnett CC et al. Laparotomy and proximal gastric vagotomy in Zollinger–Ellison syndrome: results of a 16-year prospective study. Am J Gastroenterol 1996; 91(6): 1104–11.

61. Richardson CT, Peters MN, Feldman M et al. Treatment of Zollinger–Ellison with exploratory laparotomy, proximal gastric vagotomy and H2 receptor antagonists. A prospective study. Gastroenterology 1985; 89: 357–67.

62. Jensen RT, Fraker DL. Zollinger–Ellison syndrome: advances in treatment of the gastric hypersecretion and the gastrinoma. JAMA 1994; 271: 1–7.

63. Maton PN, Miller DL, Doppman JL et al. Role of selective angiography in the management of patients with Zollinger–Ellison syndrome. Gastroenterology 1987; 92: 913.

64. Johnston D, Wilkinson AR. Highly selective vagotomy without a drainage procedure in the treatment of duodenal ulceration. Br J Surg 1970; 57: 289–95.

65. Johnston D. Operative mortality and postoperative morbidity of highly selective vagotomy. Br Med J 1975; 4: 545–7.

66. Johnston D, Humphrey CS, Walker BE et al. Vagotomy without diarrhoea. Br Med J 1972; 3: 788–90.

67. Jordan PH, Thornby J. Should it be parietal cell vagotomy or selective vagotomy antrectomy for treatment of duodenal ulcer? Ann Surg 1987; 205: 572–87.

68. Johnston D, Axon ATR. Highly selective vagotomy for duodenal ulcer – the clinical results after 10 years. Br J Surg 1979; 66: 874–8.

69. Blackett RL, Johnston D. Recurrent ulceration after highly selective vagotomy for duodenal ulcer. Br J Surg 1981; 68: 705–10.

70. Donahue PE, Bombeck T, Yoshida J, Nyhus LM. Endoscopic congo red test during proximal gastric vagotomy. Am J Surg 1987; 153: 249–55.

71. Chisholm EM, Raimes SA, Leong HT, Chung SCS, Li AKC. Proximal gastric vagotomy and anterior seromyotomy with posterior truncal vagotomy assessed by the endoscopic congo red test. Br J Surg 1993; 80: 737–9.

72. Taylor TV, Gunn AA, Macleod DAD et al. Anterior lesser curve seromyotomy with posterior truncal vagotomy for duodenal ulcer. Br J Surg 1985; 72: 950–1.

73. Raimes SA, Smirniotis V, Wheldon EJ, Venables CW, Johnston IDA. Post-vagotomy diarrhoea put into perspective. Lancet 1987; ii: 851–3.

74. Dorricott NJ, McNeish AR, Alexander-Williams J et al. Prospective randomised multicentre trial of proximal gastric vagotomy or truncal vagotomy and antrectomy for chronic duodenal ulcer: interim results. Br J Surg 1978; 65: 152–4.

75. DeVries BC, Schattenkirk EM, Smith EEJ et al. Prospective randomised trial of proximal gastric vagotomy or truncal vagotomy and antrectomy for chronic duodenal ulcer: results after 5–7 years. Br J Surg 1983; 70: 701–3.

76. Primrose JN, Axon ATR, Johnston D. Highly selective vagotomy and ulcers that fail to respond to H2 receptor antagonists. Br Med J 1988; 296: 1031–5.

77. Yunfu L, Yiding H, Shouren J et al. Experimental study of pylorus and pyloric vagus preserving gastrectomy. World J Surg 1993; 17: 525–9.

78. Bloom BS. Cross-national changes in the effects of peptic ulcer disease. Ann Intern Med 1991; 114: 558–62.

79. Bardhan KD, Cust G, Hinchliffe RFC et al. Changing patterns of admissions and operations for duodenal ulcer. Br J Surg 1989; 76: 230–6.

80. Schrumpf A, Stadaas J, Myren J, Serck-Hanssen A, Aune S, Osnes M. Mucosal

changes in the gastric stump 20–25 years after partial gastrectomy. Lancet 1977; ii: 467–9.

81. Donovan AJ, Vinson TL, Maulsby GO, Gewin JR. Selective treatment of duodenal ulcer with perforation. Ann Surg 1979; 189: 627–36.

82. Taylor H. Aspiration treatment of perforated ulcers. Lancet 1951; i: 7–12.

83. Crofts TJ, Park KGM, Steele RJC, Chung SSC, Li AKC. A randomised trial of nonoperative treatment for perforated peptic ulcer. N Eng J Med 1989; 320: 970–3.

84. Sawyers JL. Acute perforation of peptic ulcer. In: Scott Jr HW, Sawyers JL (ed) Surgery of the stomach, duodenum and small intestines, 2nd edn. Boston, Massachusetts: Blackwell Scientific, 1992; pp. 566–72.

85. Abbasakoor F, Attwood SE, McGrath JP, Stephens RB. Simple closure and follow up of H2 receptor antagonists for perforated peptic ulcer – immediate survival and symptomatic outcome. Irish Med J 1995; 88: 207–9.

86. Eggstein S, Finke M, Rickauer K, Farthmann EH. Results of simple closure of perforated peptic ulcer. Langenbeck's Archiv Chir 1996; s2: 1266–7.

87. Boey J, Wong J, Ong GB. A prospective study of operative risk factors in perforated duodenal ulcers. Ann Surg 1982; 195: 265–9.

88. Sunderland GT, Chisholm EM, Lau WY, Chang SCS, Li AKC. Laparosopic repair of perforated peptic ulcer. Br J Surg 1992; 79: 785–9.

89. Mouret P, Francois Y, Vagnal J, Barth X, Lombard-Platet R. Laparoscopic treatment of perforated peptic ulcer. Br J Surg 1990; 77: 1006.

90. Miserez M, Eypasch E, Spangenberger W, Lefering R, Troidl H. Laparoscopic and conventional closure of perforated peptic ulcer – a comparison. Surg Endosc Ultrasound Intervent Techniques 1996; 10: 831–6.

91. Mutter D, Evrard S, Keller P, Vix M, Vartolomei S, Maresaux J. Perforated peptic ulcer – the laparoscopic approach. Ann Chir 1994; 48: 339–44.

92. Munro WS, Bajwa F, Menzies D. Laparoscopic repair of perforated duodenal ulcers with a falciform ligament patch. Ann R Coll Surg Eng 1996; 78: 390–1.

93. Griffin SM, Chung SCS, Leung JWC, Li AKC. Peptic pyloric stenosis treated by endoscopic balloon dilatation. Br J Surg 1989; 76: 1147–8.

94. Chisholm EM, Chung SCS, Leung JWC. Peptic pyloric stenosis – after the balloon goes up! Gastronintest Endosc 1993; 37: 240.

95. Eypasch E, Spongenberger W, Ure B, Mannigen R, Troidl H. Laparoscopic and conventional closure of perforated peptic ulcer – a comparison. Chirurg 1994; 65: 445–50.

96. Wyman A, Stuart RC, Ng EKW, Chung SCS, Li AKC. Laparoscopic truncal vagotomy and gastroenterostomy for pyloric stenosis. Am J Surg 1996; 171: 600–3.

97. Ralphs DNL, Thomson JPS, Haynes S et al. The relationship between the rate of gastric emptying and the dumping syndrome. Br J Surg 1978; 65: 844–8.

98. Hopman WPM, Wolberink RGJ, Lamers CBHW, van Tongeren JHM. Treatment of the dumping syndrome with a somatostatin analogue SMS 201–995. Ann Surg 1988; 207: 155–9.

99. Primrose JN, Johnston D. Somatostatin analogue SMS 201-995 (octreotide) as a possible solution to the dumping syndrome after gastrectomy and vagotomy. Br J Surg 1989; 76: 140–4.

100. Cheadle WG, Baker PR, Cuschieri A. Pyloric reconstruction for severe vasomotor dumping after vagotomy and pyloroplasty. Ann Surg 1985; 202: 568–72.

101. Kelly KA, Becker JM, van Heerden JA. Reconstructive gastric surgery. Br J Surg 1981; 68: 687–91.

102. Vogel SB, Hocking MP, Woodward ER. Clinical and radionuclide evaluation of Roux-Y diversion for postgastrectomy dumping. Am J Surg 1988; 155: 57–62.

103. Karlstrom L, Soper NJ, Kelly KA et al. Ectopic jejunal pacemakers and enterogastric reflux after Roux gastrectomy: effect of intestinal pacing. Surgery 1989; 106: 867–71.

104. Mathias JR, Fernandez A, Sninsky CA et al. Nausea, vomiting and abdominal pain after Roux-en-Y anastomosis: motility of the jejunal limb. Gastroenterology 1985; 88: 101–7.

105. Raimes SA. Postvagotomy diarrhoea. MD Thesis, University of Newcastle upon Tyne, 1990.

106. Cuschieri A. Surgical management of severe intractable postvagotomy diarrhoea. Br J Surg 1986; 73: 981–4.

107. Donovan IA, Fielding JWL, Bradby H *et al.* Bile diversion after total gastrectomy. Br J Surg 1982; 69: 389–90.

108. Demeester TR, Fuchs KH, Ball CS *et al.* Experimental and clinical results with proximal end-to-end duodeno-jejunostomy for pathological duodenogastric reflux. Ann Surg 1987; 206: 414–26.

109. Herrington JL Jr, Sawyers JL. Complications following gastric operations. In: Schwarz SI, Ellis H (eds) Maingot's abdominal operations, 9th edn. Norwalk, Connecticut, Appleton and Lange, 1989, pp. 701–30.

13 The treatment of non-variceal upper gastrointestinal bleeding

Robert J. C. Steele

Introduction

Non-variceal upper gastrointestinal bleeding remains a significant problem in the Western World. A recent population based audit of upper gastrointestinal bleeding (the first in 25 years)[1] gives the incidence of acute bleeding as 103 cases per 100 000 adults per year. Of this variceal bleeding accounted for only 4% of the total. Overall mortality was 14% (11% in emergency admissions and 33% among inpatients who began bleeding).

It is interesting to compare these figures with those from two previous studies from the 1960s,[2,3] where mortality was 10% and 14% respectively. It is important to note, however, that 27% of patients from the recent audit were over the age of 80 years, as compared with less than 10% in the earlier studies, and that both incidence and mortality increased markedly with age.

Thus, although there has been little improvement in mortality over the years, this observation must be set against a dramatic shift in the age of the population at risk.

There is no room for complacency, however, and there is little doubt that the formation of specialist gastrointestinal bleeding units can minimise the morbidity and mortality of gastrointestinal bleeding.[4] Many of the therapeutic advances described in this chapter have been shown to have a significant effect, but it must be stressed that they can only be useful when employed by enthusiastic, dedicated and properly trained personnel.

Aetiology

Peptic ulcer remains by far the most common cause for upper gastrointestinal haemorrhage in the Western World. The recent audit reported by Rockall and others[1] found that peptic ulcer accounted for

Figure 13.1
Frequency of causes for upper gastro-intestinal bleeding in the United Kingdom. (From Rockall et al.[1])

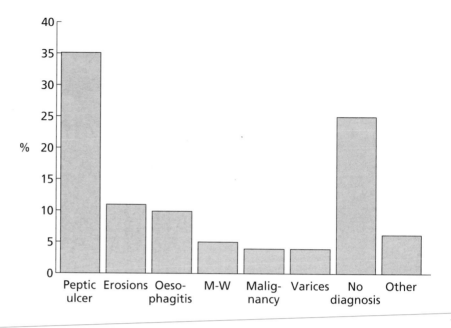

35% of cases (Fig. 13.1), and the rest of this chapter is therefore largely devoted to the management of this problem. Peptic ulcers bleed because of erosion of blood vessels, and the severity of the bleed is dependent on the size of the vessel affected. Simple oozing is caused by damage to small submucosal vessels less than 0.1 mm in diameter, but the more important arterial bleeding indicates a large vessel (between 0.1 and 2 mm in diameter) in the base of the ulcer which has been eroded by the inflammatory process.

In this case, the vessel tends to loop up to the base of the ulcer (Fig. 13.2), and when the apex of this loop becomes eroded, haemorrhage occurs. This defect in the artery may become plugged by a sentinel clot or thrombus, and it is this which is usually interpreted as a visible vessel by the endoscopist. In ulcers on the posterior wall of the duodenum or the lesser curve of the stomach the gastroduodenal or left gastric arteries can be involved, and these lesions are particularly prone to massive haemorrhage and rebleeding after initial stabilisation.[5]

Other less common but appreciably frequent causes of non-variceal upper gastrointestinal bleeding include erosions, oesophagitis, Mallory–Weiss tears and malignancy.

Erosions

Acute erosive gastritis must be distinguished from the chronic forms of gastritis as these do not bleed. Haemorrhagic gastritis is often caused by stressful stimuli such as head injury, burns, shock or hepatic failure and is probably related to impaired mucosal blood flow. Drugs may also be responsible, and the agents which are commonly

Figure 13.2 *Vessel looping up to the ulcer base.*

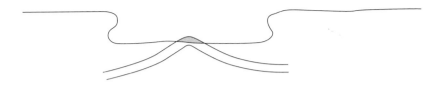

implicated include steroids, non-steroidal inflammatory agents and alcohol.

Oesophagitis

Oesophagitis is a form of peptic ulcer disease, but usually only causes minor acute bleeding. Occasionally, however, a significant vessel may be involved with consequent massive arterial haemorrhage which must be distinguished from variceal bleeding.

Mallory–Weiss tear

The Mallory–Weiss (M-W) tear occurs in the region of the gastro-oesophageal junction as a result of severe vomiting or retching, often after excessive alcohol intake. The tear is mostly in the gastric mucosa, but may extend into the oesophagus, and although bleeding is profuse, it usually stops spontaneously. Very occasionally repeated vomiting may result in a full thickness tear, 'Boerhaave's syndrome' and this is inevitably associated with sudden onset of severe pain in the upper abdomen or chest.

Malignancy

Carcinoma and lymphoma of the stomach, when at an advanced ulcerated stage, commonly bleed. This usually results in occult blood loss, but will occasionally present with acute haemorrhage.

Other diagnoses

There are several other conditions which may present as upper gastrointestinal haemorrhage and these are listed in Table 13.1.

Presentation and assessment

Patients with acute gastrointestinal haemorrhage present with haematemesis, melaena or frank rectal bleeding plus the signs and symptoms of hypovolaemia in varying degrees. Haematemesis implies vomiting of blood, either in a recognisable form or as dark brown grainy material ('coffee grounds') if the blood has been in the stomach long enough for acid to convert the haemoglobin into methaemoglobin.

Table 13.1   *Causes of upper gastrointestinal bleeding*

	Oesophagus	Stomach	Duodenum	Small bowel
Inflammation	Oesophagitis Barret's ulcer	Peptic ulcer Gastritis Dieulafoy lesion	Peptic ulcer	Peptic ulcer at stoma or Meckel's diverticulum Crohn's disease
Vascular abnormalities	Varices Aortic aneurysm	Varices Vascular malformation	Aorto-duodenal fistula	Vascular malformation
Neoplasia	Carcinoma	Carcinoma Leiomyoma Lymphoma Polyp	Carcinoma of ampulla Carcinoma of pancreas	Tumour
Other	Mallory–Weiss tear		Haemobilia Pancreatitis Post ERCP	Diverticulum

Melaena is the passage of altered blood per rectum. This is recognised as jet black liquid stool, sometimes tinged red when very fresh, which has a characteristic, pungent smell. It results from the oxidation of haem by intestinal and bacterial enzymes, and indicates that the site of bleeding is probably from the upper gastrointestinal tract, and almost certainly proximal to the ileocaecal junction. It is important to appreciate that melaena can persist for several days after the cessation of active bleeding, and its continued appearance may be misleading. It is also very important to distinguish between melaena and other causes of dark stool. Simple constipation tends to be associated with hard, dark faeces, and oral iron results in a sticky but relatively solid grey–black motion.

Fresh rectal bleeding immediately suggests a site within the colon, rectum or anal canal, but it must be remembered that brisk bleeding from the upper gastrointestinal tract can easily present in this way. Thus, in the patient with massive fresh rectal bleeding, particularly when there are signs of hypovolaemia, urgent steps must be taken to exclude bleeding from the stomach or duodenum.

When the patient with acute gastrointestinal bleeding has been identified from one of the above symptoms, the following assessment and management plan should be instituted.

1. Assess the patient rapidly to ascertain airway patency, conscious level and external signs of blood loss.

2. Measure pulse and blood pressure.
3. Establish venous access and cross-match blood.
4. If the patient is haemodynamically stable, obtain a full history, carry out a full examination and proceed with investigations promptly but within normal working hours.
5. If the patient is haemodynamically unstable, fluid resuscitation must start immediately. If an adequate pulse and blood pressure are achieved rapidly and can be maintained without aggressive fluid replacement, then it is possible to proceed as for the stable patient. However, if any difficulty is encountered in stabilisation, it is necessary to investigate the patient rapidly, often with *simultaneous* resuscitation.

Investigation

The mainstay of the investigation of acute upper gastrointestinal bleeding is flexible endoscopy. Accordingly, this section concentrates mostly on endoscopy and is divided into the following sections: (1) endoscopy equipment, (2) technique in acute bleeding; (3) endoscopic appearances in acute bleeding and (4) other diagnostic techniques.

Endoscopy equipment

Most modern endoscopy units have videoendoscopy equipment, and for routine gastrointestinal endoscopy this has major advantages. First, it affords an excellent view to all the members of the team, which is of great importance for endoscopic intervention where the assistant has to coordinate with the endoscopist, and it greatly facilitates teaching. Secondly, the head of the endoscope is held away from the endoscopist's face, which reduces the risk of blood or secretions splashing into the eyes.

Unfortunately, even the latest generation of videoendoscopy equipment is not ideal for examining the bleeding patient. In the presence of large amounts of blood the image can become very dark and fuzzy owing to saturation of the 'red channel' of the chip camera, and this can seriously hamper both diagnosis and therapy. Thus, although videoendoscopy is often suitable for upper gastrointestinal haemorrhage, it is useful to have a direct-viewing instrument to hand for the demanding situation.

The endoscope itself must be chosen with some care for the particular circumstances. The slim or 'paediatric' instrument is very manoeuvrable, but its 2.8 mm working or biopsy channel limits the use of therapeutic accessories, and does not allow good suction. The big double-channel endoscope allows good suction and washing through the unoccupied channel when an accessory is in use, but it is uncomfortable for the patient and cumbersome when trying to reach relatively inaccessible lesions. The best compromise is an endoscope with a single wide (3.7 mm) working channel, and a separate forward washing channel which allows good suction and the passage of a wide range of therapeutic instruments.

Other pieces of equipment which are important in the acute bleeding situation include a lavage tube, a pharyngeal overtube, washing devices and therapeutic accessories. *The lavage tube* is occasionally required when the stomach is full of clot, and the most useful device is a wide bore (40 Fr if possible), soft tube with an open end as well as side holes. *The pharyngeal overtube* is a 30 cm tube with a flange at one end to prevent it slipping into the mouth. This can be passed over the endoscope when lavage is needed; it both facilitates repeated changes between the endoscope and the lavage tube, while at the same time protecting the airway. The simplest *washing method* is to insert the nozzle of a 20 ml syringe filled with water directly into the working or washing channel of the endoscope and to empty its contents in one rapid action. A useful alternative is to use a dental irrigator (water toothbrush) modified by the provision of a foot switch and by attaching the outlet to the working or washing channel. Finally it is important to have all the therapeutic accessories that might be required immediately to hand; these will be described in a later section.

Endoscopy technique in acute bleeding

Even when not urgent as a life-saving procedure, endoscopy should take place within 24 h of admission, as the chance of making a diagnosis diminishes rapidly after this time.[6] Usually the endoscopy will take place in the endoscopy room under benzodiazepine sedation, but in the patient who is vomiting copious quantities of blood, general anaesthesia with cuffed endotracheal intubation should be considered. When sedation is considered adequate, careful monitoring is still required, and the patient's pulse and blood pressure should be measured regularly, preferably using an automatic device. Pulse oximetry should also be regarded as mandatory, as arterial desaturation is a particular risk during a prolonged procedure with a large diameter endoscope. For this reason it is also wise to administer oxygen throughout the procedure, either nasally or by means of a specially designed mouth guard. It is essential to have adequate staffing in the endoscopy room to cope with both the procedure and the ongoing monitoring and resuscitation of the patient.

The endoscopy should take place on a bed or trolley which can tip into either the head-up or head-down position. The examination should start with the patient in the strict left lateral position, as this encourages blood to pool in the fundus of the stomach where ulcers are uncommon (Fig. 13.3). If it becomes necessary to view the fundus, this can be done by turning the patient on to the right side, and tipping the trolley head-up so that the blood falls into the antrum. When the endoscope has been passed beyond the gastro-oesophageal junction, it is not uncommon to encounter a seeming impenetrable mass of blood and clot. However, as long as the stomach is given long enough to distend and the above guidelines are followed, a moderate amount

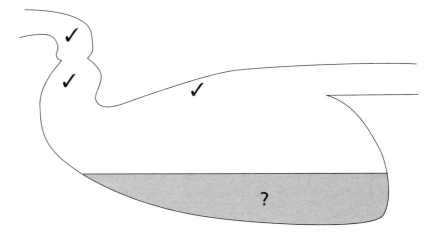

Figure 13.3 *Pooling of blood in the stomach in the left lateral position. This leaves the lesser curve, antrum and duodenum clear of blood. ✕, indicates areas visible; ?, indicates area of uncertainty.*

of blood in the stomach rarely prevents adequate visualisation of the responsible lesion. Often clot will be seen overlying an ulcer, and it is important to wash this to ascertain whether or not it is adherent; this has implications for prognosis and treatment, and gentle washing will rarely precipitate haemorrhage.

Occasionally, however, there will be too much blood in the stomach to allow an adequate examination, and lavage will be necessary. The 40 Fr lavage tube, ideally with a pharyngeal overtube in place, is passed into the stomach and direct suction is applied. This will often clear enough blood and clot to allow the examination to proceed. If not, it then becomes necessary to carry out a formal lavage, by rapidly pouring in a litre of water via a funnel. This will break up the clot, which can then be siphoned out by placing the tube in a dependent position.

Endoscopic appearances of the bleeding ulcer

The endoscopic appearance of a peptic ulcer which has bled or is still bleeding provides valuable prognostic information which can be used to predict outcome and risk of rebleeding.[7–10] Various classification systems have been used, and possibly the most popular has been that proposed by Forrest and others which distinguishes between active bleeding, a non-bleeding visible vessel and adherent clot.[6] Unfortunately, however, there is considerable interobserver variation in the interpretation of these appearances[11–13] indicating that the descriptive terms commonly employed lack sufficient precision. It is nonetheless important to have some means of describing the 'stigmata of recent haemorrhage', and the categories given below are widely recognised.

Active arterial bleeding indicates erosion of an artery or arteriole, and although studies have indicated that this type of bleeding may stop in up to 40% of cases[14], it is regarded as a clear indication for intervention.

Active non-pulsatile bleeding or oozing from the base of an ulcer implies ongoing bleeding from a partially occluded vessel and is associated with a 20–30% chance of continued bleeding. It must be distinguished from contact bleeding from the edge of an ulcer which is of no significance.

A visible vessel is best defined as a raised lesion in the base of an ulcer. This may represent either an exposed vessel or an organised thrombus plugging a hole in the underlying vessel, and is important as it carries a significant risk of rebleeding if untreated. The precise risk is difficult to ascertain because there is considerable disagreement among endoscopists as to what constitutes a visible vessel,[11–13] but it is probably in the region of 30–50%.

Adherent blood clot may be difficult to distinguish from a visible vessel, but as the underlying pathology is usually identical, making the distinction is not absolutely necessary.

Flat red or *black spots* indicate dried blood in the slough of the ulcer base, and are of little significance, with a rebleeding rate of less than 5%.

These stigmata change fairly rapidly, and a recent study from China has indicated that visible vessels disappear in a mean of four days.[15] Given the sinister implications of a visible vessel, it is unwise to discharge a patient from hospital until endoscopic evidence of fading is seen, regardless of whether or not endoscopic therapy has been delivered.

Other diagnostic techniques

When upper gastrointestinal endoscopy by an experienced endoscopist fails to provide the diagnosis, other approaches are required. If blood is not seen in the stomach, and the patient is haemodynamically unstable with continuing signs of bleeding, it is usually best to move immediately to mesenteric angiography.[16] With fresh melaena or rectal bleeding, colonoscopy is usually fruitless, and if the blood loss is more than 0.5 ml min^{-1}, on angiography the bleeding site will be seen as contrast entering the bowel lumen.

If the bleeding site is in the colon, its anatomical position will be obvious. However, when it is in the small bowel localisation can be a problem, and it is helpful for the radiologist to leave a super-selective angiogram catheter as close as possible to the lesion so that at laparotomy the affected segment of bowel can be identified by injection of methylene blue.

When the patient is bleeding intermittently, angiography may not be able to detect the blood loss, and in this case labelled red call scanning may provide useful information.[17] A blood sample is taken, the red cells labelled with an isotope such as ^{99m}Tc-methyl diphosphonate or Indium-111 and re-injected into the patient. When the bleeding occurs, a proportion of the cells will enter the gut and be seen as a distinct 'blush' on the gamma-camera image. Unfortunately, once blood has entered the intestine it rapidly moves along making local-

Figure 13.4
Algorithm for the investigation of massive rectal bleeding.

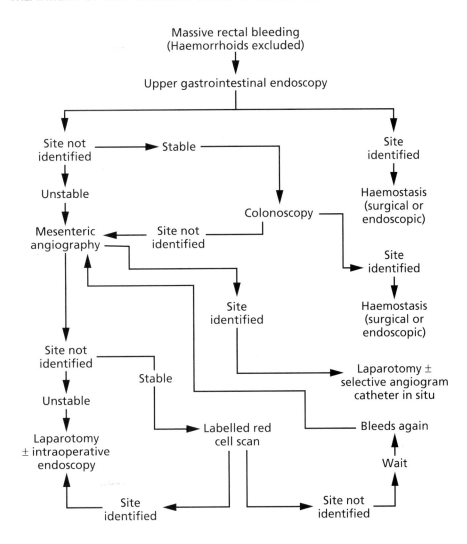

isation of the lesion imprecise. For this reason it is important for the patient to have regular, frequent scans over a prolonged period, and this is often not feasible.

Occasionally it will be impossible to localise the site of bleeding, and the surgeon will be forced into an exploratory operation. At laparotomy it is usually possible to determine whether the bleeding is originating from the small or large bowel, and an appropriate intra-operative endoscopy can be performed to pin-point the lesion.[18,19] This is done either per anum after antegrade lavage of the colon with warm saline, or through a small bowel enterotomy at the most convenient site. An algorithm for the investigation of massive melaena or rectal bleeding is given in Fig. 13.4.

Medical treatment

The majority of cases of upper gastrointestinal bleeding will resolve spontaneously, and supportive care will be all that is necessary. There is, however, little evidence that specific pharmacological intervention has any effect on peptic ulcer bleeding despite a number of well conducted trials.

Reduction of gastric acid secretion might be expected to help, as an acid environment impairs platelet function and haemostasis, and a meta-analysis of trials of H_2 receptor antagonists has suggested that such therapy might reduce mortality, especially for gastric ulcer bleeding.[20] Meta-analysis has its limitations, however, and more important data come from two large independent placebo-controlled randomised trials. The first examined the effect of the powerful H_2 receptor antagonist famotidine,[21] and the second looked at the proton pump inhibitor omeprazole.[22] Neither was able to demonstrate any effect, and it has to be concluded that acid suppression has little influence on the course of gastrointestinal haemorrhage.

Inhibition of fibrinolysis has also been explored, and in one large trial of tranexamic acid, a significant 50% reduction in mortality was seen.[23] However, there were no differences in rebleeding or operation rates, and for this reason the study has been criticised. All the trials of tranexamic acid have been put together in a meta-analysis which suggests that patients do benefit,[24] but as this conclusion was greatly influenced by the one positive study the use of fibrinolysis therapy cannot be firmly recommended.

Somatostatin has also been tested in peptic ulcer bleeding on the basis of its ability to reduce both acid secretion and splanchnic blood flow, but apart from some evidence that it may be useful in torrential bleeding from gastric erosions,[25] the trials have been disappointing. The prostaglandin analogue misoprostol appears to be promising, and there is one small trial which indicates that it may reduce the need for emergency surgery in peptic ulcer bleeding.[26]

Overall, therefore, the evidence indicates that pharmacological treatment makes little difference to the outcome in non-variceal upper gastrointestinal haemorrhage. Further studies are underway, however, and the results are awaited with interest.

Endoscopic treatment

Endoscopic haemostasis for peptic ulcer bleeding is now well established, and many randomised trials testify to the ability of several treatment modalities in reducing rebleeding and the need for emergency surgery. In this section, the various available methods will be described, and evidence relating to their efficacy will be reviewed.

Techniques of endoscopic haemostasis

Currently, the main endoscopic techniques available for controlling peptic ulcer bleeding are laser photocoagulation, bipolar diathermy, heater probe, injection sclerotherapy and adrenaline injection. Each of these will now be considered in turn.

Laser photocoagulation

Laser photocoagulation is essentially a method of delivering energy which is converted into heat on contact with tissue. The laser which is now used almost exclusively for peptic ulcer bleeding is the neodymium yttrium aluminium garnet (Nd-YAG), as this appears to achieve sufficient tissue penetration to coagulate vessels of reasonable size. A suitable laser unit has to be capable of delivering 60–100 watts, and it is best used with a double-channel endoscope. This allows adequate venting which prevents overdistension of the stomach and permits escape of the smoke generated by vaporisation of tissue.

When an ulcer is to be treated by laser therapy, it is washed clear of blood and loose clot so that the bleeding point can be clearly seen. A red helium neon aiming beam is then activated, and a test 0.5 s 70 watt pulse of the invisible Nd-YAG laser delivered to the edge of the ulcer. If the settings are correct, this should cause blanching of the mucosa but no ulceration. Ideally, the fibre should be 1 cm from the ulcer when the laser is activated.

The aim is then to coagulate the feeding vessel, but it is impossible to be sure of the course of this vessel from the external appearance of the ulcer (Fig. 13.5). For this reason it is necessary to surround the bleeding point or visible vessel with a tight ring of pulses. This will maximise the chances of delivering heat both upstream and downstream of the exposed portion of the vessel.

The main reported dangers of laser therapy are perforation of the stomach or duodenum and exacerbation of the bleeding, but these can be minimised by good technique. The laser is also hazardous for staff, and it is important for everyone involved to wear specific filter goggles to prevent possible retinal damage; the room used also has to be specifically modified. These problems, together with the cost of the

Figure 13.5
Diagram illustrating the unpredictability of the course of a vessel which becomes visible in an ulcer base.

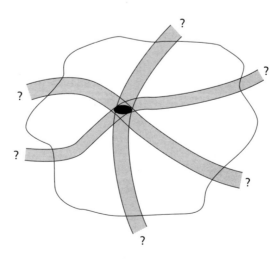

laser unit, its relative immobility and the rather indifferent results achieved in randomised trials, have resulted in laser therapy being superseded by the simpler methods described below.

Bipolar diathermy

Diathermy also relies on the generation of heat, this time by electrical current flowing through tissue near an electrode. This can be achieved by a monopolar or a bipolar system, but the former causes an unpredictably deep thermal injury and adherence of coagulated tissue to the probe can be a problem. Bipolar diathermy avoids these disadvantages to a greater extent, and has now superseded the monopolar equipment.

All contact probes, including bipolar diathermy and heat probes, rely on coaptive coagulation to achieve optimum results (Fig. 13.6). This implies that the walls of the vessel to be treated are brought into close apposition by external pressure while heat is applied. This has two advantages. First, if the pressure stops active bleeding, it means that the probe must be correctly positioned. Second, the dissipation of heat by the flow of blood ('heat sink') is minimised so that the heat has maximum effect.

The bipolar device which is now most widely used is the BICAP® probe which consists of three pairs of bipolar electrodes arranged radially around the tip. This allows current to pass into the tissue regardless of the angle of the probe tip relative to the surface of the ulcer. The current delivered to tissue is dependent on electrical resistance, and as this increases with desiccation, the current flow is decreased as the tissue heats up and dries out, thus limiting damage. The probes come in various sizes, but the best results have been reported with the largest (3.2 mm).

As for laser therapy, the ulcer must be washed to obtain a good view of the bleeding point, and if there is active bleeding this should be compressed firmly in order to obtain as much control as possible. The power and pulse length can be varied considerably, and there is some debate as to the ideal settings. Conventionally, a 50 W 2 s pulse is delivered two or three times, but it has recently been suggested that using a lower power for a longer time produces better results by allowing deeper energy penetration of the tissue.

When there is a non-bleeding visible vessel tamponade of haemorrhage is not available to provide the clue as to where to place the

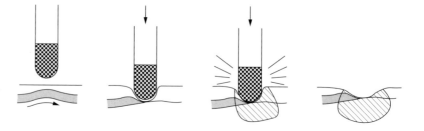

Figure 13.6
Coaptive coagulation.

probe, and it is then necessary to produce a ring of coagulation around the vessel as for laser treatment. When this has been done it is usual to treat the vessel itself in order to flatten any protruding lesion.

Heat probe

The principles of using the heat probe are very similar to that of the BICAP® device, but there are two theoretical advantages. First, because no electrical energy has to pass into the tissue, the probe can be coated by non-stick material which prevents adherence to coagulated tissue. Second, because the temperature developed is independent of tissue desiccation, the delivery of energy is not impeded by coagulum and tissue bonding may therefore be greater.

The heat probe consists of a coated hollow metal tip containing an inner heater coil which can rapidly generate a temperature of 150°C. This temperature is effective for coagulation, but avoids excessive vaporisation. The probe also incorporates channels for washing which allows better visualisation during coaptation and coagulation. As with BICAP®, the largest available probe (3.2 mm) is preferable.

The technique for using the heat probe is almost identical to that for the BICAP® device with the exception that the energy settings are graded as joules rather than watts and duration. The probe is positioned with firm pressure, and three to four pulses of around 30 J are delivered.

Both heat probe and bipolar diathermy are relatively safe, but both have been reported as causing perforations and reactivation of bleeding. It is therefore important to exercise great care in their use.

Adrenaline injection

Adrenaline injection probably achieves immediate haemostasis by virtue of the tamponade effect of the injected fluid, but the permanent effect depends on vasospasm and platelet activation encouraging the formation of platelet and fibrin thrombus within the vessel lumen.[27] A solution of 1 in 10 000 is most often used, delivered by means of endoscopic injection needle of the type used for sclerotherapy for oesophageal varices.

When an active bleeding point is identified, the ulcer is washed and the needle assembly, already flushed through with the adrenaline solution, is passed through the working channel of the endoscope with the point withdrawn into the sheath. As soon as the needle is seen emerging from the endoscope, the assistant is asked to push out the needle point. The needle is then advanced into the base of the bleeding point, and the assistant injects 0.5 ml of the adrenaline solution. A fair degree of force is required, and if the injection is very easy, the needle is probably not in the tissue. If the bleeding does not stop immediately, a further 0.5 ml should be injected at the same site and the needle moved to a slightly different site to repeat the process. When the bleeding has stopped more adrenaline should be injected around the bleeding point in four to six 0.5 ml aliquots. The non-bleeding visible vessel can be treated in the same manner.

One situation where injection therapy is particularly useful is where adherent clot obscures the bleeding point. This makes thermal coagulation difficult, but it is quite easy to pass a needle through the clot to allow injection of the ulcer base. Exacerbation of the bleeding is not a significant problem, presumably due to the combined tamponade and vasoconstriction.

Adrenaline injection appears to be very safe, with no recorded instances of perforation. Tachycardia and hypertension can occur, however, and although fatal arrhythmias have not been reported, it is a sensible precaution to use ECG monitoring in addition to pulse and blood pressure recording during the procedure.

Injection sclerotherapy

The sclerosants which have been used in non-variceal haemorrhage include absolute alcohol, 1% polidocanol, 5% ethanolamine and 3% sodium tetradecyl sulphate (STD). Alcohol acts by dehydration and fixation of tissue whereas the others are detergents which cause endothelial damage; the intended end result is obliteration or thrombosis of the feeding vessel.

If there is active bleeding it is usual to control this with adrenaline injection as above, and then to surround the bleeding point with aliquots of sclerosant – 0.1 ml for alcohol or 0.5 ml for the other sclerosants. Sclerotherapy of a non-bleeding vessel will not require adrenaline injection unless the injection precipitates active bleeding. As for adrenaline, sclerotherapy appears to be safe, although there have been a few cases of extensive necrosis of the stomach wall after injection of the left gastric artery.[28]

Results of endoscopic treatment

Because most upper gastrointestinal bleeding stops without intervention it is important for techniques of endoscopic therapy to be subjected to randomised trials before they are accepted as effective. Before drawing conclusions from these trials, however, it is important to be clear about the end points which are being studied.

Mortality is obviously the most important, but as this is likely to be around 5% in interested centres, it would take a very large trial to demonstrate a convincing improvement in death rate.[29] The next most important is probably need for emergency surgery; this can be associated with a mortality of up to 20%,[30] and any intervention which can reduce urgent operation rates is likely to be translated into a reduction in morbidity and mortality. Rebleeding is less reliable as an end point as it does not necessarily represent a clinically significant outcome if it does not result in surgery or death. In many trials, however, rebleeding is the only end point which is affected.

The available trials can be divided into those which have compared a specific form of endoscopic haemostasis with no endoscopic therapy, and those which have compared different techniques. In the remainder of this section, the trials which have examined the efficacy of each of the commonly used methods against conventional treatment will be considered, and this will be followed by an appraisal of the comparative trials.

Laser photocoagulation

Laser photocoagulation was first used for bleeding peptic ulcer in the 1970s, and since then there have been at least 12 randomised controlled trials comparing it with no endoscopic therapy.[31,32] Both the Nd-YAG and the argon laser have been used, but the former has superseded the latter owing to its superior tissue penetration qualities.

Of the nine trials of the Nd-YAG laser, four were poorly designed or were not based on sufficiently accurate definitions of the lesions being treated. Of the five remaining studies, four produced favourable results.[33–36] In the first, from Rutgeerts and colleagues, significant reduction in clinical rebleeding was seen among those who had active bleeding, but there were no differences in mortality or need for surgery.[33] Two studies have shown a reduction in the need for emergency surgery,[34,35] and one of these showed a reduction in mortality in a high-risk subgroup.[35] In both of these studies, however, relatively large numbers of patients were excluded prior to randomisation usually because of difficulties in aiming the laser beam. In another study, no benefit whatsoever was seen from laser therapy,[37] but this may have been related to selection of low-risk patients and relative lack of experience among the endoscopists.

Bipolar diathermy

Of six controlled trials of bipolar diathermy, three have been unable to demonstrate any benefit.[38–40] One showed a reduction in clinical rebleeding, but no difference in the need for emergency surgery.[41] The most impressive studies, however, were carried out by Loren Laine who performed one trial in patients with active bleeding[42] and one in patients whose ulcers exhibited non-bleeding visible vessels;[43] in both studies a reduction in the need for emergency surgery was seen. It is significant that in both of these studies the large 10 Fr probe was used and, perhaps more importantly, all the therapy was delivered by Laine himself.

Heat probe

In heat probe therapy, there have been four randomised controlled trials with 'no endoscopic treatment' arms. Two of these showed no benefit,[36,44] and one demonstrated a reduction in rebleeding but no effect on surgery rates.[45] In the 'CURE' study, however, Jensen's group demonstrated significant reduction in both rebleeding and the need for emergency surgery in high risk patients with arterial bleeding or

Table 13.2 *Comparative trials of different techniques for endoscopic haemostasis in non-variceal haemorrhage. A best result is only indicated where there was a statistically significant difference*

Study	Methods compared	Best result
Johnston *et al.* (1985)[59]	Laser vs heat probe	Heat probe
Goff *et al.* (1986)[60]	Laser vs BICAP®	No difference
Rutgeerts *et al.* (1989)[61]	Laser vs BICAP®	No difference
Rutgeerts *et al.* (1989)[62]	Laser vs adrenaline vs adrenaline + sclerosant	Adrenaline + sclerosant
Chiozzini *et al.* (1989)[63]	Ethanol vs adrenaline	No difference
Matthewson *et al.* (1990)[36]	Laser vs heat probe	No difference
Loizou *et al.* (1991)[64]	Laser vs adrenaline	No difference
Hui *et al.* (1991)[65]	Laser vs heat probe vs BICAP®	No difference
Lin *et al.* (1990)[66]	Heat probe vs alcohol	Heat probe
Jensen *et al.* (1990)[46]	Heat probe vs BICAP®	Heat probe
Laine (1990)[67]	BICAP® vs alcohol	No difference
Chung *et al.* (1991)[68]	Heat probe vs adrenaline	No difference
Waring *et al.* (1991)[69]	BICAP® vs alcohol	No difference
Choudari *et al.* (1992)[70]	Heat probe vs adrenaline	No difference
Chung *et al.* (1993)[71]	Adrenaline vs adrenaline + sclerosant	No difference
Lin *et al.* (1993)[72]	Alcohol vs glucose vs saline	No difference
Choudari *et al.* (1994)[73]	Adrenaline vs adrenaline + sclerosant	No difference
Jensen *et al.* (1994)[74]	Heat probe vs adrenaline + heat probe	No difference
Chung *et al.* (1994)[49]	Adrenaline vs adrenaline + heat probe	No difference

visible vessels.[46] In this report, the need for the large (3.2 mm) probe, firm tamponade of the vessel and the use of four 30 J pulses was stressed.

Adrenaline injection

Adrenaline injection of actively bleeding ulcers has been widely used in conjunction with other forms of treatment including laser, heat probe and injection sclerotherapy.[47–49] The rationale has been twofold: first to facilitate the delivery of the main therapeutic modality by stopping any active bleeding and secondly to reduce the heat sink effect (*vide supra*). It is now clear, however, that adrenaline injection can be effective on its own.

There has been one randomised trial of 1:10 000 adrenaline versus no endoscopic treatment in actively bleeding ulcers which showed reductions in the need for emergency surgery, blood transfusion and hospital stay in the treated group.[50] Furthermore, there have been several studies comparing adrenaline alone with adrenaline plus another form of treatment, and none of these has shown the supplementary therapy to have been of any value (Table 13.2).

Injection sclerotherapy

Although the use of absolute alcohol is very popular, especially in Japan,[51] there have been no true trials comparing it with no treatment. However, there has been one comparative study which has suggested that it can reduce emergency surgery rates,[52] and a trial which indicated that it produces better results than spraying with adrenaline and thrombin in gastric ulcers with non-bleeding visible vessels.[53]

The sclerosant polidocanol has also been widely used, and it has been tested in two randomised trials, both utilising pre-injection with adrenaline. One showed a reduction in the need for emergency surgery,[54] although the other was only able to show an effect on rebleeding.[55] In addition there have been two trials of adrenaline followed by 5% ethanolamine which showed reductions in rebleeding and non-significant trends towards less emergency surgery.[56,57]

Comparison between different methods

There is now little doubt that endoscopic haemostasis should be employed. It is effective in producing initial control of active bleeding, reducing clinical rebleeding and reducing the need for emergency or urgent surgical intervention. Whether or not it saves lives is more contentious, but a meta-analysis by Cook *et al.*[58] has indicated that endoscopic therapy can significantly reduce mortality (odds ratio 0.55; confidence interval 0.40–0.76).

Making a decision as to which type of endoscopic therapy to use is more difficult, however, and when appraising the different trials it is very important to take account of the type of lesions which have been treated. When trials in which the control patients were treated non-surgically until they fulfilled criteria which were independent of endoscopic appearances are studied, it is found that patients with active arterial bleeding came to surgery in about 60% of cases.[14] Those with active oozing or non-bleeding visible vessel required surgery in about 25% and 40%, respectively. When the results of adequately documented trials are put together, it becomes clear that whereas laser photocoagulation for active arterial bleeding is associated with an emergency surgery rate of about 40%, diathermy and injection techniques can reduce it to around 15%.[14]

In addition to this type of analysis, there have now been a very large number of trials comparing one method of endoscopic therapy with another, and these are summarised in Table 13.2. It can be seen that very few of the trials showed any difference between the techniques studied with the exception that laser therapy seems to be the least favourable. It would therefore seem that the choice of therapeutic modality remains largely personal based on training and experience. The current author's preference and reasons for his choice are given in the section on overall recommendations.

Surgical treatment

Despite the important advances in endoscopic intervention outlined above, there remains a small group of patients who will require surgical intervention as a life-saving procedure. This is becoming a major problem, as few surgeons in this country now have extensive experience of operating for peptic ulcer disease, and the emergency which does not respond to endoscopic treatment usually represents a significant surgical challenge. It is therefore vital that surgery for upper gastrointestinal bleeding is carried out by an experienced surgeon who is used to operating on the stomach and duodenum, and not delegated to a junior member of staff.

This section looks at the indications for surgery in peptic ulcer bleeding and then examines specific techniques for dealing with duodenal, gastric and oesophageal ulcers, respectively. Finally, the role of vagotomy and the choice of procedure is considered.

Indications for surgery

Before the introduction of endoscopic haemostasis the decision whether or not to operate for bleeding peptic ulcer could be difficult. When active bleeding was seen at the time of endoscopy this was usually taken as an absolute indication to proceed. However, it was more common to find that the patient had stopped bleeding at the time of endoscopy, and the surgeon had to decide between waiting for clinical evidence of rebleeding and performing 'prophylactic' surgery.

The most important factors in predicting rebleeding appeared to be the presence of significant endoscopic stigmata of recent haemorrhage, an ulcer on the posterior wall of the duodenum or high on the lesser curve of the stomach, age over 60 years and shock or anaemia on admission.[75,76] In 1984, Morris and others published the results of a randomised study comparing a policy of delayed surgery with early surgery.[77] The criteria for early surgery were one rebleed in hospital, four units of plasma expander or blood in 24 hours, endoscopic stigmata or a previous history of peptic ulcer with bleeding. In the delayed group the criteria consisted of two rebleeds in hospital or eight units of blood or plasma expander in 24 hours. For patients over the age of 60 years, early surgery was associated with a lower mortality, and despite doubts as to the appropriateness of the endoscopic stigmata chosen and the very high operation rate, this study did emphasise the need for prompt surgical intervention in high-risk elderly patients.

Since the widespread adoption of endoscopic haemostasis, it can be argued that the decision as to when to operate has become easier to make. If initial control of active bleeding is impossible endoscopically then surgery is mandatory. If re-bleeding occurs after successful delivery of endoscopic treatment then immediate surgery should be undertaken unless the patient is deemed unfit. Some endoscopists consider that re-treatment after clinical rebleeding is safe,[78] but good evidence for this is lacking. In this author's experience such a policy can be very dangerous, not infrequently leading to a patient being presented for surgery in less than optimal condition.

Some endoscopists follow a policy of routine re-endoscopy within 24 hours of endoscopic haemostasis with retreatment if indicated.[51] This policy has been tested in a small randomised trial which showed a non-significant benefit,[79] and it is possible that this approach might improve the results of endoscopic treatment. This must not, however, be confused with the re-treatment of overt clinical rebleeding.

If clinical rebleeding is to be used as an indication for surgery, it is very important to have clear definitive criteria, especially as melaena can continue for several days following a major bleed. If a patient remains haemodynamically stable without aggressive fluid replacement and does not have a fresh haematemesis or a substantial drop in haemoglobin after initial resuscitation, then rebleeding can be discounted. If there is any doubt as to whether or not a patient has rebled, then a check endoscopy should be carried out before committing the patient to surgery.

Techniques

The bleeding duodenal ulcer
The majority of bleeding duodenal ulcers which require surgery are chronic posterior wall ulcers involving the gastroduodenal artery. The first step is to make a longitudinal duodenotomy immediately *distal* to the pyloric ring, and if there is active arterial bleeding, to obtain immediate haemostasis with finger pressure. It may then be necessary to extend the duodenotomy proximally through the pyloric ring in order to obtain adequate access, but unless a vagotomy is to be carried out (see below), the pylorus should be preserved if possible.

The next stage is to clear the stomach and duodenum of blood and clot with suction to obtain an optimal view of the bleeding site. If access is still difficult, mobilisation of the duodenum laterally (Kocher's manoeuvre) may help, and taking a firm grasp of the posterior duodenal mucosa distal to the ulcer with Babcock's forceps can allow the ulcer to be drawn up into the operative field.

Regardless of whether there is active bleeding or a non-bleeding exposed artery it is then important to obtain secure control of the vessel. This is best achieved using a small (1 cm diameter), heavy, round-bodied or taper-cut semicircular needle with 0 or No. 1 size suture material. This type of needle is ideal for the relatively restricted space and the tough fibrous tissue encountered at the base of a chronic ulcer. The material can be absorbable, but of reasonable strength duration (e.g. Vicryl or Dexon). The vessel must be under-run using two deeply placed sutures – one above the bleeding point and one below (Fig. 13.7). Use of the small needle suggested above will minimise the risk of damaging underlying structures such as the bile duct.

Figure 13.7
Placement of sutures above and below a visible vessel in a posterior duodenal ulcer.

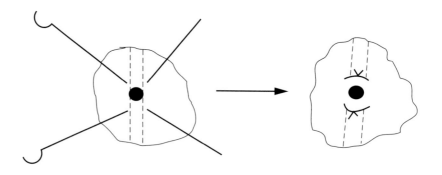

The duodenotomy may then be closed in the same direction as it was made, but if a truncal vagotomy has been performed, then a pyloroplasty should be constructed. This involves dividing the pyloric ring, if this has not already been done, and closing the defect transversely in the Heineke–Mickulicz fashion. If, however, a very long duodenotomy has been necessary, this may be impossible to achieve safely. In this case, the duodenotomy can be closed longitudinally and a gastrojejunostomy performed. Alternatively, a Finney pyloroplasty can be fashioned by approximating the adjacent walls of the first and second parts of the duodenum as the posterior wall of the new lumen (Fig. 13.8).

Occasionally, the first part of the duodenum will be virtually destroyed by a giant ulcer, and once opened, it will be impossible to repair. In this case it is necessary to proceed to a partial gastrectomy once the vessel has been secured. The right gastric and gastro-epiploic vessels are ligated and divided, and the stomach is separated from the ulcer with a combination of sharp and blunt dissection. The stomach is then divided at a level which will represent an antrectomy, and continuity restored by a gastrojejunostomy. The difficulty then lies in closing the duodenal stump.

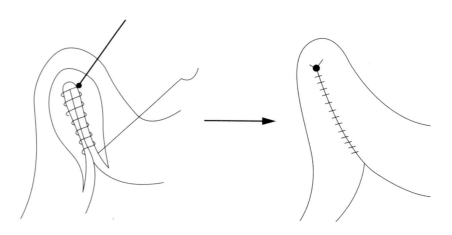

Figure 13.8 *A Finney pyloroplasty.*

Figure 13.9 *The Nissen method for closing a difficult duodenal stump.*

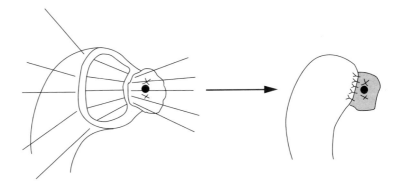

Figure 13.9 *The Nissen method for closing a difficult duodenal stump.*

Although this may be achieved by pinching the second part of the duodenum away from the ulcer to allow conventional closure, this is generally hazardous and should not be attempted. Rather, it is preferable to employ Nissen's method where the anterior wall of the duodenum is sutured on to the edge of the fibrotic ulcer base with interrupted sutures. A second layer of sutures is then inserted in the same way, rolling the anterior wall of the duodenum on to the ulcer base (Fig. 13.9). Drainage of the blind duodenal stump is then advisable, and this is most conveniently achieved by means of a T-tube brought out through the healthy side wall of the second part of the duodenum (Fig. 13.10).

The bleeding gastric ulcer

Conventionally, the bleeding gastric ulcer is treated by means of a partial gastrectomy, and for a sizeable antral ulcer this is often the best approach. However, with effective endoscopic haemostasis, by far the commonest situation requiring surgery is the chronic high lesser curve ulcer involving the left gastric artery. The important part of the procedure is then excision of the lesser curve (Pauchet's manoeuvre), and, for secure haemostasis, a formal gastrectomy may be unnecessary.

For the high lesser curve ulcer, therefore, simple ulcer excision is often the treatment of choice. This is not, however, a minor procedure, and has to be carried out with great care. The lesser curve has to be mobilised completely, often pinching the ulcer off the posterior

Figure 13.10 *The use of a T-tube for draining the duodenal stump.*

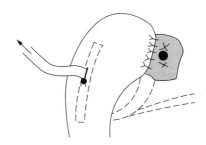

abdominal wall, and dividing the left gastric vessels. The stomach wall is then divided around the ulcer, making the incision in healthy tissue. If an anterior gastrotomy has to be made initially in order to find the ulcer or to obtain initial haemostasis, it should be made so that it can be incorporated in the excision. The defect in the lesser curve can then be closed with a continuous suture, and this is best achieved with an initial mucosal suture to obtain secure haemostasis followed by a separate serosubmucosal suture.

In a patient with a large gastric ulcer with a visible vessel, it is often tempting to merely under-run the vessel. Unless the patient will be put at risk by ulcer excision, this should be resisted as it is associated with a high risk of rebleeding. On the other hand, the tiny ulcer with an exposed vessel – the 'Dieulafoy Lesion' – can be treated very adequately in this way. In this latter condition, the ulcer can be very difficult to find at operation, even if it has been well seen at endoscopy. Rather than trying to see the lesion, it is better to feel the suspicious area with the tips of the fingers and the vessel will usually declare itself as a distinct 'bristle'.

Occasionally, with multiple erosions throughout the stomach, it will be necessary to carry out a total gastrectomy. In this case the site of bleeding is unclear, and it is important to reduce gastric blood flow as quickly as possible. The first steps should therefore be to ligate and divide the right gastric and gastro-epiploic vessels, divide the duodenum, lift up the stomach and ligate and divide the left gastric vessels. The rest of the operation can then be done at relative leisure.

The bleeding oesophageal ulcer

Arterial bleeding from the oesophagus is usually due to reflux oesophagitis or a Mallory–Weiss tear. It is very unusual for either of these to come to surgery as both tend to settle spontaneously, and even if they do not, adrenaline injection almost always achieves permanent haemostasis.[80]

However, if a Mallory–Weiss tear does require surgery, it is nearly always possible to gain access through the abdomen, certainly in a thin patient. The oesophagus is mobilised, and the gastro-oesophageal junction is opened anteriorly by means of a longitudinal incision. It is then possible to see and under-run the tear in the mucosa. In the obese patient, access to the lower oesophagus may be easier through a left thoracotomy, and this approach should certainly be used for true lower oesophageal bleeding from oesophagitis. In this case it may be possible to gain control via an oesophagotomy, but in some cases oesophagectomy may be necessary.

Choice of procedure

Vagotomy

For many years the standard treatment for a bleeding duodenal ulcer was truncal vagotomy and drainage, and when a gastrectomy was necessary, a vagotomy was often added. The rationale behind this approach was to provide definitive therapy and thereby minimise the risk of life-threatening recurrence. Over the past ten years or so, however, changes in the management of peptic ulcer disease have brought about a sea-change in attitude to this problem.

Firstly, the side effects of truncal vagotomy prompted the development of the highly selective vagotomy (HSV),[81] and it has been suggested that after local control of bleeding, HSV should be the definitive procedure.[82] However, the results of HSV are highly operator dependent, and few surgeons now have extensive experience of the operation. This, along with the time-consuming nature of the operation makes it impractical in most emergency situations.

More importantly, the medical treatment of peptic ulcer has improved immeasurably over the years. Although ineffective in stopping bleeding, anti-secretory therapy in the form of the H_2 receptor antagonists or the proton-pump inhibitors is highly effective in securing ulcer healing. In addition, the pathogenic role of *Helicobacter pylori* is now firmly established in duodenal ulcer at least, and successful eradication therapy reduces the risk of recurrent ulcer to very acceptable levels.[83]

For these reasons, the use of truncal vagotomy in acute bleeding may now be seriously questioned. It is this author's view that secure haemostasis is sufficient in the majority of patients in the acute situation. Of course it is then mandatory to ensure that the patient is properly investigated and treated postoperatively; this implies an immediate course of H_2 receptor antagonist or proton pump inhibitor followed by check endoscopy. It is then important to establish the *Helicobacter pylori* status, but this must be done when the patient is off all medication as anti-secretory agents can lead to false-negative results. The urea breath test is convenient and obviates the need for another endoscopy.

Occasionally, the surgeon will encounter the patient who has had multiple courses of treatment and attempts at *H. pylori* eradication who then bleeds from an ulcer. In this case a vagotomy is definitely indicated, but should only be carried out by a surgeon who is experienced in the technique.

Control of ulcer bleeding

In the duodenum, this inevitably involves under-running of the bleeding vessel, and, vagotomy aside, the only choice then is between closure of the duodenotomy and gastrectomy. The ideal course of action is usually obvious and determined by the size of the ulcer as outlined above. In gastric ulcer the decision can be more difficult. Two groups have found that simple under-running for bleeding gastric ulcer produced satisfactory results.[84,85] However, in a randomised trial comparing minimal surgery with conventional ulcer surgery, Poxon and others found that patients treated by under-running alone were more likely to suffer fatal rebleeding.[86]

The ideal operation for bleeding peptic ulcer is highly individual, and must vary with the clinical situation and the experience of the surgeon. The main aim is to save life; this requires secure haemostasis by whatever means are appropriate, and all other considerations are secondary.

Overall recommendations

The reasons for the following recommendations are elaborated in the main text of this chapter, but a brief outline is given with each one.

1. *A Gastrointestinal Bleeding Unit should be formed in all acute hospitals.* Interested surgeons, gastroenterologists and radiologists should be prepared to work closely together. Only in this way will patients receive optimal care, and there is good evidence that this approach reduces mortality.

2. *The patient with upper gastrointestinal bleeding should have prompt endoscopy.* This maximises the chance of making a diagnosis, provides prognostic information and allows endoscopic treatment. In the high risk patient, it is very important to document the precise location of the ulcer; ideally, the endoscopy should be carried out by the surgeon who will be operating if it becomes necessary. If videoendoscopy is available, a record of the exact ulcer location can be taken.

3. *In massive bleeding where endoscopy fails to provide a diagnosis, urgent mesenteric angiography should be arranged.* It is very important to have a clear idea of the source of bleeding before embarking on a laparotomy.

4. *Medical therapy should not be relied on for control of bleeding.* Good supportive care is obviously very important, but there is no good evidence that specific pharmacological treatment has any effect on the outcome.

5. *For active ulcer bleeding and visible vessels, endoscopic haemostasis with injection of 1:10 000 adrenaline is recommended.* Although heat probe, BICAP® and injection sclerotherapy have all been shown to be effective, adrenaline is often used with these modalities, and the available trials indicate that adrenaline alone is equally effective. In addition, adrenaline appears to be associated with the lowest incidence of adverse effects. Laser therapy cannot now be recommended.

6. *A patient with a visible vessel in an ulcer should not be discharged from hospital without endoscopic evidence of fading.* A resolving visible vessel takes about four days to disappear, and it is recommended that repeat endoscopy should provide definite evidence that the vessel

is fading before the patient is discharged from hospital. Massive rebleeding at home is more likely to be fatal.

7. *Surgical intervention is indicated when endoscopic therapy fails to control active bleeding, or at the first clinical rebleed after apparently successful endoscopic treatment.* Although routine repeat endoscopy within 24 hours with re-injection if appropriate may be of value, multiple re-injections for clinical rebleeding should be avoided if at all possible.

8. *The aim of surgery is to obtain secure haemostasis.* Unless the patient has a long history of failed medical management including attempted *H. pylori* eradication, vagotomy should be avoided. For gastric ulcer, the ideal treatment is often formal ulcer excision.

Future directions

The aims of future developments in the management of non-variceal upper gastrointestinal bleeding are to improve mortality rates and to reduce the need for emergency surgery. To this end, it is possible that improved medical treatment and new methods of endoscopic haemostasis may make contributions.

However, perhaps the most pressing immediate need is to improve the definition of stigmata of recent haemorrhage. Several studies have demonstrated that, apart from active arterial (spurting) bleeding, there is huge variation in the interpretation of the endoscopic appearances of the peptic ulcer which has bled, even among very experienced endoscopists.[11–13] This makes the results of many of the trials of endoscopic haemostasis difficult to assess, and the true value of treating a

Table 13.3 *Descriptive definitions for the endoscopic appearances of the bleeding peptic ulcer*

Definitions

Arterial bleeding – spurting blood

Oozing – blood trickling from the ulcer base

Visible vessel – a protruding discoloured lesion arising from the ulcer base, but not fleshy clot

Adherent clot – fleshy clot on the ulcer base which cannot be washed away

Stigmata
1. Arterial bleeding
2. Visible vessel with oozing
3. Adherent clot with oozing
4. Non-bleeding visible vessel
5. Non-bleeding adherent clot

NB: other appearances *not* included as too vague and of doubtful prognostic significance non-bleeding lesion is therefore still unclear. A simple, purely descriptive classification is given in Table 13.3; this has proved to be useful and reasonably reproducible, but the only way to ensure uniformity world-wide is to initiate coordinated, international consensus panels and training schemes.

Another difficult and related area is the problem of identifying those lesions which are at high risk of rebleeding after apparently successful endoscopic haemostasis. This can be fully resolved only when agreement is reached on endoscopic appearances, but there is now evidence that Doppler ultrasound may be useful in indicating the persistence of a large vessel in an ulcer.[87] This might provide a more objective measure of risk, and could be used to identify those patients who should go for early surgery.

Real improvements in the care of patients with upper gastrointestinal haemorrhage have been seen in recent years, particularly in centres which have developed bleeding units. There can be no substitute for enthusiasm and dedication in the management of this demanding problem, and the real challenge for the future is to ensure widespread cooperation between interested specialists in acute hospitals. Only in this way can a coordinated and effective response to gastrointestinal bleeding be achieved.

References

1. Rockall TA, Logan RFA, Devlin HB, Northfield TC. Incidence of and mortality from acute upper gastrointestinal haemorrhage in the United Kingdom. Br Med J 1995; 311: 222–6.

2. Schiller KFR, Truelove SC, Williams DG. Haematemesis and melaena, with special reference to factors influencing the outcome. Br Med J 1970; ii: 7–14.

3. Johnston SJ, Jones PF, Kyle J, Needham CD. Epidemiology and course of gastrointestinal haemorrhage in North-East Scotland. Br Med J 1973; iii: 655–60.

4. Dronfield MW. Special units for acute upper gastrointestinal bleeding. Br Med J 1987; 294: 1308–9.

5. Swain CP, Salmon PR, Northfield TC. Does ulcer position influence presentation or prognosis of upper gastrointestinal bleeding? Gut 1986; 27:A632.

6. Forrest JAH, Finlayson NDC, Shearmen DJV. Endoscopy in gastrointestinal bleeding. Lancet 1974; 11:394–7.

7. Foster DN, Miloszewski KJ, Losowsky MS. Stigmata of recent haemorrhage in diagnosis and prognosis of upper gastrointestinal bleeding. Br Med J 1978; i: 1173–7.

8. Griffiths WJ, Neumann DA, Welsh JD. The visible vessel as an indicator of a controlled or recurrent gastrointestinal haemorrhage. N Engl J Med 1979; 300: 1411-13.

9. Storey DW, Bown SJ, Swain CP, Salmon PR, Kirkham JS, Northfield TC. Endoscopic prediction of recurrent bleeding in peptic ulcers. N Engl J Med 1981; 305: 915–16.

10. Wara P. Endoscopic prediction of major rebleeding – a prospective study of stigmata of haemorrhage in bleeding ulcer. Gastroenterology 1985; 88: 1209–14.

11. Lau YWJ, Sung JYJ, Chan CWJ et al. Stigmata of haemorrhage in bleeding peptic ulcers: an inter-observer agreement study among international experts. In press

12. Laine L, Freeman M, Cohen H. Lack of uniformity in evaluation of endoscopic prognostic features of bleeding ulcers. Gastrointest Endosc 1994; 40: 411–17.

13. Moorman PW, Siersema PD, van Ginneken AM. Descriptive features of gastric ulcers: do endoscopists agree on what they see?

Gastrointest Endosc 1995; 42: 555–9.

14. Steele RJC. Endoscopic haemostasis for non-variceal upper gastrointestinal haemorrhage. Br J Surg 1989; 76: 219–25.

15. Yang CC, Shin JS, Lin XZ, Hsu PI, Chen KW, Lin CY. The natural history (fading time) of stigmata of recent haemorrhage in peptic ulcer disease. Gastrointest Endosc 1994; 40: 562–6.

16. Thomson JN, Salem RR, Hemingway AP et al. Specialist investigation of obscure gastrointestinal bleeding. Gut 1987; 28: 47–51.

17. Winzelberg GG, McKusick KA, Froelich JW et al. Detection of gastrointestinal bleeding with 99Tm-labelled red blood cells. Semin Nucl Med 1982; 12: 126–38.

18. Desa LA, Ohri SK, Hutton KAR, Lee H, Spencer J. Role of intraoperative enteroscopy in obscure gastrointestinal bleeding of small bowel origin. Br J Surg 1991; 78: 192–5.

19. Berry AR, Campbell WB, Kettlewell MGW. Management of major colonic haemorrhage. 1988; 75: 637–40.

20. Collins R, Langman M. Treatment with histamine H_2 antagonists in acute upper gastrointestinal haemorrhage. Implications of randomised trials. N Engl J Med 1985; 313: 660–6.

21. Walt RP, Cottrell J, Mann SG et al. Randomised, double blind, controlled trial of intravenous famotidine infusion in 1005 patients with peptic ulcer bleeding. Gut 1991; 32: A571–2.

22. Daneshmend TK, Hawkey CJ, Langman MJS et al. Omeprazole versus placebo for acute upper gastrointestinal bleeding. Results of a randomised, double-blind controlled trial. Br Med J 1992; 304: 143–8.

23. Barer D, Ogilvie A, Henry D et al. Cimetidine and tranexamic acid in the treatment of acute upper gastrointestinal tract bleeding. N Engl J Med 1983; 308: 1571–5.

24. Henry DA, O'Connell DL. Effects of fibrinolytic inhibitors on mortality from upper gastrointestinal haemorrhage. Br Med J 1989; 298: 1142–6.

25. Jenkins SA, Taylor BA, Nott DM et al. Management of massive upper gastrointestinal haemorrhage from multiple sites of peptic ulceration with somatostatin and octreotide – a report of five cases. Gut 1992; 33: 404–7.

26. Birnie GC, Fenn GC, Shield MJ et al. Double blind comparative study of Misoprostol with placebo in acute upper gastrointestinal bleeding. Gut 1991; 32: A1246.

27. Pinkas H, McAllister E, Norman J, Robinson B, Brady PG, Dawson PJ. Prolonged evaluation of epinephrine and normal saline solution injections in an acute ulcer model with a single bleeding artery. Gastrointest Endosc 1995; 41: 51–5.

28. Levy J, Khakoo S, Barton R, Vicary R. Fatal injection sclerotherapy of a bleeding peptic ulcer. Lancet 1991; 37: 504.

29. Fromm D. Endoscopic coagulation for gastrointestinal bleeding. N Engl J Med 1987; 316: 1652–4.

30. Welch CE, Rodkey GV, von Ryll-Gryska P. A thousand operations for ulcer disease. Ann Surg 1986; 204: 454–67.

31. Laurence BH, Cotton PB. Bleeding gastroduodenal ulcers: nonoperative treatment. World J Surg 1987; 11: 295–303.

32. Matthewson K, Swain CP, Bland M, Kirkham JS, Bown SG, Northfield TC. Randomised comparison of NdYAG laser, heater probe and no endoscopic therapy for bleeding peptic ulcers. Gastroenterology 1990; 98: 1239–44.

33. Rutgeerts P, Van Trappen G, Broeckaert L et al. Controlled trial of YAG laser treatment of upper digestive haemorrhage. Gastroenterology 1982; 83: 410–16.

34. MacLeod IA, Mills PR, MacKenzie JF et al. Neodymium yttrium aluminium garnet laser photocoagulation for major haemorrhage from peptic ulcers and single vessels: a single double blind controlled study. Br Med J 1983; 286: 345–8.

35. Swain CP, Kirkham JS, Salmon PR et al. Controlled trial of Nd-YAG laser photocoagulation in bleeding peptic ulcers. Lancet 1986; i: 1113–16.

36. Matthewson K, Swain CP, Bland M et al. Randomised comparison of NdYAG laser, heater probe and no endoscopic therapy for bleeding peptic ulcers. Gastroenterol 1990; 98: 1239–44.

37. Krejs GJ, Little KH, Westergaard H et al. Laser photocoagulation for the treatment of acute peptic-ulcer bleeding. N Engl J Med 1987; 316: 1618–21.

38. Goudie BM, Mitchell KG, Birnie GC et al.

Controlled trial of endoscopic bipolar electro-coagulation in the treatment of bleeding peptic ulcers. Gut 1984; 25: A1185.

39. Kernohan RM, Anderson JR, McKelvey STD et al. A controlled trial of bipolar electro-coagulation in patients with upper gastro-intestinal bleeding. Br J Surg 1984; 71: 889–91.

40. Brearly S, Hawker PC, Dykes PW et al. Per-endoscopic bipolar diathermy coagulation of visible vessel using a 3.2 mm probe – a randomised clinical trial. Endoscopy 1987; 19: 160–3.

41. O'Brien JD, Day SJ, Burnham WR. Controlled trial of small bipolar probe in bleeding peptic ulcers. Lancet 1986; i: 464–7.

42. Laine L. Multipolar electrocoagulation in the treatment of active upper gastrointestinal haemorrhage. N Engl J Med 1987; 316: 1613–17.

43. Laine L. Multipolar electrocoagulation for the treatment of ulcers with non-bleeding visible vessels: a prospective, controlled trial. Gastroenterology 1988; 94: A246.

44. Avgerinos A, Rekoumis G, Argirakis G et al. Randomised comparison of endoscopic heater probe electrocoagulation, injection of adrenaline and no endoscopic therapy for bleeding peptic ulcers. Gastoenterology 1989; 98: A18.

45. Fullarton GM, Birnie GC, MacDonald A et al. Controlled trial of heater probe treatment in bleeding peptic ulcers. Br J Surg 1989; 76: 541–4.

46. Jensen DM. Heat probe for haemostasis of bleeding peptic ulcers: techniques and results of randomised controlled trials. Gastrointest Endosc 1990; 36: S42–9.

47. Rutgeerts P, Van Trappen G, Brieckaert L et al. A new and effective technique of Yag laser photocoagulation for severe upper gastro-intestinal bleeding. Endoscopy 1984; 16: 115–17.

48. Soehendra N, Grimm H, Stenzel M. Injec-tion of nonvariceal bleeding lesions of the upper gastrointestinal tract. Endoscopy 1985; 17: 129–32.

49. Chung SCS, Sung JY, Lai CW, Ng EKW, Chan KL, Yung MY. Epinephrine injection alone or epinephrine injection plus heater probe treat-ment for bleeding ulcers. Gastrointest Endosc 1994; 40: A271.

50. Chung SCS, Leung JWC, Steele RJC et al.

Endoscopic adrenaline injection for actively bleeding ulcers: a randomised trial. Br Med J 1988; 296: 1631–3.

51. Asaki S. Endoscopic haemostasis by local absolute alcohol injection for upper gastro-intestinal tract bleeding – a multicentre study. In: Okabe H, Honda T, Ohshiba S (eds) Endoscopic surgery. New York: Elsevier, pp. 105–16.

52. Pascu O, Draghici A, Acalovachi I. The effect of endoscopic haemostasis with alcohol on the mortality rate of nonvariceal upper gastrointestinal haemorrhage: a randomised prospective study. Endoscopy 1989; 36: S53–5.

53. Koyama T, Fukimoto K, Iwakiri R et al. Prevention of recurrent bleeding from gastric ulcer with a nonbleeding visible vessel by the endoscopic injection of absolute ethanol: a prospective, controlled trial. Gastrointest Endosc 1995; 42: 128–31.

54. Panes J, Viver J, Forne M et al. Controlled trial of endoscopic sclerosis in bleeding peptic ulcers. Lancet 1987; ii: 1292–4.

55. Balanzo J, Sainz S, Such J et al. Endoscopic haemostasis by local injection of epinephrine and polidocanol in bleeding ulcer. A pros-pective, randomised trial. Endoscopy 1988; 20: 298–291.

56. Rajgopal C, Palmer KR. Endoscopic injection sclerosis: effective therapy for bleeding peptic ulcer. Gut 1991; 32: 727–9.

57. Oxner RBG, Simmonds NJ, Gertner DJ, Nightingale JMD, Burnham WR. Controlled trial of endoscopic injection treatment for bleeding from peptic ulcers with visible vessels. Lancet 1992; 339: 966–8.

58. Cook DJ, Guyatt GH, Salena BJ et al. Endoscopic therapy for acute non-variceal upper gastrointestinal haemorrhage: a meta-analysis. Gastroenterology 1992; 102: 139–48.

59. Johnston JH, Sones JQ, Long BW, Posey LE. Comparison of heater probe and YAG laser in endoscopic treatment of major bleeding from peptic ulcers. Gastrointest Endosc 1985; 31: 175–80.

60. Goff JS. Bipolar electrocoagulation versus Nd-YAG laser photocoagulation for upper gastrointestinal bleeding lesions. Dig Dis Sci 1986; 31: 906–10.

61. Rutgeerts P, Van Trappen G, Van Hootegem P et al. Neodymium-YAG laser photocoagu-lation versus multipolar electrocoagulation

for the treatment of severely bleeding peptic ulcers: a randomised comparison. Gastrointest Endosc 1987; 33: 199–202.

62. Rutgeerts P, Van Trappen G, Broechaert L, Coremans G, Janssens J, Hiele M. Comparison of endoscopic polidocanol injection and YAG laser therapy for bleeding peptic ulcers. Lancet 1989; 1: 1164–7.

63. Chiezzini G, Bortoluzzi F, Pallin D et al. Controlled trial of absolute ethanol vs epinephrine as injection agent in gastrointestinal bleeding. Gastroenterology 1989; 96: A86.

64. Loizou LA, Bown SG. Endoscopic treatment for bleeding peptic ulcers: randomised comparison of adrenaline injection and adrenaline injection + Nd:YAG laser. Gut 1991; 32: 1100–3.

65. Hui Wm, Ng MMT, Lok ASF, Lai CL, Lau YN, Lam SK. A randomised comparative study of laser photocoagulation, heater probe and bipolar electrocoagulation in the treatment of actively bleeding ulcers. Gastrointest Endosc 1991; 37: 299–304.

66. Lin HJ, Lee FY, Kang WM, Tsai YT, Lee SD, Lee CH. Heat probe thermocoagulation and pure alcohol injection in massive peptic ulcer haemorrhage: a prospective, randomised controlled trial. Gut 1990; 31: 753–7.

67. Laine L. Multipolar electrocoagulation versus injection therapy in the treatment of bleeding peptic ulcers. Gastroenterology 1990; 99: 1303–6.

68. Chung SCS, Leung JWC, Sung JY, Lo KK, Li AKC. Injection or heat probe for bleeding ulcer. Gastroenterology 1991; 100: 30–7.

69. Waring JP, Sanowski RA, Sawyer RL, Woods CA, Foutch PG. A randomised comparison of multipolar electrocoagulation and injection sclerosis for the treatment of bleeding peptic ulcer. Gastrointest Endosc 1991; 37: 295–8.

70. Choudari CD, Rajgopal C, Palmer KR. Comparison of endoscopic injection therapy versus the heater probe in major peptic ulcer haemorrhage. Gut 1992; 33: 1159–61.

71. Chung SCS, Leung JWC, Leong HT, Lo KK, Li AKC. Adding a sclerosant to endoscopic epinephrine injection in actively bleeding ulcers: a randomised trial. Gastrointest Endosc 1993; 39: 611–15.

72. Lin HJ, Perng CL, Lee FY. Endoscopic injection for the arrest of peptic ulcer haemorrhage: final results of a prospective, randomised comparative trial. Gastrointest Endosc 1993; 39: 15–19.

73. Choudari CP, Palmer KR. Endoscopic injection therapy for bleeding peptic ulcer; a comparison of adrenaline alone with adrenaline plus ethanolamine oleate. Gut 1994; 35: 608–10.

74. Jensen DM, Kovacs T, Randall G, Smith J, Freenan M, Jutabha R. Prospective study of thermal coagulation (gold probe-GP) vs combination injection and thermal (Inj + GP) treatment of high risk patients with severe ulcer or Mallory Weiss (MW) bleeding. Gastrointest Endosc 1994; 40: A42.

75. Clason AE, Macleod DAD, Elton RA. Clinical factors in the prediction of further haemorrhage or mortality in acute upper gastrointestinal haemorrhage. Br J Surg 1986; 73: 985–7.

76. Hunt PS. Bleeding gastroduodenal ulcers: selection of patients for surgery. World J Surg 1987; 11: 289–94.

77. Morris DL. Hawker PC, Brearley S et al. Optimal timing of operation for bleeding peptic ulcer: prospective randomised trial. Br Med J 1984; 288: 1277–80.

78. Palmer KR, Choudari CP. Endoscopic intervention in bleeding peptic ulcer. Gut 1995; 37: 161–4.

79. Villanueva C, Balanzo J, Torras X, Soriano G, Sainz S, Vilardell F. Value of second-look endoscopy after injection therapy for bleeding peptic ulcer: a prospective and randomised trial. Gastrointest Endosc 1994; 40: 34–9.

80. Park KGM, Steele RJC, Masson J. Endoscopic adrenaline injection for benign oesophageal ulcer haemorrhage. Br J Surg 1994; 81: 1317–18.

81. Johnston D. Operative mortality and postoperative morbidity of highly selective vagotomy. Br Med J 1975; 4: 545–7.

82. Miedema BW, Torres PR, Farnell MB et al. Proximal gastric vagotomy in the emergency treatment of bleeding duodenal ulcer. Am J Surg 1991; 162: 64–7.

83. Moss S, Calam J. Helicobacter pylori and peptic ulcers: the present position. Gut 1992; 33: 289–92.

84. Teenan RP, Murray WR. Late outcome of undersewing alone for gastric ulcer haemorrhage. Br J Surg 1990; 77: 811–12.

85. Schein M, Gecelter G. Apache II score in massive upper gastrointestinal haemorrhage from peptic ulcer: prognostic value and potential clinical applications. Br J Surg 1989; 76: 733–6.

86. Poxon VA, Keighley MRB, Dykes PW *et al.* Comparison of minimal and conventional surgery in patients with bleeding peptic ulcer: a multicentre trial. Br J Surg 1991; 78: 1344–5.

87. Fullarton GM, Murray WR. Prediction of rebleeding in peptic ulcers by visual stigmata and endoscopic doppler ultrasound criteria. Endoscopy 1990; 22: 68–71.

14 Management and surgical treatment of morbid obesity

Peter M. Sagar

Introduction

Severe obesity is a major social liability. It is a significant handicap when applying for employment, in achieving job promotion, pursuing a normal social life and in participating in sport and recreation. Unfortunately, the severely obese are subject to prejudice and abusive behaviour with a significant reduction in the quality of their lives. Such prejudice is widespread throughout society but seems to occur with extra intensity amongst physicians, nurses and paramedical personnel. In addition, although such discrimination lessens among the general population as the patients lose weight it seems to remain among medical personnel even after the patients have successfully lost weight. It would appear that physicians and nurses feel that there is something unforgivably wrong about ever being so fat. Such negative opinions are directed not only at the patients but also at the physicians and surgeons who treat the patients. Both hospital doctors and general practitioners often have little knowledge of bariatric surgery and of those who are aware of it, few would recommend surgery or refer patients for it. Indeed, in one survey, 18% of doctors would specifically advise patients to avoid such surgery. Some of this negative attitude is attributable to the misconception that jejuno-ileal bypass remains the surgical option for patients with morbid obesity. This is incorrect.

The widely held view is that fat people are totally responsible for their own weight gain and therefore should be able to lose this excess weight and stay in their new improved bodily habitus with ease. The simple concept of a balance between increased intake of calories and decreased expenditure in the form of exercise is clearly both applicable to the moderately overweight and the severely overweight. However, the morbidly obese patient on close questioning often proves to have had a period in their lives when their calorie intake has been grossly excessive with the result that their weight increased significantly over a relatively short period. Indeed, this is often related to a period of their lives when they found coping with problems somewhat difficult and resorted to eating as a means of elevating their mood. Once a patient has achieved a weight in excess of 300 lb (136 kg) simple advice to restrict calorie intake and to increase calorie expenditure is of little value. Most of us have difficulty shedding a few pounds, which can be managed with the application of willpower to avoid the tastier treats which we have become accustomed to, even then, it takes some time to notice a significant change. The morbidly obese do not even have this reward as the loss of a few pounds from a 300 lb frame will not be noticeable. In addition, the ability to take to the squash court or swimming pool or to take up jogging are not simple options when the patient is understandably over conscious of their bodily habitus. Moreover, such exercise may place unwanted demands on the myocardium which is already labouring under the strain of the excess weight.

Obesity at present is viewed in a similar way to alcoholism in the recent past, with a general feeling that the problem of obesity is a result of weak character. These attitudes and prejudices result from a failure to recognise the complex aetiology of morbid obesity and the poor outcome of both dietary and medical management of the condition.

Aetiology of morbid obesity

Genetic factors

Although it has long been recognised that obesity runs in families even careful studies have found it difficult to separate the influences of nature from those of nurture. Studies of monozygotic and dizygotic twins reared together and separately have demonstrated a clear relationship between the body mass index (BMI) (weight $\div$ height^2) (kg/m^2) of the adoptees and their biological parents but no relationship was apparent between the adoptees and their adoptive parents.[1,2] Inherited factors account for about 70% of the body mass index in adult life.[3] Genetic components are apparent in changes in body weight, body composition and the distribution of fat overall and visceral fat after periods of overeating.[4] The genetic findings apply across all body weights, from the very thin to the very fat.[5] Although the statistical distribution of obesity is consistent with polygenic inheritance, there remains the possibility that a major gene or genes for a super obesity exists.[6] To date, obesity genes have largely been studied using mouse models. In attempts to identify human obesity genes, large numbers of multigenerational families in whom extreme obesity has been shown to segregate are presently being collected, but relative risk estimates, together with models of genetic heterogeneity, suggest that at least 500 affected sibling pairs would need to be studied in order to identify major genes.[7]

Non-genetic factors

Whereas the studies cited above measured heritability, non-genetic factors also play a role in the determination of body fat. Genetically non-obese rats can be made to be obese by feeding them a fast food diet, and rats with a genetic predisposition towards obesity, although becoming obese on standard laboratory diets, become super-obese when fed fast food diets.[8] Interestingly, this super-obesity is partially reversible. Obesity and super-obesity are more prevalent in the lower socioeconomic classes, particularly among females.[9]

There is strong circumstantial evidence for hormonally driven periodic changes in female food intake. Most women eat significantly more and experience different taste preferences, particularly for sweets, during one half of their menstrual cycle.

It would appear then that obesity is the result of both genetic and environmental influences. The relative importance of these influences on obesity remains to be determined. Nevertheless the evidence supports the position that obesity is biologically determined, and as a consequence, efforts to control it solely by dietary intervention or behavioural therapy are destined to fail when the patient has become morbidly obese or super-obese. Epidemiological studies relating the prevalence of obesity to social conditions have found that obesity is 6 times more prevalent among women with lower socioeconomic status than among women with high socioeconomic status. Conversely, thinness is most prevalent among women with the highest socioeconomic status.[10] Furthermore, the prevalence of obesity is much higher among those women below the poverty line, but in contrast, American men above the poverty line, have a slightly higher prevalence of excess weight than men below the line.[11] Although genetic factors may explain much of individual variations in fatness in a society with people exposed to a similar diet, environmental influences must be invoked to account for a variation in fatness between societies, in which characteristic diets, activity levels and attitudes, concerning their physical appearance differ. The same argument applies when people who emigrate from an underdeveloped country to a developed country become fatter and when changes in diet and activity levels result in an increase in the average fatness in the society.

Arguments about the contribution of genetic and non-genetic factors towards obesity should therefore not discourage physicians and surgeons from treating obesity. The successful treatment of obesity improves quality of life and reduces the risk of a variety of illnesses, including ischaemic heart disease, hypertension, diabetes mellitus and arthritis. Longevity is improved. Indeed, it is good news that body fatness will respond to environmental conditions and is clearly controllable by a number of people concerned about their physical appearance. Within a sedentary and food-laden society the obesity prone people that wish to control their weight need to maintain a relatively high level of physical activity and eat within themselves. Those who have broken free from such control may need additional help, including surgical support.

Investigative techniques

Clinical

Patients can be chosen for operative intervention for morbid obesity according to a number of criteria. These include:

1. Body weight in excess of 100% or 45 kg over the ideal weight;
2. BMI greater than 39 kg/m²;
3. A minimum of 5 years of obesity;
4. Failure of conservative therapy. The need to justify surgical intervention based on previous failed aggressive attempts at dietary control is controversial. Indeed, this is difficult to standardise or prove and the patient needs to be given the benefit of the doubt. Frequently patients are referred after attending a number of courses of treatment for dietary control, behavioural modification or courses of drug therapy and the patient should not be made to feel they need to earn their operation. Non-surgical management of morbid obesity fails in more than 95% of patients.
5. No past medical history of a major psychiatric disorder or alcoholism. There does not appear to be a prevalence of major psychiatric disorder among the morbidly obese compared to those of normal body weight if strict well-defined criteria are used for diagnosis.[12] The mental state of the patient at the time of consideration for surgery is of greater importance than a past medical history of psychotic disorders.[13] Not surprisingly, minor psychiatric disorders, such as mild depression or anxiety, are not uncommon, but these are often the result, rather than the cause, of morbid obesity and frequently improve as the patient loses their weight in the postoperative period.

Psychological

The wishes and expectations of the patient should be discussed. Patients have often obtained information about the operations from magazine articles and television programmes and their misconceptions need to be addressed. Misunderstandings about the exact nature of the surgery and their anticipations for the postoperative period and the aims of the surgery need to be discussed in detail. Unrealistic social expectations about improving their prospects socially and at work need to be discussed. Although quality of life would be expected to be improved by successful surgical treatment of morbid obesity, unrealistic expectations of improved sexual performance and satisfaction, social acceptability and secure employment must be tempered.[14] Nevertheless, prospects of regaining employment are improved with a greater loss of excess weight, particularly among younger patients. Clearly, however, there are no guarantees.

A greater proportion of female patients with morbid obesity are referred and request surgical intervention than would be anticipated on the basis of prevalence within the population. As a rule, men tend to avoid surgical intervention unless they become physically debilitated by their excess weight, whereas women tend to proceed with referral and operation at a level when emotional distress rather than physical disability related to their obesity becomes more prominent.

Obesity-related correctable endocrine disorders such as hypothyroidism and Cushing's syndrome need to be excluded by biochemical investigations. Each patient should be assessed by a physician and dietician with an interest in morbid obesity, as well as the surgeon. Psychological profiles including the degree of motivation and cooperation of the patient can be obtained, but they often have little predictive value in terms of which patients will do well.

Not surprisingly, gallstones may be present as co-morbid pathology, as bile in the morbidly obese is supersaturated with cholesterol. Preoperative investigation of the biliary tree with an ultrasound scan is warranted, as, if gallstones are present, cholecystectomy should be carried out at the same time as the surgical procedure for morbid obesity. The patient should be advised, in the presence of gallstones, that the period of weight loss following operation is associated with increased secretion of cholesterol in the bile, which can be excessive and precipitate the formation of gallstones.

Psychological testing of the morbidly obese patient provides valuable information towards guiding a comprehensive treatment programme, which can improve behavioural and personality traits, and thus, facilitate the successful loss of weight after bariatric treatment. Although instruments such as the MMPI have not proved successful alternative questionnaires, such as the personal orientation inventory (POI), the Taylor–Johnson temperament analysis (T-JTA) and the eating disorder inventory-2 (EDI-2) have suggested that bariatric patients need to be mentally healthy and free of psychological disorders which would contraindicate surgery. Idiosyncratic attitudes, behavioural and personality traits however, can be identified using these profiles. Such attitudes should be corrected, as they may sabotage weight loss following the surgery.[15] The psychological data reassure patients that the treatment is appropriate and that they are not just 'taking the easy way out'. Patient education, support and behaviour modification are important to avoid negative attitudes should the surgery fail due to, for instance, staple line breakdown, regurgitation, food intolerance or dumping syndrome.

Management options

Jejuno-ileal bypass

Jejuno-ileal bypass became popular in the 1960s and 1970s, when it was recognised that extensive loss of small bowel as the result of trauma or disease was associated with significant loss of weight. This weight loss was maintained. Originally this was carried out by dividing the jejunum 30 cm below the ligament of Trietz with an end-to-end anastomosis onto the transverse colon. Weight loss of 60% was reported.[16] Although diarrhoea was reported to occur after this procedure, the authors suggested that this only occurred after dietary indiscretions. However, subsequent reports found the diarrhoea to be too troublesome, together with perianal discomfort. In addition, electrolyte abnormalities and hepatic failure caused excessive morbidity, and it became clear that this form of bypass was too drastic. Animal experiments and variations in the extent of the bypass resulted in the classic operation of a 14 and 4 in operation, in which malabsorption was induced by anastomosing 35 cm (14 in) of the proximal jejunum to the distal 10 cm (4 in) of the terminal ileum.[17] The rest of the jejunum and ileum was bypassed, but the ileocaecal valve was preserved. This resulted in the severity of diarrhoea being reduced to more acceptable levels. The operative mortality was low (2.5%) given the significant pre-existing pathology and 60% of patients found that their weight fell to within 10 kg of their ideal body weight.[18] In many respects this procedure was ideal with patients, who by their disposition were gluttonous, were able to eat merrily, and yet all of the excess calories would be swept away in the stool. In reality, patients would actually reduce their intake, particularly of carbohydrate, because such overeating was associated with the passage of large volumes of flatus, with an unpleasant smell and liquid stool. It subsequently became recognised that the weight loss was achieved by fat malabsorption and significant disturbances of the enterohepatic circulation were apparent. Weight loss stabilised 1 to 2 years after the procedures. Nevertheless, patients did indeed acquire a new body image, which pleased them, and impressed their medical and psychiatric staff.[19] There followed a relative explosion in the practice of this procedure, particularly in the USA, but the extent of the associated complications gradually became apparent, with up to one third of patients having a stormy post-operative course, which would often require in-hospital treatment, additional nutritional support and also the reversal of the jejuno-ileal bypass, because of the electrolyte and hepatic disturbances. Most worryingly, a number of deaths occurred, which were attributable to hepatocellular dysfunction. Up to 7% of patients developed progressive histological changes within the liver, or frank cirrhosis[20,21] and subsequently developed ascites, oedema and jaundice. Such liver failure would sometimes be attributed to excessive consumption of alcohol (wrongly) and usually occurred within 24 months of operation. It carried a mortality rate of 50%.[23] Patients in whom such liver failure did not occur suffered the later sequelae of bypass enteritis, deficiencies of fat-soluble vitamins, osteomalacia, reduced bony mineral content, due to depleted vitamin D[23] and polyarthritis, due to immune complex deposition,[24] which all helped in the demise of this procedure, which was abandoned[25] in the early 1980s. The relevance of this procedure to modern day practice is that patients are still presenting with problems relating back to their jejuno-ileal bypass and requesting reversal. Although much time has elapsed since their operation, they clearly need to be warned about the possibility of regaining their weight, should they continue to take in significantly more calories than they burn off. A technical point to note, if embarking on reversal of a jejuno-ileal bypass, is that the bypassed small bowel, proximal to the jejuno-ileal anastomosis, is often markedly atrophic and even appendiceal-like in diameter and texture, and constructing a jejunojejunal anastomosis onto such bowel, can be technically challenging!

Current surgical options

The ideal surgical option for correction of morbid obesity would be one in which there was an acceptable reduction in weight to levels in which premature death would not be significantly different from the rest of the population and in which the weight loss was maintained and associated with low morbidity and mortality rates in the postoperative period. Long-term sequelae should be minimal. Current surgical treatment of morbid obesity centres on three types of procedure. Each leads to gastric restriction, with a small capacity gastric reservoir or pouch, with a restricted, carefully measured outlet. These operations result in the restriction of solid food intake, but not liquids. The weight loss is thus achieved by reducing calorie intake.

Vertical gastroplasty

This involves the stapling of a vertical partition to create a tube along the lesser curve of the stomach, down to about the incisura. The outlet of this tube into the gastric antrum can be restricted by the use of foreign prosthetic material. The fundus and much of the body of the stomach are thus excluded from the meal, while being allowed to drain into the antrum.[26]

Horizontal gastroplasty

This works by similarly creating a restricted gastric pouch, involving the fundus and upper body of the stomach. This pouch can be created either by a stapled horizontal partition, or by enclosing the upper stomach with a calibrated piece of prosthetic material.[27] Both vertical gastroplasty and horizontal gastroplasty achieve weight loss by inducing a feeling of fullness after a small meal.

Gastric bypass

This achieves weight loss by both restricting intake, by having a gastric pouch, but also inducing some malabsorption, which is not as extensive as after jejuno-ileal bypass, by permitting drainage from the gastric pouch into a jejunal loop in a Roux-en-Y arrangement.[28] Randomised studies have demonstrated that gastric bypass will achieve significantly greater weight loss than that seen with either vertical gastroplasty or horizontal gastroplasty.[29,30] It is, however, more technically demanding and associated with higher rates of morbidity. In addition, patients may experience the dumping syndrome following this procedure, which does not occur after vertical or horizontal gastroplasty.

Operative procedures

Vertical gastroplasty

Vertical banded gastroplasty combines relatively low morbidity and mortality rates (less then 1%) with significant and maintained reduction of weight.[26,31,32]

Surgical technique

With the patient under general and epidural anaesthesia, in the supine position, on a suitable reinforced operating table a long upper mid line incision is made. A size 32, 15 mm, French bougie is passed by the anaesthetist through the mouth into the stomach. This can be achieved by the passage of the bougie after the endoscopic placement of a guidewire, as for fundoplication. This allows measurement of the volume of the gastric pouch together with the outlet of the gastric pouch. In addition, it protects the oesophagus and aids identification. A window is created opposite and just above the incisura, in the stomach, by means of a circular stapling device (such as 25 or 28 mm EEA Auto Suture, Ascot, UK). This is introduced from the back wall of the stomach, by the lesser sac, by advancing the spike of the instrument through first the back wall and then the front wall of the stomach, while maintaining pressure to keep the two walls of the stomach in close proximity. The spike is removed and the head of the stapling gun attached. The stapling gun is then closed and fired, creating a circular window in the stomach. A window is then made above the gastro-oesophageal junction, above the fundus, taking care to protect the short gastric vessels. A 24 French Foley catheter can then be passed around the longitudinal axis of the stomach, such that the open end of the catheter emerges through the circular window in the stomach, and is then attached to the toe of the linear stapling device. This catheter is then manipulated to allow the base of the stapling device to be manipulated into position behind the stomach, such that the toe emerges through the peritoneal window, adjacent to the cardia. This allows the staples to be correctly and safely positioned, having taken care to stretch the greater curve of the stomach out laterally to prevent bunching of the gastric tissue. Linear stapling devices with either two or four rows of parallel staples can be used. The advantage of the four-row stapler is that this requires only one pass of the instrument behind the stomach and also avoids possible necrosis, caused by crossover of staple lines, rendering part of the gastric tissue ischaemic.[33] The presence of the 32 Fr bougie in the gastric pouch and careful adjustment of the stapler gun before firing, such that it is in close proximity, but not tight on this bougie, should allow the correct size gastric pouch to be made.

It is debatable as to whether the stomach needs to be divided between these rows of staples. No randomised studies exist, comparing the safety and efficacy of division versus no division. The advantage of leaving the staple lines intact is that it reduces the risk of gastric leakage. The disadvantage is that there is the potential for late disruption of the staple line. In the author's opinion, the latter is the lesser of the two evils.

The size of the gastric pouch can be assessed visually or measured accurately by instilling saline down a nasogastric tube connected to a manometer. The volume of the pouch is measured at a pressure of 25–30 cm of saline above the level of the cricoid cartilage, when the operating table is horizontal. A sling placed around the oesophagus prevents reflux and obviously such measurement is made before the stomach is completely stapled to allow for adjustments of position.

When constructed in this fashion the outlet of the gastric pouch measures about 12 mm in diameter and can be reinforced with the use of a 1.5 cm wide strip of either polypropylene Marlex mesh (C. R. Bard, Billerica, Massachusetts, USA) or Gore-Tex (W.L. Gore, Woking, UK), which should be secured to itself with two rows of polypropylene sutures, measured to give a collar circumference of 5 cm. The placement of two rows of polypropylene sutures allows for dilatation of the stoma, should it prove to stenose, by breaking the first row of sutures by dilatation, while leaving the second row intact. If the stoma is too tight, this may lead to inadequate weight loss because of dehiscence of the vertical staple line[34] and if the stoma is too wide insufficient weight loss will result because of the inability of the gastric pouch to induce sufficient satiety.[35] Stenosis of the gastric outlet may occur in up to 10% of patients, but is successfully treated endoscopically in up to 90% of patients.

Prospective randomised trials comparing the incidence of wound seromas, haematomas and wound infections have shown similar rates of complications in patients in whom wound drainage has been used, with those in whom it has not.[36] Similarly, sutures designed to eliminate the subcutaneous dead space in the mid line abdominal wounds in morbidly obese patients, seem to offer no significant advantage in the prevention of wound infections and other complications.[37] Ultrasound examination of the wounds suggests that the potential dead space within the subcutaneous fat does not in fact occur, contrary to conventional surgical teaching.[38] Meta-analysis of 21 trials suggested that monotherapy with amoxicillin-clavulanic acid was as effective as other comparative regimens, including combination regimens of gentamycin and metronidazole in the prevention of the low incidence of wound infections. One shot amoxicillin-clavulanic acid has benefits in terms of convenience, tolerance and cost.[39]

Postoperative management

Patients are ideally managed on a high dependency unit for the first 24–48 h. The use of an epidural should permit adequate pain relief and, critically, allow early mobilisation and good postoperative breathing exercises. Movement of the patient in the early postoperative period requires well motivated and strong nursing staff. An orthopaedic trapeze over the bed greatly aids early mobilisation. For the first 4–6 weeks after surgery, patients should receive a fluid diet. This encourages early loss of weight and gives the patient an incentive. Thereafter soup, jelly and ice-cream may be gradually reintroduced together with liquidised or puréed food for the following 4–6 weeks. Mineral and vitamin supplements should be added.[40] A light food diet should be introduced after 10–12 weeks. Close supervision of the patient by a dietician with an interest in surgery for the morbidly obese is required to prevent patients over-restricting their calorie intake. Dieticians should aim to achieve a food intake of about five meals, each of 50 g a day.[31] Foods rich in protein are to be recommended. Patients should be informed that their loss of weight is most marked in the first 12 months, but continues thereafter to 18–24 months. Up to 50% of patients would be expected to lose 50% of their excess weight in the first 12 months and most studies report that 70–80% of patients fall to within 50% of their ideal body weight at 2 years. The loss of weight is maintained in the long term.[41]

Postoperative morbidity

Gastric leakage is uncommon (less than 1%).[42,43] If there is concern about the longitudinal staple line (if it has been divided) at the time of operation then it should be tested by installation of methylene blue, via the nasogastric tube, at the time of operation. Oversewing of this staple line with reinforcement with an omental patch may be required. The most common complication in the early postoperative period is vomiting, caused by rushed intake. Patients should be encouraged to build up their fluid intake gradually, over a period of 3 to 5 days, and expect some regurgitation.

Vertical gastroplasty leads to an increase in the lower oesophageal sphincter pressure, with the gastric pouch and stoma acting as a high pressure zone. This leads to a strengthening of the mechanism to prevent reflux of gastric acid. Interestingly, vertical plication of the stomach has been suggested as a treatment for reflux oesophagitis.[44] Uncommonly, the functional reserve of the lower oesophageal sphincter can be overcome by distal obstruction of the stoma. In a small group of patients the clearance of the lower oesophagus becomes inadequate and such patients, although small in number, develop severe ulcerative oesophagitis.[45] This may respond to the usual medical treatment, using proton pump inhibitors, H_2 receptor antagonists etc, but may be unresponsive to such treatment and require conversion to a Roux-en-Y bypass.

The digestion and absorption of food are unaffected by vertical gastroplasty. The patients in whom weight loss is not achieved to any significant extent, or patients in whom, after an early loss, subsequently regain their weight, may have experienced disruption of the staple line or dilatation of the gastric pouch and stoma, which becomes increasingly accommodating to food intake. Patients may learn that meat and vegetables will fill the gastric pouch promptly and empty slowly, and also learn that highly refined food will empty more promptly. They can thus bypass the gastric restrictive procedure by maintain a high calorie liquid intake and a number of patients have discovered that the recently marketed ice cream sweets negotiate the restrictive procedure very well and thousands of calories can be taken relatively quickly and presumably quite pleasurably. Patients need to be warned that such manoeuvres will quickly negate the value of their surgery and make the whole procedure worthless.

Horizontal gastroplasty

This procedure also restricts oral intake and thereby achieves significant loss of weight.[46] Several technical variations of the procedure have been described, using strands of nylon sutures, bands of polytetrafluoroethylene, Gore-Tex or Marlex or two or four rows of staples, each to create an upper gastric pouch above a horizontal restricted outlet, with the volume of the pouch measuring 50–60 ml and a 1 cm stoma into the lower stomach. One putative benefit of this procedure, as against the vertical procedure, is that it avoids dissection around the gastro-oesophageal junction, thereby avoiding possible trauma to the oesophagus and upper short gastric vessels. One putative disadvantage of the procedure, against the vertical procedure, is a hypothetical increased risk of dehiscence of the horizontal staple line, subjected to the gravitational effects of the food bolus within the upper gastric pouch and the direction of the propulsive waves through the stomach, being perpendicular to the horizontal staple line and tangential to the vertical staple line. Operatively the procedure is perhaps most easily achieved by use of a linear staple device, from which four staples have been removed from the middle (such as the TA90 linear stapling device Auto-Suture, Ascot, UK). The firing of this stapling device, from the greater to the lesser curve, thus creates two staple lines with a central gap, to allow slow emptying from the upper gastric pouch, into the lower stomach. Transverse position of this stapling device on the body of the stomach determines the size of the pouch, while 50 ml is optimal, in practice attempts to create a larger pouch would actually be met with the stapling device not reaching across the whole body of the stomach, with the resultant bunching of the gastric wall.

Postoperative management is similar to that described in vertical gastroplasty and again, patients should not be encouraged to take large quantities of food or liquid in the early postoperative period for fear of disrupting the stapling line. This is most likely to occur at the point at which the staple line abuts onto the gastric outlet.[47] This area may be reinforced with interrupted sutures.[48] In addition, there is a small risk of devascularisation of the upper gastric pouch, which can lead to perforation.[49]

The use of an encircling band of prosthetic material, as opposed to a staple line to create the restriction of the stomach, has been found to be associated with erosion, and less commonly, chronic infection.

Indeed, the prosthetic material may erode completely through the gastric wall and be visible in the stomach and there have been rare cases of the material being passed with the stool. An alternative to prosthetic material, which eliminates this risk, is by using ligementum teres, in which the blood supply is maintained by leaving it attached at the hepatic end.[50]

Reflux oesophagitis, which can be severe, is not uncommon after horizontal gastroplasty.[51] In patients in whom satisfactory weight loss has been achieved, but are troubled with reflux oesophagitis, the horizontal gastroplasty may be converted into a vertical banded gastroplasty.[52] This may also be carried out in patients in whom satisfactory weight loss has not been achieved. In general, horizontal gastroplasty is considered mechanically less reliable than vertical banded gastroplasty, with the relatively thin-walled gastric fundus being permitted to overdistend with inadequate loss of weight.[47]

Gastric banding-stoma adjustable gastric banding

The stoma adjustable silicone gastric banding procedure has been favoured by some surgeons on the basis that the material used is unstretchable, the size of the outlet is adjustable, there is no gastric incision and the operation can be reversed. In one series of 111 patients (mean body mass index $46.4 \pm 6.3 \, kg/m^2$) at a median follow-up of 18 months (range 12–44) the percentage excess weight loss was $52 \pm 23\%$. Late complications included band slippage, stomal stenosis with pouch dilatation, band erosion and reservoir band erosion. Surgical revision was performed in 10 patients. Proponents of this procedure have suggested that this technique is suitable for laparoscopic applications.[53]

Comparison of vertical-banded gastroplasty versus adjustable silicone gastric banding, in a series of 40 patients (19 VBG, 21 ASGB) found a similar degree of excess weight loss of 62% in both groups.[54]

Gastric bypass

It is well recognised that Billroth II gastrectomy is associated with loss of weight when used to treat peptic ulcer disease. This procedure has been used effectively in the surgical treatment of morbid obesity as a form of biliopancreatic bypass.[55] Several variations have been described, which include a complete division of the stomach and the construction of a short retrocolic gastrojejunostomy, a small upper gastric pouch, in which there is preservation of a long but narrow greater curve, with a gastrojejunostomy, anterior gastrojejunostomy, with the stomach stapling continuity, with a Roux-en-Y reconstruction, again with the stomach stapled in continuity.[56] With each of these procedures, there is restriction of volume of ingested food together with altered absorption of nutrients, especially fat. These two factors contribute to achieve the weight loss. The size of the stoma in such gastric bypass procedures is not as important as in the previously described vertical banded gastroplasty or horizontal gastroplasty. As a result, it would appear that patients are able to eat a wider choice of foods.[30]

Such procedures are more technically demanding, particularly when the size of the patient is considered. Not surprisingly these more complex operations are associated with a higher incidence of morbidity. The main worry after gastric bypass is anastomotic leakage, which in large series may reach 5%.[56] In addition, although the parietal cell mass is small, stomal ulceration remains a problem. Although such ulceration may respond to proton pump antagonists and H2 receptor blockers, revisional surgery may be required.[56] Serum gastrin levels may become excessive and the excluded stomach may require resection. 'Sweet-eaters' constitute a subgroup of patients in whom gastric bypass procedures may be advantageous over gastroplasty, in so much as consumption of highly refined foods, high calorie sweets and drinks may result in dumping syndrome with the sudden onset of light headedness and abdominal colic, caused by the rapid movement of water into the bowel.[27]

A combination procedure of vertical banded gastroplasty with distal gastric bypass involves a conventional vertical-banded gastroplasty, after which the mid body of the stomach is stapled transversely 2–3 cm below the outlet stoma of the gastroplasty, with a Roux-en-Y jejunal loop being brought up to the gastric pouch. Such a gastro-jejunostomy is thus constructed in a relatively more accessible part of the operative field and the weight loss is superior to that obtained with vertical banded gastroplasty alone.[57] In patients in whom weight loss has been inadequate after vertical-banded gastroplasty, distal gastric bypass may be added at a subsequent operation,[51] particularly in patients who are super-obese (over 150 kg).[58] Repeat procedures of this kind carry an increased morbidity.

Most surgeons active in the field of morbid obesity surgery consider that gastric bypass procedures are associated with greater weight loss than that obtained by either vertical or horizontal gastroplasties,[30] but carry the cost of increased morbidity, the dumping syndrome,[59] nutritional deficiencies and the requirement for vitamin B_{12} injections.[60]

The biliopancreatic bypass

Although jejuno-ileal bypass has been abandoned, the malabsorption procedures have not been completely discarded. Scopinaro[55] has described a biliopancreatic bypass procedure in which the pancreato-biliary secretions from the duodenum are diverted into the ileum or colon, and the remaining small intestine is anastomosed to the stomach, after antrectomy. Although the operation produces significant weight loss, there is the potential for serious nutrition and other complications. It is not reversible.

Current areas of research

Laparoscopic procedures

The recent application of laparoscopic techniques to general surgical procedures has led to the early development of laparoscopic surgery for morbid obesity.[61] Before embarking on laparoscopic techniques for morbid obesity surgeons need to be experienced in the surgical treatment of obesity. As discussed above, the operations for the treatment of morbid obesity require special attention to technical detail. Undoubtedly there is a learning curve, and a skilled laparoscopist, who has never either performed the standard operations for obesity nor taken care of the severely obese, should not undertake such procedures before carefully reviewing the experience and difficulties which have arisen with the open procedures. An awareness of the time required to evaluate differences in operative techniques and the significance of seemingly minor variations in technique in the lifelong success or failure of such procedures is required.

Operative technique

Briefly, with the patient in the lithotomy position (reverse Trendelenburg), four trocars (10 mm) are introduced through the abdominal wall, with three placed centrally through the linea alba and a fourth under the right costal cartilage. A fifth 15 mm trocar is inserted in the left upper quadrant. After mobilisation of the stomach, a Penrose drain is passed around behind the oesophagus. A large, curved needle, joined to the anvil of a circular stapler head is passed through the posterior and anterior gastric wall, about 6 cm below the cardiac incisura and 3 cm on the lesser curve. A trocar of this anvil is then pulled through the wall and the shaft of the stapler, having been introduced through the abdominal wall, is aligned with the trocar. As usual a bougie is used to size the gastric pouch and correctly position the neogastric window. An endo GIA-60 stapler is manipulated into position and placed vertically parallel to the lesser curve and fired to create the gastric pouch. Finally, a Marlex mesh band is placed around the outlet of the gastric pouch. This can be fixed with the help of a standard stapler gun used in laparoscopic hernia repairs. It is important that spatial orientation, the avoidance of damage to the cardia and lower oesophagus and ensuring an ideal pouch volume, should remain a critical part of the laparoscopic procedure as they are in the open method.

In one series of 25 patients treated by this technique, the loss of weight was similar to that seen with conventional open vertical banded gastroplasty. There was no mortality.[62]

Gastric banding can also be performed laparoscopically. Windows are created in the gastrosplenic and gastrohepatic ligaments. A tunnel is made behind the stomach by blunt dissection.[63] The anaesthetist passes a 25 ml balloon catheter into the stomach, via the oesophagus. The balloon is then inflated and a silicone band, introduced into the peritoneal cavity, is wrapped around the stomach, with the help of an Endograsper (US surgical, Norwalk, Connecticut, USA), and this is tightened onto the intragastric balloon. Presently only small series of patients have been reported with short follow-up. Long-term follow-up of complete series of laparoscopic surgery in morbid obesity is as yet unavailable.

Overall results | ## Follow-up after surgical treatment of morbid obesity

Follow-up of patients after surgical treatment for obesity is important to determine the success of the procedure. It has been suggested that patients lost to follow-up should be considered to be failures. Summation of data from 34 series of patients found that follow-up data were available at 1 year in only 61% of patients.[64] The most reliable estimate of weight loss requires that follow up is complete. This is not always possible in clinical practice, particularly when the referral practice may be tertiary in nature, as is often the case with morbid obesity surgery. Although patients may default from follow-up because they were unhappy with their assumed failure, it is equally possible that patients who have an excellent response to treatment become so involved with work and other activities that they simply do not return. It should not be assumed then that inadequate follow-up implies poor results in the patients in whom data are not available. Assessment of reported studies should use patients followed as the denominator of each group reported.

Improvements in obesity-related medical conditions after surgery for morbid obesity

The pulmonary complications affecting the morbidly obese can often be incapacitating. The obesity–hypoventilation syndrome is largely due to an increase in chest and abdominal wall mass, which causes a decrease in chest wall compliance, with restrictive pulmonary sequelae. The improvement in pulmonary function can allow patients who were formally incapacitated, to lead normal, productive lives. Almost all patients with morbid obesity of long duration will suffer degenerative bone disease as an effect of the large body mass upon a relatively small skeletal structure. Hips, knees and lumbar vertebrae are most frequently affected. It is painful and results in chronic disability. Morbidly obese individuals develop arthritis at a relatively young age compared with the general population. It is more difficult to treat without marked weight loss and in addition to osteoarthritis the morbidly obese are prone to herniation of the intravertebral discs. Loss of weight from successful morbid obesity surgery results in substantial amelioration of these bony conditions.

Encouraging reports have been published on improvement in medical conditions associated with morbid obesity after surgical treatment of the morbid obesity. In a series of 39 patients who underwent either vertical-banded gastroplasty ($n = 23$) or Roux-en-Y gastrointestinal bypass ($n = 16$) the mean blood pressure of the group fell from 148/83 mmHg preoperatively to 121/77 mmHg at 1 year after operation ($P < 0.05$). These results were consistent with those of Brolin[65] and Foley,[66] who reported that hypertension generally improves and often resolves following successful bariatric surgery. The reduction in hypertension can be predicted from the amount of weight lost. In the same series, diabetes mellitus resolved in seven of nine patients ($P < 0.05$) and dermatitis was significantly improved in eight of nine patients. Shortness of breath was reported by two-thirds of patients preoperatively, but was absent postoperatively in all of the 26 patients who had the condition. In addition, Pickwickian symptoms, particularly postprandial somnolence, resolved in all four patients in whom they were present preoperatively. Sleep apnoea resolved in six of eight patients.[67]

Data for different techniques

Outcome following the various available procedures for the surgical treatment of morbid obesity is shown in Table 14.1. Inevitably different authors have reported their results differently, but it is important that patients are aware of the targets for weight loss. A suitable goal is to aim for the patients, weight to come to within 50% in excess of the ideal body weight within 18 months of their surgery. Since, if achieved, this target is associated with improvements in co-morbid pathology, including management of diabetes mellitus, ischaemic heart disease, hypertension, the slowing of the changes of arthritis and improved life span, the obesity-related health hazards are thus avoided. Most published studies discuss results at 1–2 years and long-term follow-up 10, 15 or 20 years after such procedures are presently lacking. Variation in outcomes with similar operative procedures is probably due to variations in patient population and variable sizes of the gastric pouch and gastric outlets.

Although weight and weight loss are easy to measure and provide definable end points, the quality of life of patients after successful surgery for morbid obesity is usually improved. Clearly, however, this is difficult to measure. Nonetheless, the depth of the unhappiness of the morbidly obese patient is often most noticeable when the excess weight has been shed and the patients find a new enthusiasm for life. They are usually delighted about their loss of weight, the ability to buy normal-sized clothing and to participate in recreational activities without ridicule. Successful surgery for morbid obesity does, however, generate further need for operative intervention, with patients requiring apronectomy to remove the fatty drape from around the abdomen, and the correction of the skin flaps which hang like flying squirrel's wings from the undersurface of the upper arms. Such operations are best deferred for at least 18–24 months after surgical intervention for the morbid obesity, to prevent the need for further repeat procedures.

The assessment of outcome following surgical treatment of morbid obesity is not simply a case of balancing the extent weight loss and patient satisfaction, against postoperative morbidity and mortality. Indeed, cost-effectiveness assessment needs to include an estimation of the possible savings which result from correction of hypertension, improved cardiac status, resolution or amelioration of diabetes

Table 14.1 *Results of various surgical options in the surgical treatment of morbid obesity.*

Reference	Operation	No.	Weight loss	Complication	Morbidity Rate (%)	Mortality Rate (%)
Salmon[68]	Jejuno-ileal bypass (10-inch and 2-inch)	120	63% within 10 kg of ideal body weight	Diarrhoea	22	4
Scott et al.[18]	Jejuno-ileal bypass (12-inch and 8-inch)	200	70% within ideal body weight at 1 year	Hepatic failure	2.5	2.5
Ashley et al.[32]	Vertical banded gastroplasty	42	59% lost more than 50% excess weight	Gastric	2.6	0
Owen et al.[35]	Vertical banded gastroplasty	60	80% within 40% of ideal body weight at 1 year	Staple line	7	
				Stomal stenosis	8	3
				Band erosion	2	
Morino et al.[69]	Vertical banded gastroplasty	124	53% loss of excess body weight at 1 year	Stomal stenosis	4	0
				Band erosion	1	
Sintenie et al.[70]	Vertical banded gastroplasty	40	63% of excess weight lost at 1 year	Gastric perforation	2.5	0
MacLean et al.[30]	Vertical banded gastroplasty	54	57% within 50% ideal body weight	Stomal stenosis	22	0
Pace et al.[71]	Horizontal banded gastroplasty	115	30 kg weight loss	Failure at 1 year	15	1
Knol et al.[47]	Horizontal banded gastroplasty	77	62% of excess weight lost at 1 year	Stomal stenosis	25	0
Mason et al.[56]	Gastric bypass	138	29% of excess body weight lost at 1 year	Gastric perforation	5	0
MacLean et al.[30]	Gastric bypass	52	77% within 50% ideal body weight	Staple line fistula	23	0
Zimmerman et al.[59]	Gastric bypass	14	42 kg weight lost at 1 year	Dumping syndrome	7	0
				Anaemia	7	0
Näslund et al.[52]	Vertical banded gastroplasty after failed horizontal gastroplasty	36	Body mass index to 37 kg/m^2	Gastric	3	0
				Staple line dehiscence	3	0
Salmon and McArdle[57]	Vertical banded gastroplasty with distal gastric bypass	263	87% of excess weight lost at 1 year	Band removal	9	0
				Stomal ulcer	6	0
				Staple line dehiscence	5	0

mellitus and respiratory function, in terms of the cost, in health care terms, to the ongoing treatment of these conditions. There are also cost benefits to society and the state, in terms of gainful employment, avoidance of state benefits and avoidance of death of the patient, who may arguably be in their prime.

Conclusions

Surgical treatment of morbid obesity at present is a crisis-driven form of therapy – a final option, after all other possibilities for treatment have failed. Medical and behavioural therapies to correct morbid obesity have low rates of success. Such patients who are not offered surgical intervention would tend to lead a non-productive life. At present, it would appear that surgical interventions of a mechanical nature, to induce early satiety, with or without concomitant impaired absorption of nutrients, offer the best solution.

References

1. Stunkard AJ, Harris JR, Pedersen NL *et al*. The body mass index of twins who have been reared apart. N Engl J Med 1990; 322: 1483–7.
2. MacDonald A, Stunkard A. Body-mass indexes of British separated twins. N Engl J Med 1990; 322: 1530 (Letter).
3. Sims EAH. Destiny rides again as twins overeat. N Engl J Med 1990; 322: 1522–4.
4. Bouchard C, Tremblay A, Despres JP *et al*. The response to long-term overfeeding in identical twins. N Engl J Med 1990; 322: 1477–82.
5. Stunkard AJ, Sorensen TIA, Harris *et al*. An adoption study of human obesity. N Engl J Med 1986; 314: 193–8.
6. Sorensen TIA, Price RA, Stunkard AJ *et al*. Genetics of obesity in adult adoptees and their biological siblings. BMJ 1989; 298: 87–90.
7. North M, Jacobs MS, Murphy Leo *et al*. Identification of genes predisposing to clinically severe obesity: an approach. Obes Surg 1995; 319.
8. van Itallie TB. Bad news and good news about obesity. N Engl J Med 1986; 314: 239–40 (Editorial).
9. Goldblatt PB, Moore ME, Stundard AJ. Social factors in obesity. JAMA 1965; 192: 1039–44.
10. Goldblatt PB. Editorial. N Engl J Med 1986; 192: 1039–44.
11. Van Itallie TB. Health implications of overweight and obesity in the United Stated. Ann Intern Med 1985; 103: 983–8.
12. Halmi KA, Long M, Stunkard AJ, Mason E. Psychiatric diagnosis of morbidly obese gastric bypass patients. Am J Psychiatry 1980; 137: 470–2.
13. Cowan GSM Jr. The future of bariatric surgery. Obes Surg 1992; 2: 169–76.
14. Rabner JG, Dalton S, Greenstein RJ. Obesity surgery: dietary and psychosocial expectations and reality. Mt Sinai J Med 1993; 60: 305–10.
15. Gaye Andrews. A psychological profile of the bariatric patient with implications for treatment. Obes Surg 1995; 5: 330.
16. Lewis LA, Turnbull RB Jr, Page IH. 'Short-circuiting' of the small intestine. Effect on concentration of serum cholesterol and lipoproteins. JAMA 1962; 182: 77–9.
17. Payne JH, DeWind LT. Surgical treatment of obesity. Am J Surg 1969; 118: 141–7.
18. Scott HW, Dean RH, Shull HJ, Gluck F. Results of jejunoileal bypass in 200 patients with morbid obesity. Surg Gynecol Obstet 1977; 145: 661–73.
19. Abrams HS, Meixel SA, Webb WW, Scott HW. Psychological adaptation to jejunoileal bypass for morbid obesity. J Nerv Ment Dis 1976; 162: 151–7.
20. Halverson JD, Wise L, Wazna MF, Ballinger WF. Jejunoileal bypass for morbid obesity. A critical appraisal. Am J Med 1978; 64: 461–75.
21. Hocking MP, Duerson MC, Alexander RW,

Woodward ER. Late hepatic histopathology after jejunoileal bypass for morbid obesity. Relation of abnormalities on biopsy and clinical course. Am J Surg 1991; 141: 159–63.

22. Anderson T, Juhl E, Quaade F. Fatal outcome after jejunoileal bypass for obesity. Am J Surg 1981; 142: 619–21.

23. Arnaud SB, Goldsmith RS, Lambert PW, Go VLW. 25-Hydroxyvitamin D_3: evidence of an enterohepatic circulation in man. Proc Soc Exp Biol Med 1975; 149: 570–2.

24. Wands JR, LaMont JT, Mann E, Isselbacher KJ. Arthritis associated with intestinal-bypass procedure for morbid obesity. Complement activation and characterization of circulating cryoproteins. N Engl J Med 1976; 294: 121–4.

25. Griffen WO Jr, Bivens BA, Bell RM. The decline and fall of the jejunoileal bypass. Surg Gynecol Obstet 1983; 157: 301–8.

26. Mason EE. Vertical banded gastroplasty for obesity. Arch Surg 1982; 117: 701–6.

27. Kuzmak LI. Silicone gastric banding: a simple and effective operation for morbid obesity. Contemp Surg 1986; 28: 13–18.

28. Alden JF. Gastric and jejunoileal bypass. A comparison in the treatment of morbid obesity. Arch Surg 1977; 112: 799–804.

29. Sugarman HJ, Starkey JV, Birkenhauer R. A randomized prospective trial of gastric bypass versus vertical banded gastroplasty for morbid obesity and their effect on sweets versus non-sweet eaters. Ann Surg 1987; 205: 613–24.

30. MacLean LD, Rhode BM, Sampalis J, Forse RA. Results of surgical treatment of obesity. Am J Surg 1993; 165: 155–62.

31. Anderson T, Backer OG, Stockholm KH, Quaade F. Randomized trial of diet and gastroplasty compared with diet alone in morbid obesity. N Engl J Med 1984; 310: 352–6.

32. Ashley S, Bird DL, Sugden G, Royston CMS. Vertical banded gastroplasty for the treatment of morbid obesity. Br J Surg 1993; 80: 1421–3.

33. Whiteley GSW, Baildam AD, Walter DP et al. Technical points in vertical gastroplasty for morbid obesity. Obes Surg 1992; 2: 101–3.

34. MacLean LD, Rhode BM, Forse RA. Late results of vertical banded gastroplasty for morbid and super obesity. Surgery 1990; 107: 20–7.

35. Owen ERTC, Abraham R, Kark AE. Gastro-

plasty for morbid obesity: technique, complications and results in 60 cases. Br J Surg 1989; 76: 131–5.

36. Shaffer D, Benotti PN, Both A Jr et al. A prospective, randomized trial of abdominal wound drainage in gastric bypass surgery. Ann Surg 1987; 206: 134–7.

37. Chung RS, Schertizer M, Fromm D et al. Effect of wound closure technique on wound infection in morbidly obese: results of a randomized trial. Obes Surg 1991; 1: 33–5.

38. Halstead WS. The treatment of wounds with special references to the value of blood clot in the management of dead spaces. Johns Hopkins Hosp Rep 1890–1891; 2: 255–80.

39. Wilson AP, Shrimpton S, Jaderberg M. A meta-analysis of the use of amoxicillin-clavulanic acid in surgical prophylaxis. J Hosp Infect 1992; 22 (Suppl A): 9–21.

40. Owen ERTC, Abraham R, Kark AE. Dietary deficiencies after vertical banded gastroplasty (VBG). Int J Obes 1987; 11 (Suppl 2): 123 (Abstract).

41. Mason EE, Doherty C, Scott DH et al. Vertical banded gastroplasty (VBG) for treatment of obesity: an eight year review. Int J Obes 1989; 13: 593–9.

42. Dietal M, Jones BA, Petrov I et al. Vertical banded gastroplasty: results in 233 patients. Can J Surg 1986; 29: 322–4.

43. Buckwalter JA, Herbst CA Jr. Leaks occurring after gastric bariatric operations. Surgery 1988; 103: 156–60.

44. Taylor TV, Knox RA, Pullan BR. Vertical gastric plication: an operation for gastro-oesophageal reflux. Ann R Coll Surg Engl 1989; 71: 31–6.

45. Downie JRF. Observations on nine personal cases where oesophagitis has appeared as a complication of a functioning vertical gastroplasty. Obes Surg 1992; 2: 75–8.

46. Gomez CA. Gastroplasty in morbid obesity. Surg Clin North Am 1979; 59: 1113–20.

47. Knol JA, Strodel WE, Eckhauser FE. Critical appraisal of horizontal gastroplasty. Am J Surg 1987; 153: 256–61.

48. Linner JH. Comparative effectiveness of gastric bypass and gastroplasty: a clinical study. Arch Surg 1982; 117: 695–700.

49. MacLean LD, Rhode BM, Shizgal HM. Gastroplasty for obesity. Surg Gynecol Obstet 1981; 153: 200–8.

50. Broadbent R. Use of the round ligament as a natural living gastric band for weight loss surgery: a preliminary report. Obes Surg 1992; 2; 185–8.
51. Sapala JA, Bolar RJ, Bell JP, Sapala MA. Technical strategies for converting the failed vertical banded gastroplasty to the Roux-en-Y gastric bypass. Obes Surg 1993; 3: 400–9.
52. Näslund E, Granström L, Stockeld D, Backman L. Vertical banded gastroplasty: one treatment for oesophagitis and/or weight gain after gastric banding. Obes Surg 1993; 3: 365–8.
53. Lise M, Favretti F, Belluco C et al. Stoma adjustable silicone gastric banding: results in 111 consecutive patients. Obes Surg 1994; 274.
54. Taskin M, Apaydin B, Carkman S et al. Comparison of two gastric restrictive procedures: vertical banded gastroplasty vs adjustable silicone gastric banding. Obes Surg 1995; 5: 274.
55. Scopinaro N, Gianetta E, Civalleri D et al. Two years of clinical experience with biliopancreatic bypass of obesity. Am J Clin Nutr 1980; 33: 506–14.
56. Mason EE, Printen KJ, Blommers R et al. Gastric bypass in morbid obesity. Am J Clin Nutr 1980; 33 (Suppl): 395–405.
57. Salmon PA, McArdle MO. The rationale and results of gastroplasty/distal gastric bypass. Obes Surg 1992; 2: 61–8.
58. Salmon PA. Gastroplasty/distal gastric bypass: an operation producing excellent and prolonged weight loss in the super obese. Obes Surg 1993; 3: 391–6.
59. Zimmerman V, Campos CT, Buchwald H. Weight loss comparison of gastric bypass and Silastic ring vertical gastroplasty. Obes Surg 1992; 2: 47–9.
60. Smith CD. Herkes SB, Behrns KE et al. Gastric acid secretion and vitamin B_{12} absorption after vertical Roux-en-Y gastric bypass for morbid obesity. Ann Surg 1993; 218: 91–6.
61. Catona A, Gossenberg M, La Manna A, Mussini G. Laparoscopic gastric banding: preliminary series. Obes Surg 1993; 3: 207–9.
62. Catona A, Gossenberg M, Mussini G et al. Videolaparoscopic vertical banded gastroplasty. Obes Surg 1995; 323.
63. Cadière GB, Bruyns J, Himpens J, Favretti F. Laparoscopic gastroplasty for morbid obesity. Br J Surg 1994; 81: 1524.
64. Renquist KE, Cullen JJ, Barnes D et al. The effect of follow up on reporting success for obesity surgery. Obes Surg 1995; 5: 285–92.
65. Brolin RE. Results of obesity surgery. Gastroenterol Clin North Am 1987; 2: 317–38.
66. Foley EF, Benotti PN, Borlage BC et al. Impact of gastric restrictive surgery on hypertension in the morbidly obese. Am J Surg 1992; 163: 294–7.
67. Bourdages H, Goldenberg F, Phuong Nguyen et al. Improvement in obesity-associated medical conditions following vertical banded gastroplasty and gastrointestinal bypass. Obes Surg 1994; 4: 227.
68. Salmon PA. The results of small intestine bypass operations for the treatment of obesity. Surg Gynecol Obstet 1971; 132: 965–79.
69. Morino F, Toppino M, Fronda et al. Weight loss and complications after vertical banded gastroplasty. Obes Surg 1992; 2: 69–73.
70. Sintenie JB, Tuinebreijer We, Kreis RW et al. Results of vertical banded gastroplasty for treatment of morbid obesity. Obes Surg 1992; 2: 181–4.
71. Pace WG, Martin EW Jr, Tetirick T et al. Gastric partitioning for morbid obesity. Ann Surg 1979; 190: 392–400.

Index

Page numbers in *italics* refer to illustrations and tables; **bold** page numbers indicate a main discussion.

Abdominal oesophagus, 113
Achalasia, 279, *292*, **293–4**
  oesophageal cancer association, 20, 40
  oesophageal cancer screening, 40, 50
  oesophageal scintigraphy, 290
Acid reflux provocation test (ARPT), 289
Adenoid cystic carcinomas, **251**
Adenomatous polyps, 12, 13, **257–8**, *258*, 259
  familial adenomatous polyposis (FAP), 13
Adenomyoma (myoepithelioma), 259
Adjuvant chemotherapy *see* Postoperative chemotherapy
Adjuvant radiotherapy *see* Postoperative radiotherapy
Adrenaline injection, bleeding peptic ulcer, **373–4**, **376**, 377, 384
Adriamycin, 205
Aerodigestive fistula, 216, **234–5**
Airway evaluation, preoperative, 95
AJC gastric cancer staging, **79**, *80*
AJC oesophageal cancer staging, *84*
Alcohol intake
  Barrett's oesophagus conversion to malignancy, 24
  oesophageal cancer, 20, 22, 192
Alginates, 276, 300
Ambulatory manometry, 280, **283**
Ambulatory oesophageal pH measurements, 284, 285
Ambulatory oesophageal scintigraphy, 290
Amoxycillin, 333
Anaemia, 216, 235
Anaesthesia, **97–104**
  endobronchial intubation, 98–9
  oesophageal surgery, **100–4**
  peroperative monitoring, 99–100, *100*
  premedication, 97
  preoperative anaesthetic management, 100
  preoperative assessment, **89–95**, *90*
    airway evaluation, 95
    anaesthetic history, 90
    family history, 90
    gastro-oesophageal reflux, 94–5

    medical history, 90–3
    smoking, 93–4, *94*
  preoperative investigations, **95–7**, *96*
  preoperative preparation, 97–8
  rapid sequence induction, 98
Anastomotic leak
  post-gastric surgery, **180–1**
  post-oesophagectomy, 135, **137**
Aneuploidy, 8, 28
Angina, 92
Angle of His, 273
Antacids, 276, 300
Antibiotic prophylaxis
  laser oesophageal stricture treatment, 227
  postoesophagectomy, 136, 137
  postsplenectomy infections, 182
Antibiotic therapy
  bacterial overgrowth, 185
  Helicobacter pylori eradication, **333**
Anticoagulants, 97
Antireflux mechanism, **271[–]5**, *272*
  angle of His, 273
  diaphragmatic crus, 273
  duodenogastric reflux, 275
  failure, 275, *276*
  gastro-oesophageal reflux disease, 278
  gastric acid secretion, 274–5
  gastric emptying, 274
  gastric motility, 274
  lower oesophageal sphincter, 272–3
    vagal reflex, 274
  mucosal rosette, 273
  oesophageal motility, 273
  saliva secretion, 274
Antireflux surgery, 278, **301–16**
  Barrett's oesophagus management, 41, 319
  with cholecystectomy, 304
  complications, 315–16
    slipped Nissen, 316
  with Heller's myotomy, 313
  indications, 302–4, *302*
  laparoscopic, 313–14, 315
  mechanism of action, 306

Antireflux surgery *cont*
  patient counselling, 305–6
  postoperative care, 314
  preoperative investigations, 304–5
  techniques, **307–14**
Antithromboembolic stockings, 98, 115
Antral exclusion, 348
Arterial blood gases, preoperative assessment,
    96, 97
ASA assessment of physical status, *89*
Aspiration pneumonia, 73, 216
  following laser treatment, 228
  following oesophageal prosthesis insertion,
    221–2
  gastro-oesophageal reflux disease, 303
  oesophageal motility disorders, 291
Asthma, 95
Atkinson prosthesis, 218, *219*, 222
  fistula prosthesis, 235
Atropine, 95
Auerbach's (myenteric) plexus, 268
Automatic calf compressors, 98

B-cell lymphoma of MALT type, **16–19**, *17*,
    254, 256
  genetic abnormalities, 18
  lymphoepithelial lesion, 17, *18*
  prognosis, 18–19
Bacterial overgrowth
  diarrhoea, 184–5, 351, 352
  fat malabsorption, 354
  post-gastrectomy vitamin deficiency, 186
Barrett's oesophagus, 1, *24*, **316–18**, 320,
    321
  antireflux surgery, 41
  benign complications, 316–17
  duodenogastric reflux, 275
  dysplasia, 25, *26*, 318
  endoscopy, 68, 280
  epidemiology, 317
  gastro-oesophageal reflux disease, 23, 40,
    275, 278, 303, 317
  oesophageal adenocarcinoma, **23–4**, *25*, 40–1,
    140, 317–18
    following cessation of reflux, 319
    predisposing factors, 41
    risk assessment, 318
  oesophageal cancer epidemiology, 192
  oesophageal scintigraphy, 290
  oesophageal squamous carcinoma, 21
  p53 mutations, 30

surveillance endoscopy/screening, 24, 50,
    318
treatment, **318–19**
  ablation of mucosa, 319
Belsey 'Mark IV' partial fundoplication,
    309–10
Benign anastomotic stricture, 138–9
Benign epithelial tumours, **252**
Benign oesophageal stricture, 20
Beta-carotene, 193
BICAP *see* Bipolar electrocoagulation
Bile reflux, 275
  antireflux surgery preoperative assessment,
    305
  post-gastrectomy, 185
Biliopancreatic bypass, **403**
Biopsy
  gastric ulcer, 330, 344
  gastro-oesophageal reflux disease, 279
Bipolar electrocoagulation, **231–2**
  bleeding peptic ulcer, *372*, **372–3**, **375**, 377,
    384
  complications, 231–2
  dysphagia relief, 232
  endoscopic technique, 231
  laser therapy comparison, 232
Bleomycin, 199
Blood pressure measurements, preoperative,
    92
Blood transfusion, 106
Boerhaave's syndrome, 363
Brachytherapy (intracavitary radiation),
    dysphagia palliation, **233–4**
Bronchoscopy, preoperative, 97
Brush cytology
  gastric cancer, 68–9
  oesophageal cancer, 67
Bupivacaine, 107, 108
Burkitt-like lymphoma, 19
Burkitt's lymphoma, 19

c-erb B2 overexpression, 29
C-met, 29
c-myc overexpression, 29
Caffeine consumption, 327
cag A gene, 11
Calcium supplements, post-gastrectomy,
    186
Cape Town gastric cancer study, 162–3
Carbohydrate absorption, post-gastrectomy,
    186

Carcinoid syndrome, 20, 257
Carcinoid tumours
  oesophagus, **249**
  stomach, 2, 19–20, **256–7**
Carcinoma-in-situ, 1, 2
Carcinosarcoma
  oesophagus, 250
  stomach, 260
Cardia *see* Gastro-oesophageal junction
Cardiac dysrhythmias, 101, 106
Cardiac risk assessment, 91–2, *91*
Cardiopulmonary preoperative assessment,
  95
  anaesthetic risk, 91–2
    Goldman risk index, *91*
  exercise testing, 97
  pulmonary function tests, 96–7
Cardiorespiratory illness
  anaesthetic risk, 91–2, *91*
  postoperative hypoxia, 105
Cardiovascular instability
  oesophageal surgery, 100–1, 104
  postoperative care, 106
Cardiovascular monitoring, 99–100
Carney's triad, 16
CD44, 29
Celestin tube, 219, *219*, 222
Cerebral vascular episodes, 137
Cervical oesophagus, 80, **112**, *113*
  lymph nodes, 82, *82*, *114*
  pharyngolaryngo-oesophagectomy, **129**
Chemotherapy, **191–209**
  gastric cancer, **204–7**, 214
    immunochemotherapy, 207
  gastric carcinoids, 257
  gastric lymphoma, 255
  gastric outflow obstruction palliation,
    237
  hyperthermic, 195–6, **205**
  oesophageal cancer, 214
    adenocarcinoma, **202**
    squamous cell carcinoma, **198–9**, 201
  treatment strategies, **194–6**
Chemotherapy-radiotherapy combination,
  196
  gastric cancer, **207–8**
  gastric lymphoma, 255
  oesophageal adenocarcinoma, **202–3**
  oesophageal squamous cell carcinoma,
    201
    followed by surgery, **200–1**
    without surgery, **199**

Chest pain
  gastric cardia cancer, 216
  gastro-oesophageal reflux disease, 278, 280
  oesophageal cancer, 216
  oesophageal motility disorders, 290, 291,
    294, 295
Chinese University of Hong Kong gastric
  cancer study, 163
Cholecystectomy
  with antireflux surgery, 304
  with obesity surgery, 395
Cholestyramine, 352
Chondroma, 262
Chondrosarcoma, 247
Choriocarcinoma, 2, 262
Chylothorax, 137–8
Cimetidine, 300
Cisapride, 138, 301
Cisplatin, 198, 199, 200, 202, 203, 205, 237
Clarithromycin, 333
Coeliac disease, 21
Collis Nissen partial fundoplication, 311, *312*
Colloidal bismuth, 333
Colon, oesophageal reconstruction, *127*, **127–8**
Computed tomography (CT)
  gastric cancer, 65–6
  gastrinoma localisation, 338
  gastro-oesophageal junction carcinoma,
    63–4
  intracranial metastases, 73
  oesophageal cancer
    distant metastases, 64–5
    local spread, 62–4, *63*
  preoperative assessment, **62–6**, 74
Correa hypothesis, 43–4, *43*
Corrosive strictures
  oesophageal cancer epidemiology, 39
  oesophageal cancer screening, 50
  progression to squamous carcinoma, 20
Cowden's disease, 259
cripto expression, 29
Cronkhite-Canada syndrome, 259
Cyclophosphamide, 255
Cytological atypia, 1, 2

Deleted in colorectal cancer (DCC), 30
Diaphragmatic crus, 273
Diaphragmatic resection, 101
Diarrhoea
  post-gastrectomy, **184–5**
  post-peptic ulcer surgery, **351–2**

Dietary advice
  advanced cancer, 217
  oesophageal prostheses, 220
  post-gastrectomy, 183, 184
  post-peptic ulcer surgery dumping
    syndrome, 349
  post-vertical gastroplasty, 400, 401
  postvagotomy diarrhoea, 351
Dietary factors
  chronic (atrophic) gastritis, 9
  gastric cancer, 9, 12, **45–7**, 192–3
  gastro-oesophageal reflux disease, 299
  oesophageal cancer, 20, 192
    premalignant conditions, 39, 40
  peptic ulcer disease, 327
Dieulafoy lesion, 382
Diffuse leiomyomatosis, 246
Diffuse oesophageal spasm, *292*, 294
Distal pancreatectomy, 176
Domperidone, 301
Dor partial fundoplication, 310
Double lumen endobronchial tube, 95, 98, *99*
Doxorubicin, 204, 205, 206, 257
Dumping syndrome
  diarrhoea, 184, 351
  gastric bypass, 403
  post-gastrectomy, **183–4**, 185
  post-oesophagectomy, 138
  post-peptic ulcer surgery, **348–9**, *349*, **351**,
    353
    medical treatment, 349
    surgery, 349, *350*
Duodenal bypass, 177, *178*
Duodenal stump leak, **180**
Duodenal switch procedure, *353*
Duodenal ulcer
  blood group O association, 329
  control of bleeding, 383
    surgical technique, **379–81**, *380*, *381*
  gastric acid secretion, 327
  management protocol, *331*
  surgery, **339–43**
    refractory ulcers, 341–3
Duodenogastric reflux, 275
  see also Bile reflux
Dutch gastric cancer study, 163
Dynamic CT, 66
Dyspepsia, gastric cancer screening, 53–4,
  146
Dysphagia
  following antireflux surgery, 305, 315–16
  gastric cardia cancer, 216

gastro-oesophageal reflux disease, 278,
  280
oesophageal cancer, 216
  survival, 215
oesophageal motility disorders, 290, 291,
  294, 295
premedication, 97
pulmonary aspiration risk, 94, 98
recurrent following oesophageal prosthesis
  insertion, 222
Dysphagia relief, **217–34**
  bipolar electrocoagulation, 231–2
  ethanol induced tumour necrosis, 232–3
  intubation, 218–26
  laser treatment, 226–30
  oesophageal dilatation, 217–18
  photodynamic therapy, 230
  radiotherapy, 233–4
Dysplasia, 1, 2
  in gastric adenomas, 13
  in gastric remnant, 13
  Ménétrier's disease (hypertrophic
    gastropathy), 14

EAP chemotherapy, 205
Early gastric cancer, 2, **7–8**, 36
  classification, *62*
  computed tomography (CT), 66
  curative limited resections, 169
  detection through screening, 51, *52*, 147
    dyspepsia screening, 53–4
  DNA analysis, 8
  endoscopic ultrasonography, 69
  in gastric remnant, 13
  histology, 7
  intramucosal types, 7, 8
  macroscopic classification, 7, *8*, 52, *52*
  perigastric nodal metastases, 8
  prognosis, 2, 7–8
  radiological contrast examinations, 62–3
  recurrence, 8
  survival after early detection, 54, *54*
Early satiety, 216
  post-gastrectomy, 183, 185
  post-peptic ulcer surgery, 353
Eating disorder inventory-2 (EDI-2), 395
Edrophonium (tensilon) testing, 290
Elderly patients
  anaesthetic risk, 92, 93
  fitness for treatment, 215
  oesophageal cancer treatment, 111

oesophageal surgery objectives, 116
postoperative hypoxia, 105
preoperative assessment, 114
Endobronchial intubation, **98–9**
Endoluminal ultrasound (EUS), 232
early gastric cancer, 53
Endoprostheses *see* Expandable metal stents;
    Non-expandable plastic endoprostheses
Endoscopic ultrasonography
lymph node metastases, 69–70, 119
oesophageal cancer staging, 119, 141
preoperative assessment, **69–71**, 74
Endoscopy
antireflux surgery
    postoperative assessment, 314
    preoperative assessment, 304–5
Barrett's oesophagus surveillance, 318
bipolar electrocoagulation for dysphagia
    relief, 231
early gastric cancer, 52, *52*
ethanol induced tumour necrosis, 232
gastric cancer, 68–9, **170**
    screening, 51–2, 53, 54, 146
gastro-oesophageal reflux disease, **279**
laser oesophageal stricture treatment, 227
oesophageal cancer, 67–8
    screening, 50
oesophageal motility disorders, **293**
oesophageal prosthesis placement, 218
    aerodigestive fistulae, 234
    non-expandable plastic endoprostheses,
        220
oesophagectomy techniques, **134**
peptic stricture dilatation, 319, 320
peptic ulcer disease, 330
    persistent symptoms, 334
    recurrence following surgery, 347
preoperative assessment, **66–9**, 74
pyloric stenosis treatment, **345**
upper gastrointestinal bleeding, **365–8**
    acute bleeding, 366–7, *367*
    definition of appearances, 367–8, 385–6,
        385
    equipment, 365–6
    intraoperative, 369
    routine re-endoscopy/retreatment, 379
    techniques, 370–4
    treatment, **370–7**, *376*, 384
    washing method, 366
Enflurane, 95
Enteral nutrition, 136
Enterogastric reflux, **352–3**, *353*

Epidemiology, 35–56
advanced disease, 213–14
gastric cancer, **41–9**, **192–3**
Helicobacter pylori infection, **329**
oesophageal cancer, 35, **36–41**, *37*, **192**
    adenocarcinoma, **40–1**
peptic ulcer disease, **325–6**
Epirubicin, 237
Epithelial growth factor (EGF), 29
Epithelial growth factor receptor (EGFR), 30
erb-B2 overexpression, 30
Erosive gastritis, 362–3
Erythromycin, 138
ESKA-Buess tube, 219
fistula funnel, 235
EsoPhacoil, *223*, 224
Ethanol induced tumour necrosis, **232–3**
Etoposide, 202, 205
Exercise testing, preoperative, 97
Expandable metal stents, *223*, **223–6**
complications, 224–5
gastric outflow obstruction palliation, 237
implantation, 224
non-expandable stent comparative trial,
    225–6
Extradural analgesia, **107–8**, *108*

FAM chemotherapy, 205
Familial adenomatous polyposis (FAP), 30, 259
gastroduodenal polyps, 12–13
Famotidine, 300, 370
FAMTx chemotherapy, 204, 205
Fat malabsorption, 354
post-gastrectomy, 185, 186
Fat-soluble vitamin deficiency, post-
    gastrectomy, 186–7
Feeding jejunostomy, 115, 136
Feeding tubes, 237
Fibroma, 262
Fibrosarcoma, 247
Finney pyloroplasty, 380, *380*
Flat adenoma, 13
Fluid balance
peroperative, 100
postoperative, 106, 135
upper gastrointestinal bleeding, 364, 365
5-Fluorouracil, 199, 200, 202, 203, 204, 205,
    206, 207, 208, 237, 257
Food preservation techniques, gastric cancer
    epidemiology, 47, *47*, 193
Fundic gland polyps, 12, 13, **258–9**

Gardner's syndrome, 259
Gastrectomy, 154, *155*
  bleeding gastric ulcer, 382
  gastric nitrite metabolism, 46
  gastric outflow obstruction palliation, **236–7**
  peptic ulcer recurrence following surgery, 348
  postoperative care, 105
  stump cancers, 354
  see also Gastric cancer surgery
Gastric acid secretion
  gastro-oesophageal reflux, 274–5, 277–8
  incomplete vagotomy, 348
  peptic ulcer disease, 327
Gastric acid suppression
  peptic ulcer disease, **333–4**
    perforation, 344
  pyloric stenosis, 345
  upper gastrointestinal bleeding, 370
Gastric adenocarcinoma, 1–2
Gastric adenoma, depressed, **259**
Gastric adenomyoma (myoepithelioma), 259
Gastric adenosquamous carcinoma, 7
Gastric antireflux mechanisms, **274–5**
Gastric banding, 402
  laparoscopic procedure, 404
Gastric bypass, 397, **397**, **402–3**
Gastric cancer
  advanced, **2–7**, 213, 214, **216–17**
    classification, 3–5, *4, 5*
    histological features, 3–5, *5, 6*
    macroscopic features, 2–3, *3, 4*
    prognostic features, 5–7
    survival, 214, 215
  aetiology, 45–9, 193
    Correa hypothesis, 43–4, *43*
  chemotherapy, **204–7**
    immunochemotherapy, 207
    intraoperative chemohyperthermia, 205
    intraperitoneal, 205
    postoperative (adjuvant), 205–7, *207*
    preoperative (neoadjuvant), 205
    radiotherapy combination, 207–8
  dietary factors, **45–7**, *47*
  diffuse type, 2, 3, *4, 5*, 43, 69, 154, 193
  direct extension, 150
  distant metastases, 72, *72*
  early *see* Early gastric cancer
  environmental influences, *9*, 45
  epidemiology, 35–56, **41–9**, **192–3**
    incidence trends, 41–2, *42*
  geographic variation, *9*, 44

haematogenous spread, 151
Helicobacter pylori association, 11–12, **47–8**
intestinal type, 3, *4*, *5*, *6*, *9*, 43, 44, 69, 154, 193
  Japan versus West, 148
intraoperative investigations, **74–5**, 171–2
Japanese treatment programmes, 145–6
liver metastases, *79*
locoregional disease, 151–2
  recurrence, 193, 194
lymph node involvement, 69, 73, *77*, 157, *157, 158*, 193
  PHNS staging, *77, 78, 79*
  tiers of lymph nodes, 157–8, *159*
lymphatic spread, 150–1
metastatic pathways, 150–1, 154
molecular aspects, 27, 28–9, *28*
occupational risk, 45
palliative treatment, **236–7**, 238, *238*
pathology, **1–20**
peritoneal seeding, 151, 153
  PHNS staging, *79*
post-peptic ulcer surgery, 354
precursor lesions, 1, **8–15**, *9*, **42–4**
  classification, 42–3
preoperative assessment, **59–85**, 74
  computed tomography (CT), 65–6
  endoscopic ultrasonography, 69, **70–1**, *71*
  endoscopy, 68–9
  laparoscopy, 72–3, *72*
  radiological contrast examinations, 60, 61–2
prognosis, 193
proximal, 148, *149*
radiotherapy, **203–4**
  intraoperative, 204
  postoperative (adjuvant), 204
  postoperative plus chemotherapy, 207–8
  preoperative, 203
recurrence, 151, 152–3, **187**, 193
resection margins, 172
screening, 35–6, 49, **51–5**, 145
  asymptomatic, 51–3, 146, *147*
  Helicobacter pylori, 55
  symptomatic, 53–5, 146
  tumour markers, 54
  in West, 146–7
serosal invasion, 151, 152
  PHNS staging, *79*
socioeconomic factors, 44–5, 48

staging, **76–80**, 147–8
  International Unified TNM staging
    system, 159–60
  intraoperative, 171
  lymph node involvement, 147–8
  PHNS, 76–9, *76*, *77*
  stage migration phenomenon, 147–8
  TNM, 6, **80**, *81*
  upper gastrointestinal bleeding, 363
  Western treatment programmes, 146–50
Gastric cancer surgery, **145–87**
  distal pancreatectomy, **166–7**
  extended resections, **168–9**
  extent, 154–6, *155*
    distal third cancer, 154
    extensive cancers, 155
    middle third cancer, 155
    proximal third cancer, 155
    total gastrectomy 'de principe', 156
  implantation of free cancer cells, 152–3
  limited resections, **169–70**
  lymphadenectomy, 152, **156–64**
  pancreas-preserving gastrectomy, 167–8
  patient selection, 215
  postoperative complications
    early, **179–82**
    late, **182–7**
  principles, **153–70**
  radical, 152, 153
    Japanese practice, 146
    perioperative mortality, 148–9
    in Western practice, 149–50, *149*
  reconstruction, **176–8**
    duodenal bypass, 177, *178*
    duodenal continuity, 177, *178*
    jejunum pouch, 178
  recurrence of cancer, **187**
  resection margins, 152, 154, 156
  splenectomy, **165–6**
  technique, **170–6**
    incision, 170–1
    initial dissection, 172–4
    intraoperative investigations, 171–2
    intraoperative staging, 171
    subtotal gastrectomy, 174–5, *175*
    total gastrectomy, 175, *175*
    total gastrectomy with splenectomy and
      distal pancreatectomy, 176
  see also Gastrectomy
Gastric carcinoids, 2, 19–20, **256–7**
Gastric carcinosarcoma, 260
Gastric cardia *see* Gastro-oesophageal junction

Gastric chondroma, 262
Gastric choriocarcinoma, 262
Gastric emptying, 274
Gastric epithelial dysplasia, 14–15, 44
  gastric cancer association, 14
  grades, 14
  Helicobacter pylori, 48
  surveillance protocol, 15
Gastric fibroma, 262
Gastric glomus tumour, 262
Gastric granular cell tumour (myoblastoma),
  262
Gastric haemangioendothelioma, 262
Gastric haemangioma, 262
Gastric haemangiopericytoma, 262
Gastric leiomyoblastoma, 261
Gastric leiomyoma, 260, *261*
Gastric leiomyosarcoma, 260–1
Gastric lipoma, 261–2
Gastric lymphangioma, 262
Gastric lymphoma, 2
  in gastric remnant, 13
  primary, **253–6**, *255*
  secondary, 256
  upper gastrointestinal bleeding, 363
Gastric metastatic tumours, 262
Gastric motility, 274
Gastric mucoepidermoid carcinoma, 259
Gastric mucosal polyps, 12–13
Gastric myxoma, 262
Gastric neurogenic tumours, 260
Gastric osteoma, 262
Gastric outlet obstruction, 216, **236–7**
  palliative treatment, 217
  peptic ulcer disease, 345
  postoesophagectomy, 138
Gastric polyps, **257–9**
Gastric pseudolymphoma (lymphoid
  hyperplasia), 256
Gastric remnant
  benign histological changes, 13
  gastric carcinoma risk, 13–14
Gastric rhabdomyoma, 262
Gastric small-cell carcinoma, 262
Gastric smooth muscle tumours, 2
Gastric squamous cell carcinoma, 2, 259
Gastric teratoma, 262
Gastric ulcer
  biopsy, 330
    perforated ulcers, 344
  control of bleeding, 383–4
    surgical technique, **381–2**

Gastric ulcer *cont*
  gastric acid secretion, 327
  management protocol, *332*
  pathogenesis, 327
  surgery, **343**
Gastric wedge excision, 170
Gastrin, gastric cancer screening, 54, 55
Gastritis, chronic (atrophic), 43–4
  carcinoid tumours, 20
  gastric cancer pathogenesis, **8–12**, *9*
  in gastric remnant, 13
  gastric ulcers, 327
  Helicobacter pylori, 47, 48
Gastritis cystica profunda, 13
Gastritis, superficial, 43
Gastro-oesophageal junction (cardia), 113, *113*,
    267
  anatomical factors influencing gastro-
      oesophageal reflux, **273**
Gastro-oesophageal junction (cardia) cancer, 1,
    2
  advanced, **216**
  computed tomography (CT), 63–4
  distant metastases, 71
  dysphagia *see* Dysphagia relief
  endoscopic appearance, 67
  epidemiology, 2, 48–9
  palliation, **217–36**
  resection margins, 118
  staging, 81–2
Gastro-oesophageal reflux, 275
  antireflux mechanism, **271–5**, *272*
  LOS relaxation, 271
  in newborn, 277
  oesophageal adenocarcinoma association,
      40
  pathological, 271
  physiological, 271
  preoperative assessment, 94–5
  sliding hiatus hernia, 272, *273*
Gastro-oesophageal reflux disease, **267–95**
  aetiology, 277
  antireflux mechanism failure, 278
  antireflux surgery, 278, 320
  Barrett's oesophagus, 23, 40, 275, 278, 303,
      317
  clinical presentation, 276, **278**, *279*
  complications, 275, 278, **316–20**
  endoscopy and biopsy, 280
  gastric acid secretion, 277–8
  life-style advice, 299
  manometry, *288*, 280–3

medical therapy, 276, 278, **300–1**, 320
  oesophageal pH measurements, *285*, *286*,
      283–9, *287*, *288*
  oesophageal scintigraphy, 289
  pathophysiology, 277–8
  post-horizontal gastroplasty, 402
  post-vertical gastroplasty, 400
  prevalence, 276, 277
  provocation tests, 288–89
  radiology, 279–80
  respiratory complications, 303
  surgical therapy *see* Antireflux surgery
Gastroduodenal polyps, 12–13
Gastroenterostomy, *350*
Gastrointestinal Bleeding Unit, 384
Gastrointestinal stromal tumours (GIST),
    15–16, *16*
Genetic abnormalities
  gastric carcinoma, 27, 28–9, *28*
  morbid obesity, 392
  oesophageal cancer, 27, 29–30, 40
German gastric cancer study, 162, *162*
Gianturco Z stent, *223*, *224*, *225*
Glomus tumour, 2, 262
Glycopyrrolate, 95
Goldman Cardiac risk index, *91*
Granular cell tumours
  oesophagus, 252
  stomach, 262

H$_2$-receptor antagonists, 276, 353
  gastro-oesophageal reflux disease, **300–1**
  peptic ulcer disease, 325, 332, 333, 383
  preoperative preparation, 97
  upper gastrointestinal bleeding, 370
h-ras overexpression, 30
Haemangioendothelioma, 262
Haemangioma
  oesophagus, 252
  stomach, 262
Haemangiopericytoma, 262
Haematemesis, 363
Haemophilus influenzae vaccination, 182
Haemorrhage
  post-gastric surgery, **179–80**
  postoesophagectomy, 137
  see also Upper gastrointestinal haemorrhage
Halothane, 95
Heart failure, 92
Heartburn, 278
  persistent after antireflux surgery, 315

Heat probe, **373**, **375–6**, 384
Heineke-Mickulicz technique, 380
Helicobacter pylori, 11
 cytotoxin-associated gene A (*cagA*) strains, 329
 diagnosis of infection, 331
 epidemiology, 329
 epithelial cell Lewis antigen binding, 329
 gastric cancer, 193
  epidemiology, **47–8**
  screening marker, 55
 gastric MALT lymphomas, 17–18, 256
 gastric mucosal effects, 47
  endocrine cell proliferation, 19
  mechanism of injury, 330
  mutagenic mechanisms, 11–12
 host responses, 329–30
 peptic ulcer disease, 326, **328–30**, 333, 383
  with NSAIDs use, 332
  recurrence following surgery, 347
 persistent infection, 334
 stump cancers, 354
 subgroup-disease associations, 329
 transmission, 328–9
Helicobacter pylori eradication, **333**
 gastro-oesophageal reflux disease, 301
 peptic ulcer disease, 325
  perforation, 344
  pyloric stenosis, 345
Heller's myotomy with antireflux surgery, 313
Heparin thromboprophylaxis
 oesophageal surgery, 115, 136
 preoperative, 98
Hepatoid carcinoma, 259–60
Hiatal manipulation, 100
 cardiovascular instability, 100–1
Hiatus hernia, 95, 272, 273, 280, 305
High dependency unit, 104, 105, 107
Highly selective vagotomy, 340, 341, 383
Hill partial fundoplication, 311
Hodgkin's lymphoma
 oesophagus, 247
 stomach, **256**
Horizontal gastroplasty, **397**, **401–2**
5-HT$_3$ blockers, 208
Human papilloma virus, 20
Hydroxycobalamin supplements, 186
Hypergastrinaemia, 19, 20
Hyperplastic polyps, 12, 13, 257, 259
Hypertension, anaesthetic risk, 92
Hyperthermic chemotherapy, 195–6, **205**

Hypertrophic gastropathy (Ménétrier's disease), 14
Hypoglycaemic attacks, reactive, 184
Hypopharynx, 112, *113*
 pharyngolaryngo oesophagectomy, **129**
Hypothermia, peroperative, 100
Hypovolaemia, upper gastrointestinal bleeding, 364, 365
Hypoxic pulmonary vasoconstriction response, 101–2

Imidazole carboxamide, 257
Immunochemotherapy, **207**
Incomplete vagotomy, 348
Influenza vaccination, 182
Inhalational anaesthetics, 95, 105
Injection sclerotherapy
 oesophageal tumour bleeding palliation, 235
 peptic ulcer bleeding, **374**, 377, **377**, 384
Intensive care unit, 104, 105, 107
Interleukin 1α, 29
Intestinal metaplasia
 complete (type II), 10
 gastric cancer pathogenesis, **8–12**, *9*, *10*
 gastric cancer precursor lesions, 44
 gastric epithelial dysplasia, 14
 Helicobacter pylori, 48
 incomplete (type III), 10
Intra-abdominal sepsis, post-gastric surgery, **181–2**
Intracavitary radiation (brachytherapy), dysphagia palliation, **233–4**
Intracranial metastases, 73
Intraoperative assessment, **74–5**
Intraoperative chemohyperthermia, **205**
Intraoperative investigations, gastric cancer, 171–2
Intraoperative lymph node frozen-section, 171–2
Intraoperative radiotherapy, 194, 204
Intraperitoneal chemotherapy, 153, 171, **195–6**, **205**
Intrathoracic oesophagus, 80–1, *113*, **113**
 lymph nodes, 82, *82*, 114
 surgical approach, **129–33**
Intravenous cannulae, 100
Intubation *see* Oesophageal prosthesis placement
Invasive cardiovascular monitoring, 99–100
Iron absorption, post-gastrectomy, 187
Ischaemic heart disease, 92–3

Japanese Research Society for Gastric Cancer (JRSGC), **146**
Jejuno-ileal bypass, **395–7**
Jejunum in oesophageal reconstruction, **127**
Jejunum pouch reconstruction, 178, *178*
Juvenile polyposis, 259

K-sam, 29
Kaposi's sarcoma
    oesophagus, 247
    stomach, 262

Labelled red cell scanning, 368–9
Lanzoprazole, 300
Laparoscopic surgery
    antireflux surgery, **313–14**, 315
    limited gastric resection, 170
    obesity procedures, **403–4**
    peptic ulcer disease, 343
        perforation, 344–5
        pyloric stenosis, 346
    stomach mobilisation, 134
Laparoscopy
    preoperative assessment, **71–3**, 74
Laparsocopic ultrasound, 73
Laser treatment
    bipolar electrocoagulation comparison, 232
    dysphagia relief, **226–30**, 229
        complications, 228–9, *228*
        endoscopic technique, 227
        radiotherapy combined treatment, 229–30
    gastric cancer, 170
    oesophageal recanalisation, 214
    oesophageal tumour bleeding palliation, 235
    peptic ulcer bleeding, *371*, **371–2**, *375*, 377, 384
Lateral oesophageal lymph nodes, 114, *114*
Lavage tube, 366
Left upper quadrant evisceration, 169
Left-sided thoracoabdominal approach, 132
Leiomyoblastoma
    oesophagus, 247
    stomach, 261
Leiomyoma
    oesophagus, 245–6, *246*
    stomach, 260, *261*
    see also Gastrointestinal stromal tumours (GIST)

Leiomyosarcoma
    stomach, 260–1
    see also Gastrointestinal stromal tumours (GIST)
Leucovorin, 202, 203
Lewis antigens, 329
Lind partial fundoplication, 309, *310*
Linitis plastica, *4*
Lipoma, 261–2
Liposarcoma, 247
Liver biopsy, 172
Liver metastases, 71, 72, *72*, *73*, 74
    gastric cancer, 151
        PHNS staging, *79*
    intraoperative assessment, 75
    intraperitoneal chemotherapy, 195
Local analgesia, 107, *108*, **108**
Loperamide, 352
Low-molecular weight heparin, 98
Lower oesophageal sphincter, *269*, **269–70**
    antireflux mechanism, 272–3
    endoscopy, 280
    intra-abdominal length, 272–3
    intrinsic pressure, 272
    manometry, *279*
        pressure measurement, 282–3
        pull-through techniques, 282
        static measurement technique, 281–2
    in newborn, 277
    total length, 272
    transient relaxations
        during swallowing, 271
        gastro-oesophageal reflux, 271, 277
    vagal reflex, **274**
Lower oesophagus, 81, 113, *113*
    left-sided subtotal oesophagectomy, 132
    transhiatal oesophagectomy, 132–3
    two stage subtotal oesophagectomy, 129–30
Lymph node frozen-section, 171–2
Lymph node involvement
    computed tomography (CT), 64, 65, 66
    gastric cancer, 5, 6, 65, 66, 73, 77, 150–1, 157, *157*, *158*, 193
        endoscopic ultrasonography, 69
        intraoperative frozen-section histology, 171–2
        staging, *77*, *78*, *79*, 147–8
        tiers of lymph nodes, 157–8, *159*
    intraoperative assessment, 75
    laparoscopy, 71, 73

oesophageal cancer, 21, 22, 64, 71, 73, 192
  endoscopic ultrasonography, 69–70, 119
  staging, 82, *82*, 121
  radiotherapy rationale, 194
Lymphadenectomy
  gastric cancer surgery, 152, **156–65**
    absolute/relative curative surgery, 159
    Cape Town study, 162–3
    Chinese University of Hong Kong study, 163
    Dutch study, 163
    extended (D3), 158–9, 163, 169
    German study, 162, *162*
    International Unified TNM staging system, 159–60
    Japanese experience, 160–1, *161*
    limited (D1), 158, 160, 162–3, 164
    MRC trial (ST01), 164
    nomenclature, 158–9
    pancreas-preserving gastrectomy, 167–8
    splenectomy, 165, 166
    station 10 node clearance with splenic preservation, 166
    station 11 (splenic artery) node removal, 167
    systematic (D2), 158, 159, **160–4**, 165
  oesophagectomy, 84, **118–22**, *120*
    locoregional tumour control, 121–2
    outcome, 122
    staging, 121
Lymphangioma, 262
Lymphoid hyperplasia (pseudolymphoma), 256
Lymphoma, **16–19**
  classification, *17*, 255
  gastric, **253–6**, *255*
    B-cell of MALT type, 16–19, *17*, *18*, 254, 256
    secondary, 256
    treatment, 255–6
    upper gastrointestinal bleeding, 363
  oesophageal, **247**
  small intestinal disease, 19
  see also Hodgkin's lymphoma
Lymphomatous polyposis, 19

Magnetic resonance imaging (MRI)
  gastric cancer, 66
  oesophageal cancer, 65
  preoperative assessment, **65**, 74

Malignant fibrous histiocytoma
  oesophagus, 247
  stomach, 2
Malignant granular cell tumour, 247
Malignant hyperpyrexia, 90
Malignant melanoma, 248–9, *249*
Malignant schwannoma, 247
Mallory-Weiss tear, 363
  surgery, **382**
Malnutrition, 114
  dyphagia, 216
  gastric bypass, 403
  gastric cancer, 216
  post-gastrectomy, 176, 183, 185, **185–7**
  post-peptic ulcer surgery, 354
Manometry
  antireflux surgery preoperative assessment, 305
  gastro-oesophageal reflux disease, **280–3**
  lower oesophageal sphincter, *281*, **282**
  motility measurement techniques, 281–3
  oesophageal motility disorders, **293**
  with oesophageal pH recording, 288–9, *288*
  prolonged ambulatory recordings, 282
  static, 280–1
  upper oesophageal sphincter, 282
Mediastinal manipulation, 100–1
Mediastinoscopic techniques, 134
Medical history, anaesthetic risk, 90–3
Medication, preoperative preparation, 97–8
Meissner's (submucosal) plexus, 268
Melaena, 363, 364
  investigations algorithm, *369*
Ménétrier's disease (hypertrophic gastropathy), 14
Mental preparation, oesophageal surgery, 115
Mesenteric angiography, 368, 384
Metabolic bone disease, 187
Metaclopramide, 138, 301
Methotrexate, 199, 204
Methyl-CCNU, 206, 208
Metronidazole, 185, 333, 334
Microepidermoid tumours, **251**
Middle oesophagus, 81, 113, *113*
  left-sided subtotal oesophagectomy, 132
  three stage subtotal oesophagectomy, 131
  two stage subtotal oesophagectomy, 129–30
Misoprostol, 334, 370
Mitomycin C, 195, 199, 200, 205, 206, 208

Monoamine oxidase inhibitors, 97
Morbid obesity, **391–408**
  aetiology, 392–3
  biliopancreatic bypass, 403
  clinical investigations, 394
  dietary management option, 391–2
  endocrine disorders, 395
  follow-up after surgery, 405
    medical conditions improvement, 405–6
  with gallstone disease, 395
  gastric banding, 402
  gastric bypass, 397, **402–3**, 405
  genetic factors, 392
  horizontal gastroplasty, 397, **401–2**
  jejuno-ileal bypass, 395–7
  laparoscopic procedures, 403–4
  psychological investigations, 394–5
  social attitudes, 391, 392
  socioeconomic factors, 393
  vertical gastroplasty, 397, **398–401**, 405
Morphine, 106
Mousseau-Barbin tube, 220
MRC gastric cancer surgical trial (ST01), 164
Mucosal protectants, **301**
Multiple endocrine neoplasia (MEN I)
  carcinoid tumours, 20
  Zollinger-Ellison syndrome, 337, 339
Mutated in colorectal cancer (MCC), 30
Myoblastoma (granular cell tumour), 262
Myocardial infarction, 92
Myocardial ischaemia, 137
Myoepithelioma (adenomyoma), 259
Myxoma, 262

N-nitroso compounds, 11, 46, 193
Nasal polyps, 95
Nasogastric intubation
  antireflux surgery aftercare, 314
  gastric outflow obstruction palliation, 237
  postoesophagectomy management, 136
  pyloric stenosis, 345
Nasotracheal intubation, 95, 98
Nd:YAG laser, 226, 227, 371
Neomycin, 185
Neoplastic gastric polyps *see* Adenomatous
    polyps
Neurofibroma
  oesophagus, **252**
  stomach, 260
Neurofibromatosis, 252, 260
Neuroma, 260

Nissen duodenal stump closure, 381, *381*
Nissen fundoplication, **307**, *308*
  comparative aspects, 311–13
  complications, 315, 316
Nitrite intake, 46
Nitrosamines, 39, 192, 193, 354
Nitrosating bacteria, 11
Nitrous oxide, 105
Nizatidine, 300
nM23, 29
Non-expandable plastic endoprostheses,
    218–23, *219*
  complications, 221–2, *221*
  dysphagia relief, 222–3
  expandable metal stents comparative trial,
    225–6
  gastric outflow obstruction palliation, 237
  insertion method, 220
  introducing devices, 220
  postoperative management, 220, *221*
  removal, 222
Non-specifice oesophageal motility disorder,
    292, 295
Non-steroidal anti-inflammatory drugs
    (NSAIDs)
  peptic ulcer disease, 326, **328**, 332
    medical treatment failure, 335
    recurrence following surgery, 347
    treatment, **332**
Nutcracker oesophagus (symptomatic
    oesophageal peristalsis), *292*, 294–5
Nutritional support, 114–15

Oat cell carcinoma *see* Small cell carcinoma
Obesity
  gastro-oesophageal reflux disease, 299
  postoperative hypoxia, 105
  pulmonary aspiration risk, 94
  see also Morbid obesity
Obesity genes, 392
Obstructive airway disease, chronic (COAD)
  anaesthetic risk, 93
  postoperative complications, 97
  preoperative pulmonary function tests, 96–7
Occupational gastric cancer risk, 45
Octreotide, 19, 349
  scintigraphy, 338
Oesophageal adenocarcinoma, 112, 140, 141,
    247–8
  in Barrett's oesophagus *see* Barrett's
    oesophagus

chemotherapy, **202**, 203
  postoperative, 202
  preoperative, 202
  radiotherapy combination, 191, **202–3**
epidemiology, 35, 37, 38, **40–1**, 192, 201
lymph node resection, 119, 121
radiotherapy, **201**, 203
  chemotherapy combination, 191, **202–3**
  postoperative, 201
  preoperative, 201
rare variants, *253*, **253**
staging, 81
Oesophageal adenoid cystic carcinoma, 26,
  251
Oesophageal adenoma, 252
Oesophageal anatomy, *267*, **267–70**
  blood supply, 113–14, 268
  innervation, 268
  lower sphincter (LOS), 269–70, *269*
  surgical anatomy, **112–14**
  upper sphincter (UOS), 268–9
Oesophageal benign epithelial tumours, **252**
Oesophageal bleeding
  cancer palliation, 235–6
  surgical technique, **382**
Oesophageal cancer
  advanced, 213, 214, **216**
    classification, 67–8
    survival, 214, 215
  age of onset, 38
  demography, 37–8
  distant metastases, 62, 64–5, 71, 72, *72*, 74,
    82
  endoscopy
    early cancer, 67
    in vitro dye staining, 50, 67
    preoperative, 67–8
  epidemiology, 35, **36–41**, *37*, **192**
    incidence, 36–7, *37*
  genetic predisposition, 40
  geographical variation, 36, 37–8
  intraoperative assessment, **74–5**
  locoregional recurrence, 194
  lymph node involvement, 64, 69–70, 71, 82,
    82, 192
  lymphadenectomy fields, 84
  mediastinal invasion/local spread, 62–3, *63*,
    65, 82
  molecular aspects, 27, 29–30, 50
  palliation, **217–36**, 238, *238*
    aerodigestive fistulae, **234–5**
    bleeding, 235–6

dysphagia *see* Dysphagia relief
  recurrent laryngeal nerve palsy, 235
pathology, 1, **20–7**
precursor lesions, 1, 2, 23, **38–41**
preoperative assessment, **59–85**, 74, 117
  computed tomography (CT), 62–5
  endoscopic ultrasonography, 69, *70*, **70**
  laparoscopy, 71–3, *72*
  magnetic resonance imaging (MRI), 65
  radiological contrast examinations,
    60–1
radiotherapy, 194
screening, **49–51**, 61
staging, **80–4**, 117
  anatomical description, 80–2, *113*
  clinical, 83
  clinicopathological, 84
  endoscopic ultrasonography, 141
  histopathological, 83
  lymphadenectomy, 121
  TNM classification, 83–4, *83*, *84*, 112, *113*
superficial spreading, 68
surgery *see* Oesophagectomy
surgical pathology, 112
Oesophageal carcinoid tumours, 249
Oesophageal carcinoma-in-situ, 23
  asymptomatic screening follow-up, 49, 50
·Oesophageal carcinosarcoma, 23, 250
Oesophageal chondrosarcoma, 247
Oesophageal diffuse leiomyomatosis, 246
Oesophageal dilatation, **217–18**
Oesophageal dysplasia, 1, 2, 23
  asymptomatic screening follow-up, 49–50
  in Barrett's oesophagus, 25, *26*
    classification, *26*
  oesophageal squamous cell carcinoma, 38,
    39
Oesophageal fibrosarcoma, 247
Oesophageal granular cell tumours, **252**
Oesophageal haemangioma, 252
Oesophageal histology, 268
Oesophageal leiomyoblastoma, 247
Oesophageal leiomyoma, 245–6, *246*
Oesophageal lymph nodes, *82*, *114*
Oesophageal lymphatics, 113–14
Oesophageal lymphoma, 247
Oesophageal malignant melanoma, 248–9,
  249
Oesophageal metastases, 247
Oesophageal microepidermoid tumours,
  251
Oesophageal motility, 273

Oesophageal motility disorders, **290–5**, *291*
  classification, 291
  investigations, *292*, 293
Oesophageal mucosal rosette, 273
Oesophageal neurofibroma, **252**
Oesophageal perforation, 221, 222, 225, 228
Oesophageal pH recording, **283–9**, *285*, *286*
  ambulatory measurements, 284, *285*
  antireflux surgery, 305, 314
  with manometry, 288–9, *288*
  multichannel, 285
  procedure, 284
  recorders, 283
  sensors, 283
Oesophageal polyps, 251–2
Oesophageal prosthesis placement, **218–26**
  contraindications, 218
  expandable metal stents, **223–6**
  intravenous sedation, 218
  non-expandable plastic endoprostheses,
    218–23, *219*
Oesophageal pseudoepitheliomatous
    hyperplasia, 23
Oesophageal reconstruction, **122–8**
  with colon, 127–8, *127*
  with jejunum, 127
  posterior mediastinal route, *123*, 124
  presternal route, 122–3, *123*
  retrosternal (anterior mediastinal) route,
    123–4, *123*
  with stomach, 124–6, *125*
    gastric drainage, 126
    stomach lengthening methods, 126
Oesophageal rhabdomyosarcoma, 247
Oesophageal sarcomatous lesions, 246–7
Oesophageal scintigraphy, **289**
Oesophageal small cell (oat cell) carcinoma,
    27, *27*, **248**
Oesophageal spasm, 279, 280
  diffuse, *292*, 294
  provocation tests, 289–90
Oesophageal squamous cell carcinoma, 1,
    20–3, *22*, 112, 140, 141
  chemotherapy, **198–9**, 201
    postoperative (adjuvant), 198, 199
    preoperative, 198, 199
  chemotherapy-radiotherapy combination,
    191, 201
    followed by surgery, **200–1**
    without surgery, **199**
  endoscopic appearance, 67
  epidemiology, 35, *37*, 38

histology, 22–3, *22*
  incidental second tumours, 22
  lymph node resection, 119, 121
  metastatic potential, 21–2
  predisposing factors, 20, *21*
  premalignant conditions, **38–40**
  radiotherapy, **196–8**, 201
    postoperative, 197–8
    preoperative, 197
  rare variants, *253*, **253**
Oesophageal squamous papilloma, 23, 252
Oesophageal verrucous carcinoma, **250–1**
Oesophagectomy, **111–41**
  anaesthesia, **100–4**
  anastomosis technique, **134–5**
  cardiovascular instability, 100–1
  epidemiology, 214
  extended radical surgery, 116
  lymph nodes resection, **118–22**, *120*
  mental preparation, 115
  nutritional support, 114–15
  objectives, **115–16**
  oesophageal reconstruction, **122–8**
  one lung anaesthesia, 101–3, *102*
    anaesthetic techniques, 103–4, *103*
    cardiac output, 104
  outcome, 116, *116*, 122, **139–40**
    residual disease, 122
  patient selection, 215
  peroperative hypoxia, 101, *101*
  postoperative complications, **136–9**
  postoperative management, 105, 106, *135*,
    135–6
  preoperative preparation, 114–15
  principles, **117–34**
  resection margins, 117–18, *118*
  surgical approach, **128–34**
    combined synchronous two team
      oesophagectomy, 131
    endoscopically assisted techniques,
      134
    left-sided subtotal, 132
    pharyngolaryngo oesophagectomy,
      129
    three stage subtotal, 131
    transhiatal, 132–3
    two stage subtotal via right thoracotomy,
      129–30
  total/subtotal, 116
Oesophagitis, 40, 61, 95, 271, 275, 278
  endoscopy, 280
  medical treatment, 300

mucosal rosette reflux barrier, 273
oesophageal squamous cell carcinoma
  epidemiology, 38, 39
  post-vertical gastroplasty, 400
  upper gastrointestinal bleeding, 363
Oesophagogastric junction see Gastro-
  oesophageal junction (cardia)
Oesophagorespiratory fistulas, 216, **234–5**
Omeprazole, 300, 302, 338, 370
Oncogenes, 29, 30
One lung anaesthesia
  anaesthetic techniques, *103*, **103–4**
  cardiac output, 104
  endobronchial intubation, 98–9, *99*
  oesophageal surgery, **101–3**, *102*
  peroperative hypoxia, 101, *101*
  peroperative monitoring, 99–100
  preoperative investigations, 95, 96
Opiate analgesia, 95, 106
  extradural, 107, 108, *108*
  patient controlled analgesia (PCA), 106–7
  postoperative hypoxia, 105
Oral hypoglycaemics, 97
Orodental hygiene, 115
Oropharynx, 112
Osteoma, 262
Osteomalacia, 186
Osteosarcoma, 247
Oxygen therapy, postoperative, 105

p53 mutations, 11
  Barrett's oesophagus, 30
  gastric cancer, 28
  oesophageal cancer, 29, 30
Pain, postoperative hypoxia, 105
Palliative treatment, 59, 71, **213–39**
  aerodigestive fistulae, **234–5**
  bleeeding, 235–6
  chronic blood loss from gastric tumours,
    237
  dysphagia relief, **217–34**
  epidemiology, 213–14
  gastric outflow obstruction, **236–7**
  patient selection, **215–16**, 239
  recurrent laryngeal nerve palsy, 235
  survival, 214–15
Pancreas-preserving gastrectomy, **167–8**
Pancreatic enzyme supplements, 185
Pancreatic fistula, 182
Pancreatic resection, **166–7**
Paraoesophageal lymph nodes, *82*, 114, *114*

Parenteral feeding, 115
Partial fundoplication, **308–11**
  complete fundoplication comparison,
    311–13
Partial gastrectomy, 154, *155*, 170
  refractory duodenal ulcers, 342, *342*
  technique, 174–5, *175*
Patient controlled analgesia (PCA), **106–7**
Patient treatment preferences, 216, 303–4
Patterson Brown Kelly (Plummer Vinson)
    syndrome, 20–1, 40
Penicillin, 182
Pepsinogen, 54–5
Peptic stricture, 40, 41, 275, 278, **319–20**
  endoscopy, 280
  oesophageal scintigraphy, 290
Peptic ulcer disease, **325–54**
  aetiology, 326–30
  bleeding, 361–2, *363*
    endoscopic appearances, 367–8
    endoscopic haemostasis, **370–7**
    indications for surgery, 378–9
    surgical haemostasis, **379–84**
    see also Upper gastrointestinal bleeding
  disease associations, 328
  endoscopic confirmation, 330
  epidemiology, 325–6
  malignant transformation, 14
  management protocols, *331*, *332*
  non-steroidal anti-inflammatory drugs
    (NSAIDs), 326, **328**, 332, 335
  pyloric stenosis, **345–6**
  recurrence following surgery, **346–8**
  resistant ulcers, **334–6**, 341–3
    management protocol, *335*
  treatment, **332–4**
Peptic ulcer perforation, **343–5**
  conservative management, 343–4
  laparoscopic surgery, 344–5
  open surgery, 344
Peptic ulcer surgery
  abdominal pain following, *347*
  complications management, **346–54**
  diarrhoea, **351–2**
  dumping syndrome, 348–9, *349*, **351**
  elective surgery, **339–43**
  enterogastric reflux, **352–3**
  laparoscopic, 343
  nutritional problems, 354
  small stomach syndrome, **353–4**
Perfused tube manometry, 280
Perioesophageal lymph nodes, 114, *114*

Peritoneal metastases, 71, 72, *72*
  intraoperative assessment, 75, 171
  intraperitoneal chemotherapy, 171, 195
  PHNS staging, *79*
Peritoneal seeding, 151, 153
  during surgery, 153
  intraoperative investigations, 171
  intraperitoneal chemotherapy, 171
Pernicious anaemia, 9, 44
  gastric cancer screening, 53
  gastric nitrite metabolism, 46
  neuroendocrine tumours, 19
Peroperative monitoring, **99–100**, *100*
Personal orientation inventory (POI),
  395
Peutz-Jegher's syndrome, 259
pH monitoring *see* Oesophageal pH
  recording
Pharyngeal overtube, 366
Pharyngo-oesophageal (Zenker's)
  diverticulum, 21
Pharyngolaryngo oesophagectomy, **129**
PHNS gastric cancer staging, 76–9, *76, 77*
  anatomical description, 77
  pathological description, 77–9, *77, 78*
Photodynamic therapy, **230**
Photosensitising drugs, 230
Physiotherapy, 105, 115, 135, 136
Pirenzepine, 334
Plain chest radiography, 73
Plasmacytomas, 247
Plummer Vinson (Patterson Brown Kelly)
  syndrome, 20–1, 40
Pneumococcal vaccination, 182
Polya gastrectomy, *350*
Polyposis syndromes, **259**
Polyps
  gastric, **257–9**
    adenomatous, 12, 13, 257–8, *258*, 259
    fundic gland, 12, 13, **258–9**
    hyperplastic, 12, 13, 257, 259
    polyposis syndromes, **259**
  oesophagus, **251–2**
Porphyria, 90
Postoperative (adjuvant) chemotherapy,
  196
  gastric cancer, **205–7**, *207*
    multiagent, 206–7
    single agent, 205–6
  oesophageal adenocarcinoma, 202
  oesophageal squamous cell carcinoma, **198**,
    199, 201

Postoperative (adjuvant) radiotherapy, 194
  gastric cancer, 204
    chemotherapy combination, **207–8**
  oesophageal adenocarcinoma, 201
  oesophageal squamous cell carcinoma,
    197–8, 201
Postoperative care, **104–8**
  antireflux surgery, **314**
  cardiovascular instability, 106
  oesophagectomy, *135*, **135–6**
  pain relief, 106–8, 135
  postoperative hypoxia, 105
Postoperative complications
  gastric cancer surgery, **182–7**
    early, **179–82**
  oesophagectomy, **136–9**
  pulmonary, **105**, 115, 136, 316
  smoking, 93–4
Postoperative hypoxia, **105**
Postoperative pain relief, **106–8**, 135
Postoperative staging, 59
Postsplenectomy infections, 182
Prednisolone, 256
Premedication, 97
Preoperative assessment, 59, **60–74**, **95–7**, *96*
  anaesthesia *see* Anaesthesia
  antireflux surgery, **304–5**
  computed tomography (CT), 62–6, 74
  endoscopic ultrasonography, 69–71, *70, 71*,
    74
  endoscopy, 66–9, 74
  laparoscopy, 71–3, 74
  magnetic resonance imaging (MRI), 65, 74
  plain chest radiography, 73
  radiological contrast examinations, 60–2, 74
Preoperative (neoadjuvant) chemotherapy, **195**,
  205
  oesophageal adenocarcinoma, 202
  oesophageal squamous cell carcinoma, **198**,
    199, 201
Preoperative preparation
  anaesthetic management, 100
  oesophageal cancer, **114–15**
Preoperative radiotherapy, 194
  gastric cancer, 203
  oesophageal adenocarcinoma, 201
  oesophageal squamous cell carcinoma, **197**,
    201
Presbyoesophagus, *292*
Prokinetic agents, 138, **301**
Proster-Livingston tube, 219
Protein absorption, post-gastrectomy, 186

Proton pump inhibitors
  Barrett's oesophagus management, 319
  gastro-oesophageal reflux disease, 276, 278,
    300–1, 302
  peptic ulcer disease, 325, 332, 333, 334,
    383
    recurrence following surgery, 348
  side effects, 301
  upper gastrointestinal bleeding, 370
  Zollinger-Ellison syndrome, 338
Provocation tests, **288–89**
Proximal gastric vagotomy, 340
Pseudocholinesterase deficiency, 90
Pseudolymphoma (lymphoid hyperplasia),
    256
Pulmonary aspiration
  anaesthesia-associated risk factors, 94–5
  preventive measures, 97, 98
Pulmonary function tests, 96–7
Pulmonary metastases, 74
Pyloric stenosis, **345–6**
  endoscopic treatment, 345
  surgery, 345–6
Pyloroplasty, *350*
  oesophageal reconstruction with stomach,
    126
Pylorus-preserving gastrectomy, 170, 342–3,
    342

Quality of life
  antireflux surgery, 304
  palliative treatment, 238, 239
  post-gastrectomy, 182, 183

Radiological contrast examinations, **60–2**, 74
  gastric cancer, 60, 61, *61*
    early cancer detection, 61–2, *62*
  gastro-oesophageal reflux disease, **279–80**
  oesophageal cancer, 60
    early cancer detection, 60–1
  oesophageal motility disorders, **293**
Radiotherapy, **191–209**
  dysphagia palliation, **233–4**
  fitness for treatment, 215
  gastric cancer, **203–4**
  gastric outflow obstruction palliation, 237
  gastric primary lymphoma, 255
  laser treatment combined dysphagia
    palliation, 229–30
  oesophageal adenocarcinoma, **201**

oesophageal squamous cell carcinoma, 21,
    196–8, 201
  oesophagectomy resection margins, 118
  treatment strategies, **194**
  see also Chemotherapy-radiotherapy
    combination
Ranitidine, 300
Reactive hypoglycaemic attacks, 184
Rectal bleeding, 363, 364
  investigations algorithm, *369*
Recurrent laryngeal nerve palsy, 138, 216,
    235
Regurgitation, 291
Resection margins
  gastric cancer surgery, 152, 154, 156
    frozen-section histology, 172
  oesophagectomy, **117–18**, *118*
    postoperative radiotherapy, 194
Retinoblastoma (Rb), 29–30
Rhabdomyoma, 262
Rhabdomyosarcoma, 247
Rigid bronchoscopy, preoperative, 73
Robertshaw double lumen endobronchial
    tube, *99*
Rosetti-Nissen fundoplication, **307–8**, *309*
Roux-en-Y reconstruction, 177, 183
  dumping syndrome alleviation, 351
  enterogastric reflux alleviation, 353
  with selective vagotomy and antrectomy,
    340
  with subtotal gastrectomy for refractory
    duodenal ulcers, 342, *342*
Roux-en-Y syndrome, 351

Saliva secretion, gastro-oesophageal reflux
    influence, 274
Salt intake, 46, 192–3
Sarcomatous oesophageal lesions, 246–7
Schwannoma, 260
Screening, 35–56
  gastric cancer, 49, 51–5
    asymptomatic, 52–3, 146, 147
    dyspeptic patients, 53–4, 146
    Japanese programme, 145
    population awareness, 147
    shift to the left phenomenon, 147
    in West, 146–7
  oesophageal cancer, 49–51, 61
Selective vagotomy and antrectomy, 340, 341,
    342
  refractory duodenal ulcers, **341–2**

Sleeve sensor manometry, 280–1
Sliding hiatus hernia, 272, 273
Small cell (oat cell) carcinoma, 2
  oesophagus, **248**
  stomach, 262
Small intestinal lymphoma, 19
Small stomach syndrome, **353–4**
Smoking
  Barret's oesophagus malignant
    transformation, 24, 41
  effects of stopping, 94, *94*
  gastro-oesophageal reflux disease, 299
  oesophageal cancer, 192
  oesophageal squamous carcinoma
    pathogenesis, 20, 22, 39
  oesophageal surgery, 115
  peptic ulcer disease, 327–8, 335
  postoperative complications, 93–4, 105
  preoperative assessment, 93–4
Socioeconomic factors
  gastric cancer, 44–5, 48
  morbid obesity, 393
  peptic ulcer disease, 326
Somatostatin, 370
Splenectomy
  complicating antireflux surgery, 316
  gastric cancer surgery, **165–6**
  indications, 165, 166
  postoperative infections, 182
  technique, 176
Splenic hilar node dissection, 166
Squamocolumnar junction (SCJ; Z line), 267,
  280
Staging, **75–85**
  gastric cancer, 76–80, 147–8
    International Unified TNM system,
      159–60
    intraoperative, 171
    lymph node involvement, 147–8
    stage migration phenomenon, 147–8
  oesophageal cancer, 80–4, 117
    endoscopic ultrasonography, 141
    patient selection for palliative treatment,
      215
Standard acid reflux test (SART), 289
Stapling devices, 134–5, 139
Steatorrhoea, 185
Stoma adjustable gastric banding, 402
Stomach in oesophageal reconstruction, **124–6**,
  125
  gastric drainage, 126
  stomach lengthening methods, 126

Strain gauge manometry, 280
Subtotal gastrectomy *see* Partial gastrectomy
Sucralfate, 301
Super-extended radical gastrectomy, 169
Swallowing, **270–1**
Symptomatic oesophageal peristalsis
    ('nutcracker' oesophagus), *292*, 295
Synovial sarcoma, 247

T-cell lymphomas, 19
Taylor-Johnson temperamental analysis
    (T-JTA), 395
Teratoma, 2, 262
Tetracycline, 333
Thermal injury, 39
Thiopentone, 95
Thoracoscopic antireflux surgery, 313
Thoracoscopic chest dissection, 134
Thoracotomy
  combined two team oesophagectomy, 131
  left-sided subtotal oesophagectomy, 132
  peroperative monitoring, 99–100
  postoperative care, 105
  postoperative pulmonary complications,
    115
  two stage subtotal oesophagectomy,
    129–30
Thromboembolic complications, 136–7
Thromboprophylaxis
  antireflux surgery, 314
  oesophageal surgery, 115
  postoesophagectomy management, 136
  preoperative preparation, 98
TNM gastric cancer staging, **80**, *81*
  AJC modification, 79, *80*
  International Unified system, 159–60
  UICC modification, 79
TNM oesophageal cancer staging, 80, 83–4, *83*
  UICC and AJC system, *84*
Total gastrectomy, 154, *155*
  gastric outflow obstruction palliation, 236,
    237
  perioperative mortality, 148, 149
  with splenectomy and distal
    pancreatectomy, 176
  technique, 175, *175*, 176
Toupet partial fundoplication, 308–9, *310*,
  312–13
Tracheobronchial tree assessment, 73
Tracheo-oesophageal fistula, 218
Tranexamic acid, 370

Transhiatal approach
  gastric cancer surgery, 171
  oesophagectomy, 132–3
Tumour growth factor-α (TGFα), 29, 30
Tumour markers, 54
Tumour suppressor gene abnormalities, 28, 29–30
Two team oesophagectomy, 131
Tygon prosthesis, 218
Tylosis, 20, 40, 50

UICC gastric cancer staging, **79**
UICC oesophageal cancer staging, *84*
Ultraflex stent, *223*, *224*, *225*
Upper gastrointestinal bleeding, **361–86**
  aetiology, 361–3, *362*, *364*
  assessment/immediate management, 364–5
  chronic blood loss, 216
    gastric tumours, **237**
  endoscopy, **365–8**, 384
    definition of appearances, 385–6, *385*
    treatment, **370–7**
  epidemiology, 361
  investigations algorithm, *369*
  labelled red cell scanning, 368–9
  laparotomy, 369
  management recommendations, **384–5**
  medical treatment, 370, 384
  mesenteric angiography, 368, 384
  oesophageal cancer palliation, **235–6**
  presentation, 363–4
  surgery, **378–84**
    control of bleeding, 383–4
    indications, 378–9, 385
    techniques, **379–84**
    vagotomy, 383, 385
Upper oesophageal sphincter (UOS), **268–9**
  manometric assessment, **283**
Upper oesophagus, 80, 113, *113*
  transhiatal oesophagectomy, 132–3

Vagotomy
  diarrhoea following, **351–2**
  dumping syndrome following, **348–51**, *350*
  upper gastrointestinal bleeding, 383
Verrucous carcinoma, **250–1**
Vertical gastroplasty, **397**, **398–401**
  postoperative management, 399–400

postoperative morbidity, 400–1
  surgical technique, 398–9
Video-assisted thoracic surgery (VATS), 313
Videoendoscopy, 365
Videofluoroscopy, **279**
Vinblastine, 199, 200
Vincristine, 255
Vital staining
  gastro-oesophageal reflux disease, 280
  oesophageal cancer, 50, 67
Vitamin A deficiency, 186
Vitamin A protective effect, 46
Vitamin B complex deficiency, 186
Vitamin B_{12} deficiency, 186
Vitamin C, 11, 187
  gastric cancer protective effect, 46, 47, 193
  oesophageal carcinoma protective effect, 39
Vitamin D deficiency, 186
Vitamin deficiencies, 39, 40
Vitamin E protective effect, 46
Vocal cord palsy, 216
von Recklinghausen's neurofibromatosis, 252

Wallstent, 223–4, *223*, 225
Watson partial fundoplication, 310, *311*
Weight loss
  post-antireflux surgery, 305
  post-gastrectomy, 185–6
Wilson-Cook prosthesis, 219, *219*
  fistula prosthesis, 234–5

Xanthomas, 13

Z line (squamocolumnar junction), 267, 280
Zenker's diverticulum, 21
Zollinger-Ellison syndrome, **336–9**
  carcinoid tumours, 20
  clinical features, 336
  diagnosis, 337
  pathology, 336–7
  peptic ulcer disease recurrence, 347
  preoperative tumour localisation, 338
  treatment, 337–9
    gastric secretion suppression, 338
    gastrinoma excision, 339
    parietal cell vagotomy, 338